Ultrasound
and Infertility

PROGRESS IN OBSTETRIC
AND GYNECOLOGICAL
SONOGRAPHY SERIES

SERIES EDITOR: ASIM KURJAK

Ultrasound and Infertility

Edited by

S. KUPESIC and D. de ZIEGLER

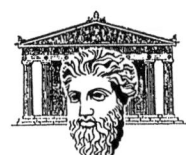

The Parthenon Publishing Group

International Publishers in Medicine, Science & Technology

NEW YORK   LONDON

Library of Congress Cataloging-in-Publication Data
 Data available on request

British Library Cataloguing in Publication Data
Ultrasound and infertility (Progress in obstetric and
 gynecological sonography series)
 1. Infertility - Ultrasonic imaging 2. Generative
organs, Female - Ultrasonic imaging
 I. Kupesic, S. II. Ziegler, D. de
 618'.1'78'07543

ISBN 1-85070-620-4

Published in the UK and Europe by
The Parthenon Publishing Group Limited
Casterton Hall, Carnforth
Lancs., LA6 2LA, UK

Published in the USA by
The Parthenon Publishing Group Inc.
One Blue Hill Plaza, PO Box 1564,
Pearl River, NY 10965, USA

Copyright © 2000 Parthenon Publishing Group

Typesetting by Siva Math Setters, Chennai, India
Printed by T. G. Hostench S. A., Spain

Contents

List of principal contributors

A. H. Balen
Clarendon Wing
The General Infirmary at Leeds
Belmont Grove
Leeds LS2 9NS
UK

C. Battaglia
Department of Obstetrics and Gynecology
University of Modena
Via Del Pozzo 71
41100 Modena
Italy

M. M. Biljan
Department of Obstetrics and Gynecology
McGill Reproductive Centre
Royal Victoria Hospital
Women's Pavilion
687 Pine Avenue West
Montreal, Quebec H3A 1A1
Canada

B. Cacciatore
Department of Obstetrics and Gynecology
Helsinki University Central Hospital
Helsinki PL 140
00029 Helsinki
Finland

U. Deichert
Frauenklinik
Stadtkrankenhaus Cuxhaven
Altenwalder Chaussee 10–12
D-27474 Cuxhaven
Germany

D. de Ziegler
Reproductive Endocrinology and Infertility
Hôpital de Nyon
CH-1260 Nyon
Switzerland

V. H. Eisenberg
Department of Obstetrics and Gynecology
Hadassah University Hospital
Kiryat Hadassah
PO Box 12000
Jerusalem 91120
Israel

H. Fernandez
Department of Obstetrics and Gynecology
Hôpital Antoine Béclère
157 Rue De La Porte de Trivaux
F-92141 Clamart Cedex
France

S. Kupesic
Department of Obstetrics and Gynecology
Medical School University of Zagreb
Sveti Duh 64
10000 Zagreb
Croatia

A. Kurjak
Department of Obstetrics and Gynecology
Medical School University of Zagreb
Sveti Duh Hospital
Sveti Duh 64
10000 Zagreb
Croatia

A. Lewin
Department of Obstetrics and Gynecology
Hadassah-Hebrew University Hospital
PO Box 12087
Ein Kerem
Jerusalem 91120
Israel

D. Moeglin
28 Route de Cannes
Le Neroli
06130 Grasse
France

D. Nugent
School of Medicine
Division of Obstetrics and Gynaecology
University of Leeds
Belmont Grove
Leeds LS2 9NS
UK

S. L. Tan
Department of Obstetrics and Gynecology
McGill Reproductive Centre
Royal Victoria Hospital
Women's Pavilion
687 Pine Avenue West
Montreal, Quebec H3A 1A1
Canada

I. E. Timor-Tritsch
New York University Medical Center
Department of Obstetrics and Gynecology
550 First Avenue, Room 9E2-NB
New York, NY 10016
USA

M. Toth
Department of Obstetrics and Gynecology
The New York Hospital-Cornell
  Medical Center
328 East 75th Street
New York, NY 10021
USA

J. Zaidi
Department of Obstetrics and Gynecology
Conquest Hospital
The Ridge
St. Leonards on Sea
East Sussex
TN37 7RD
UK

Preface

Some of the most important advances in medically-assisted conception have resulted from developments in ultrasonography. Ultrasound has simplified oocyte retrieval techniques enabling the procedure to be performed under sedation and has completely replaced laparoscopic oocyte collection under general anesthesia. It is also the method of choice for monitoring follicular growth and the assessment of ovarian and uterine perfusion by Doppler methods. In addition, it seems that the recent introduction of three dimensional and power Doppler will be an additional useful parameter.

Ultrasound has a permanent advantage over other imaging and diagnostic techniques, including laparoscopy, by being rapid, safe, and non-invasive. It is, therefore, time to produce a book which will serve as a useful guide for the optimal use of ultrasound in an infertility clinic, containing most of the information necessary for practical work, and bringing ultrasonographers and clinicians up-to-date information on the current knowledge and special problems for the future.

S. Kupesic

Applied sonographic imaging in the evaluation of the infertile couple

V. H. Eisenberg and A. Lewin

INTRODUCTION

Infertility is defined as the inability to conceive after 1 year of intercourse without contraception[1]. Half of all couples attempting conception will conceive in 3 months, 75% will conceive in 6 months, and about 85% will conceive by the end of 1 year[2]. Thus, infertility occurs in 10–15% of couples[3], with its incidence varying in different socioeconomic groups and certain geographic areas and races, and increasing with increasing age of the woman. Maximal fertility occurs at age 24 years, and fertility decreases rapidly after age 35 years, due to an increase in the frequency of anovulatory cycles and early abortions. The main causes of infertility are: anovulation in 10–30% of cases, tubal factor in 15%, male factor in 20–30%, cervical factor in 5%, endometriosis in 5–25%, and unexplained causes of infertility in 15–30% of cases[1,4], some of which are related to nutritional imbalance, stress and exposure to chemical and physical factors. For 10–30% of couples there is more than one cause of infertility[2,5]. About one-half of couples with primary infertility and one-fifth of couples with secondary infertility seek medical treatment[6]. During recent decades there has been an increase in the rate of couples seeking medical assistance for infertility. This is the result of the general increase in the number of women of child-bearing age, the increased incidence of sexually transmitted diseases, increased occupational exposure to chemicals and toxins and the growing trend of career-related postponement of parenthood.

Primarily, timing of ovulation with coitus must be optimized, and the couple should be informed that there is only about a 20% chance of conceiving in each ovulatory cycle even with optimal timing of coitus in fertile couples[1]. Cigarette smoking and possibly caffeine consumption independently decrease the chances of conception[7,8]. The initial diagnostic evaluation of the infertile couple comprises a complete history, physical examination, and laboratory tests, which include a complete blood count, urine analysis, Pap smear, and fasting blood glucose. The presence and quality of ovulation is assessed by measurements of daily basal body temperature and serum progesterone level on day 21 of the cycle. A progesterone level of at least 10 ng/ml confirms ovulation and is positively correlated with conception[9]. A possible male factor should be investigated at an early stage, by semen analysis, usually after 1 to 4 days of abstinence. The next step is a postcoital test for a preliminary evaluation of the cervical and immunological factors, followed by assessment, when necessary, of antisperm antibodies. Hysterosalpingography (HSG) is usually performed in the follicular phase of the next cycle, if the first three tests are all normal. This cycle could also be the right timing for endometrial sampling for dating, performed on day 22–26. Laparoscopy is performed when the HSG or history raise the possibility of endometriosis, pelvic adhesions or tubal occlusion. It should also be considered in the presence of normal HSG findings, after several treatment cycles have failed to achieve pregnancy. Preferably at least 3 months should pass between the HSG and the laparoscopy, because up to 20% of women conceive after HSG[10]. Dilatation and curettage at the time of laparoscopy is unnecessary and inadvisable, as it may cause uterine adhesions[11]. A concomitant hysteroscopy should always be performed during laparoscopy and not only if an abnormality has been found in the HSG, as a discrepancy of up to 30% between HSG and hysteroscopic findings may exist[12]. The above initial evaluation can be completed within a few months, and usually uncovers the cause of infertility in 70–85% of couples[2].

An extended evaluation is warranted when the cause of infertility remains unexplained after the initial work-up. Genital tract infection with *Chlamydia trachomatis* is often asymptomatic, but may cause tubal damage and obstruction. Infection by *Ureaplasma urealyticum* and *Mycoplasma hominis* are more common in infertile couples than in fertile couples, and may be a cause of unexplained infertility[4]. Infection is a rare cause of male factor infertility, which warrants antibiotic treatment of both partners[13]. Morphologic evaluation of sperm is valuable in cases of suspected male factor infertility even in the presence of a normal sperm count[14].

The applications of sonography in the assessment of the infertile couple are varied and expand over time. The ultrasonic picture is a faithful demonstration of the anatomy being scanned. Correct interpretation depends on the quality of the ultrasound equipment and the proficiency of the person performing the examination. According to the American Institute of Ultrasound in Medicine there are no confirmed biologic adverse effects on patients or instrument operators caused by exposure at currently used intensities[15]. In this chapter we review the application of ultrasound to the assessment of the infertile couple. Other imaging modalities are briefly discussed.

ASSESSMENT OF THE FEMALE REPRODUCTIVE TRACT

Imaging is essential in the evaluation and treatment of infertility patients. Various modalities

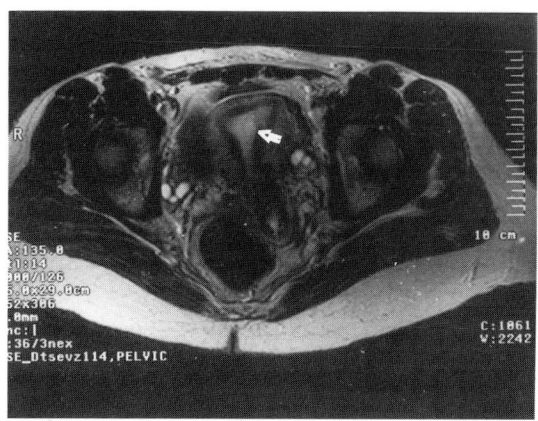

Figure 1 Magnetic resonance imaging of normal uterus and uterine cavity. Arrow = uterine cavity

are used for the anatomical and functional diagnosis of the female genital tract. Hysterosalpingography is a minimal outpatient procedure useful in the diagnosis of uterine and tubal disease, which may also suggest peritoneal pathology[16]. Magnetic resonance imaging (MRI) enables clear delineation of uterine anatomy (Figure 1) and is the best imaging modality for the diagnosis of endometriosis, but is of no value in examination of the Fallopian tubes[17]. Ultrasonography has an increasingly important role in the evaluation and treatment of infertility patients, being an efficient and cost-effective modality for studying the female reproductive organs and for monitoring functional changes during spontaneous and induced cycles[18,19] (Figure 2). Recently hydrosonography, or sonohysterography, has been applied for uterine cavity and tubal patency evaluation[20,21].

Cervical factor infertility

The uterine cervix is the first obstacle that the spermatozoa, deposited in the vagina, have to pass on the way to the oocyte. Proper function of the cervical glands, under estrogen stimulation, secretes an alkaline, nonviscous mucus, that assists the passage of sperm and its capacitation, prevents phagocytosis, and provides an environment rich in energy supply. Some 5–10% of infertility causes are related to cervical factors, which include anatomical and

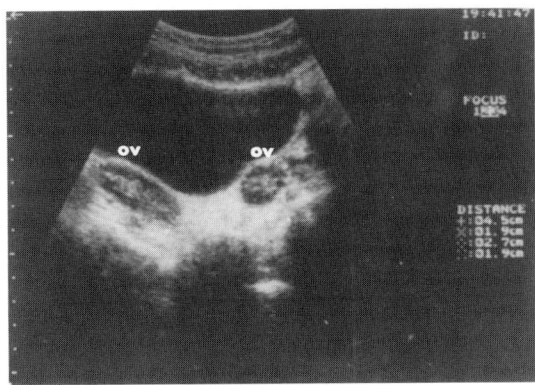

Figure 2 Transabdominal sonography of uterine agenesis. Note two polycystic ovaries (OV)

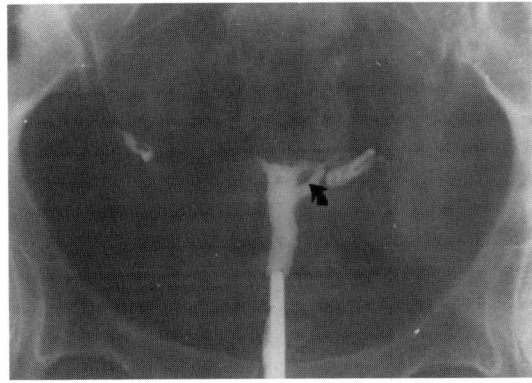

Figure 3 Hysterosalpingograph of intrauterine adhesions

functional problems. Congenital malformations include those resulting from diethylstilbestrol (DES) exposure *in utero*, cervical agenesis and cervical stenosis. Acquired causes are cervical conization, coagulation or infection.

The postcoital test evaluates the interaction between sperm and cervical mucus 2–8 h after intercourse. Accurate timing with ovulation is essential, as the cervical mucus has optimal physical and chemical properties for penetration and survival of sperm at maximal estradiol levels, prior to the progesterone rise. An abnormal test may indicate an abnormality in the characteristics of the cervical mucus, oligoasthenospermia, or the presence of anti-sperm antibodies. An error of interpretation often results from inappropriate timing, yielding negative test results[22]. Ultrasonographic monitoring of ovarian follicles is far more accurate in timing ovulation than clinical determinants that rely on the progesterone rise, such as basal body temperature. Thus, the reliability of the postcoital test can be increased by sonographic timing of ovulation[23,24].

Uterine factor infertility

Uterine factors causing infertility interfere with two main reproductive processes, namely embryo implantation and continuation of pregnancy. These factors comprise intrauterine adhesions, leiomyomas, polyps, congenital uterine malformations, inappropriate

endometrial growth and secretory transformation during the ovulatory cycle.

The adult uterus is normally 6–10 cm in length and 3–5 cm in width, with a central linear echo, which represents the endometrial cavity. Various modalities are available for the assessment of the uterine cavity, such as hysteroscopy, HSG, ultrasonography, hydrosonography and MRI. Hysteroscopy is performed most often as an outpatient procedure not requiring anesthesia. When performed under general anesthesia, it has the advantage that abnormal findings, such as fibroids, synechiae or polyps, can be removed under vision. Hysteroscopy is considered to be more accurate than HSG for the evaluation of intrauterine causes of infertility, due to high false-positive and false-negative rates in HSG[25].

Intrauterine synechiae may be caused by infection or trauma to the endometrium, such as curettage or myomectomy. These may obliterate the endometrial cavity and obstruct the cervical canal. Diagnosis can be made by hysteroscopy or HSG, while sonography is less widely used. Recently, hydrosonography was introduced for this application. The characteristic findings on HSG are irregular filling defects within the endometrial cavity (Figure 3). Transvaginal sonography (TVS) may reveal echogenic serpiginous endometrial bridges. To date, there are no reports which systematically compare these methods for this application[22].

Leiomyomas may cause infertility by impairing the patency of the reproductive tract by occluding the cervical canal or Fallopian tubes, by obstructing the uterine cavity and diminishing available endometrium for implantation, and by interfering with oocyte and sperm transport. Detection and localization of myomas has clinical importance only when these obstruct the reproductive tract. When HSG is used for pelvic screening, small noncalcified lesions may be missed, while calcified myomas are easily detected. However, noncalcified submucous myomas will be detected when distorting the uterine cavity or when causing filling defects in the endometrial contour. Subserous myomas are likely to go undetected with HSG until they cause displacement of the uterus or tubes. Intramural myomas should be suspected when enlargement of the uterine cavity is visualized (Figure 4), but their precise localization cannot be achieved if there are no accompanying filling defects.

Ultrasonography is the most useful clinical tool in screening for leiomyomas. Common findings include an enlarged uterus, abnormalities in contour, and focal masses with different echogenicity. Small lesions may be missed if they are not of different echogenicity from that of the normal myometrium. Since more than 99% of leiomyomas are benign, a conservative medical approach is usually warranted. As ultrasound is a non-invasive and inexpensive tool it can be offered for the lengthy conservative follow-up.

MRI is considered to be the most accurate imaging technique available for detection and localization of myomas, being more accurate and sensitive than either sonography or HSG[22]. One series compared MRI, sonography and HSG for preoperative localization of myomas[26], reporting an 85% sensitivity and 94% accuracy for MRI compared to a 69% sensitivity and 87% accuracy with sonography, and 18% sensitivity and 72% accuracy with HSG. The specificity for the three techniques was not significantly different, ranging between 98 and 100%. In cases where leiomyomas are found to be the primary cause of

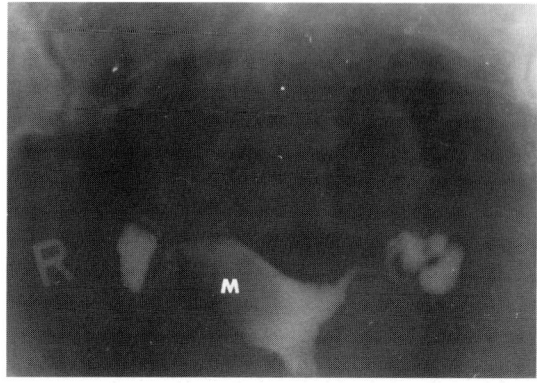

Figure 4 Hysterosalpingograph of myomatous uterus. The uterine cavity is distorted by a submucous myoma (M)

infertility, and a myomectomy is indicated, MRI is recommended for preoperative surgical planning and assessment, because of its superiority in this application[26]. It is also possible to assess whether the myoma has undergone degeneration based on differences in signal intensity[27]. MRI is likewise valuable in distinguishing adenomyosis from leiomyomas. The diffuse form of adenomyosis manifests as an enlarged uterus with a decreased signal intensity of the myometrium[17].

Congenital uterine malformations may be diagnosed in 0.1–0.4% of women, and are mainly due to a defect in the differentiation of the Mullerian system. They are an important factor causing fertility problems and habitual spontaneous abortions[28,29], although more than 80% of women with congenital malformations will have no difficulty in conceiving. Uterine malformations are considered to be responsible for about 20% of habitual abortions, most commonly caused by septate and bicornuate uteri[30]. The techniques used to detect anomalies are HSG, sonography, MRI, hysteroscopy and laparoscopy. HSG is commonly used to visualize a defect, but it is unable to show the external morphology of the uterus (Figures 5–8). In order to differentiate between a bicornuate and septate uterus, for example, an additional modality may be necessary. On HSG, a bicornuate uterus has a bilobar fundal configuration with convex lateral margins and a wide separation between

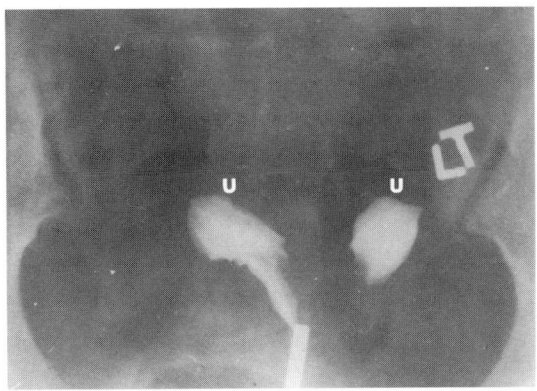

Figure 5 Hysterosalpingograph of double uterus (U)

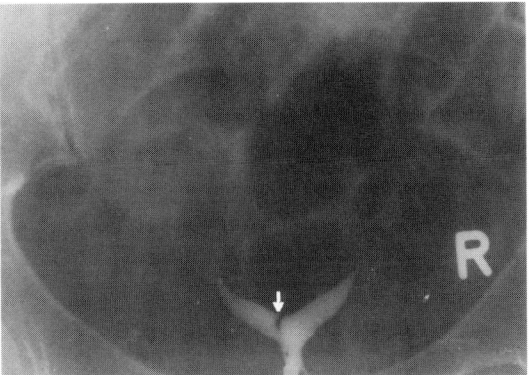

Figure 8 Hysterosalpingograph demonstrating arcuate uterus with small septum. R = right

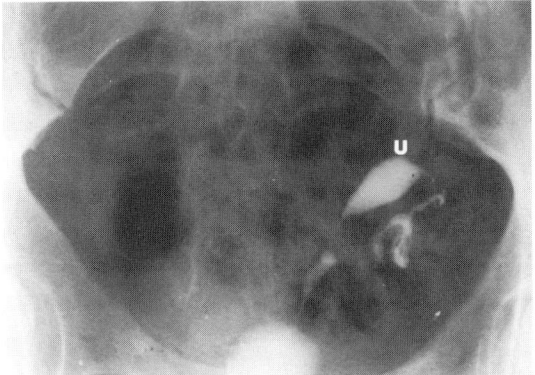

Figure 6 Hysterosalpingograph of unicornuate uterus (U)

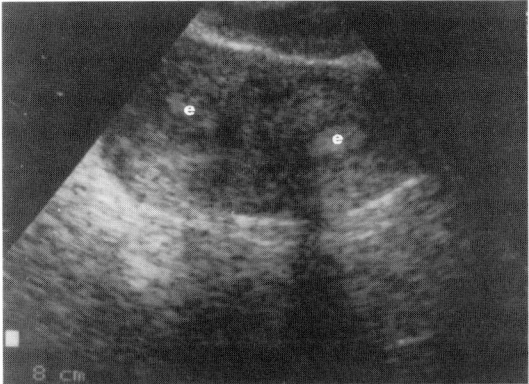

Figure 9 Transvaginal sonography demonstration of bicornuate uterus. Note two separate endometrial echoes (e)

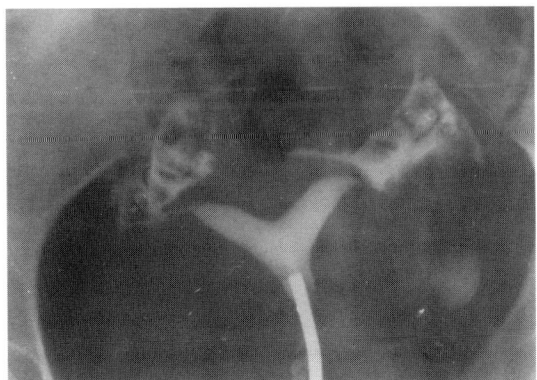

Figure 7 Hysterosalpingograph of bicornuate uterus

the horns, whereas a septate uterus usually has an angle of less than 75° between its two cavities. Nevertheless, there is wide overlap, contributing to errors in diagnosis. The diagnostic accuracy of HSG alone in differentiating between the two is around 55%. Combining HSG with sonography, that to some extent allows visualization of the external uterine contour, achieves an accuracy of 90% in the diagnosis of uterine malformations[31,32] (Figure 9). Sonography alone may misdiagnose an intrauterine septum, and adnexal masses may be confused with an additional uterine horn. Existing technical limitations may be overcome in many cases with the use of TVS, which allows better determination of external uterine contour and detection of uterine anomalies[33]. Here too, MRI is the most accurate technique for diagnosis[33,34] (Figure 10). A bicornuate uterus appears as two high signal intensity endometrial regions, surrounded by a low signal junctional zone,

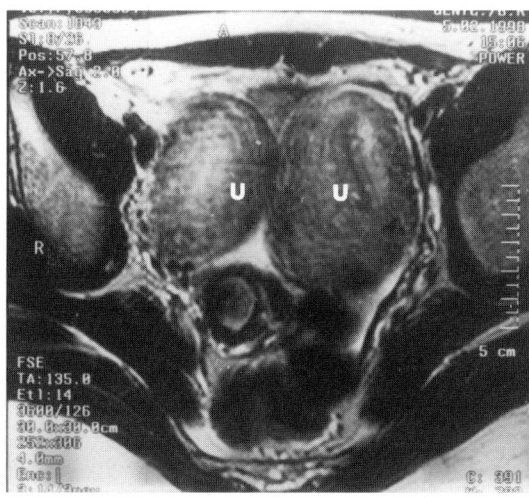

Figure 10 Magnetic resonance imaging of uterus didelphys (U)

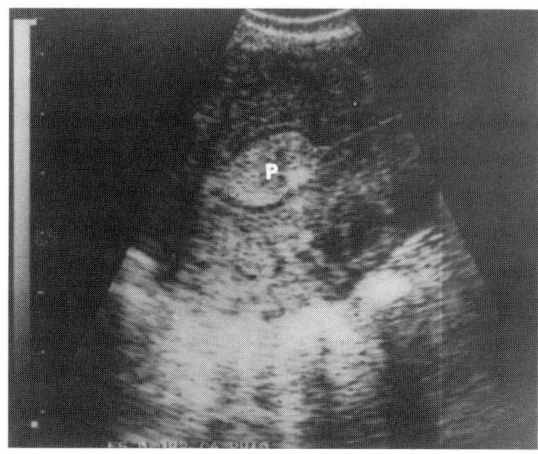

Figure 11a Transvaginal sonography of endometrial polyp (P)

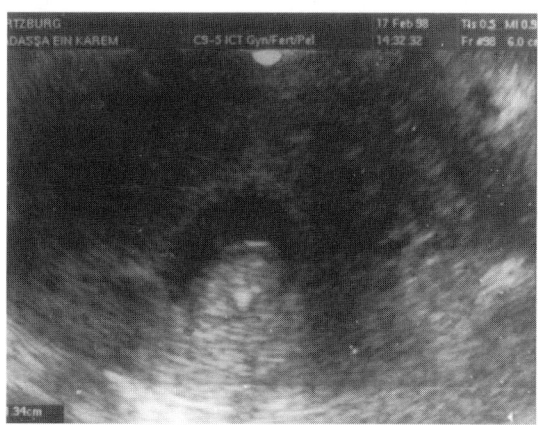

Figure 11b Hydrosonographic evaluation of the uterine cavity, demonstrating an endometrial polyp

further surrounded and separated by a medium signal myometrial band. The latter is not present in a septate uterus. MRI is extremely valuable in the preoperative evaluation of cases requiring reconstructive surgery, as it enables estimation of the length of the septum[17].

Sonohysterography, or hydrosonography, which involves the instillation of sterile saline into the uterus under continuous sonographic visualization, enables assessment of the uterine cavity without the use of radiation or contrast agents. In a normal uterus the endometrium appears symmetric, surrounding the anechoic, saline-distended cavity. Adhesions appear as bridging bands of tissue distorting the cavity or as very thin undulating membranes. Polyps can be seen surrounded by anechoic fluid and the thickness of the stalk can be determined (Figure 11). Leiomyomas can be located, as intramural lesions do not distort the cavity, whereas submucosal lesions often do. Focal areas of endometrial thickening can be identified in women with abnormal uterine bleeding[20]. Sonohysterography is highly sensitive, specific and accurate for screening the uterine cavity[35], and can be more advantageous than hysterosalpingography in patients with early pregnancy loss[36,37].

Another important application of sonography is as an aid in evaluating systemic hormonal levels apparent through serial changes in the endometrium during the menstrual cycle[31,38] (Figures 12–14). The endometrium changes in thickness and reflectivity. Smith and colleagues[38] described reflectivity as a means to grade the endometrium. This is based on a comparison of the gray-scale appearance of endometrial texture with that of myometrial texture. Drugan and associates described four patterns of sonographic endometrial appearance[39]. Grade D is defined as an almost anechoic endometrium with a prominent midline echo, which is consistent with the early follicular phase. Grade C is defined as a solid area of reduced reflectivity which appears darker than the surrounding

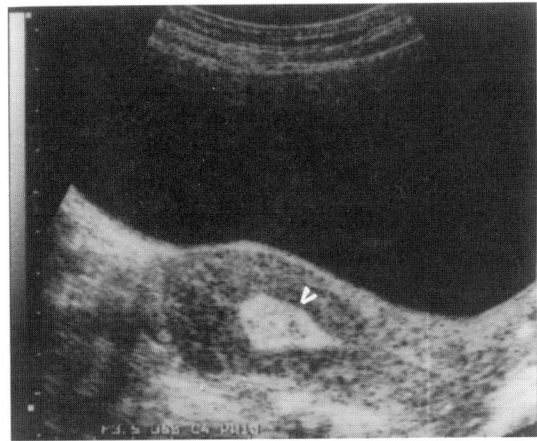

Figure 12 Transabdominal sonography of hyperechogenic endometrium

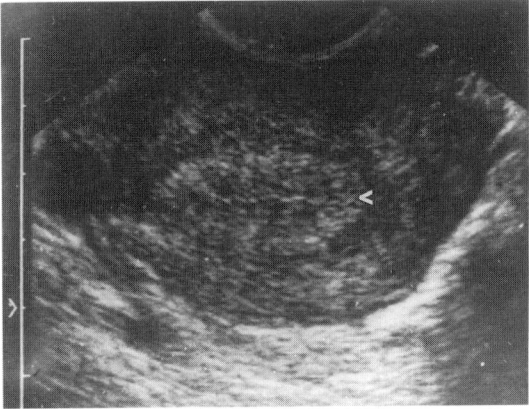

Figure 13 Transvaginal sonography of endometrium in early secretory phase

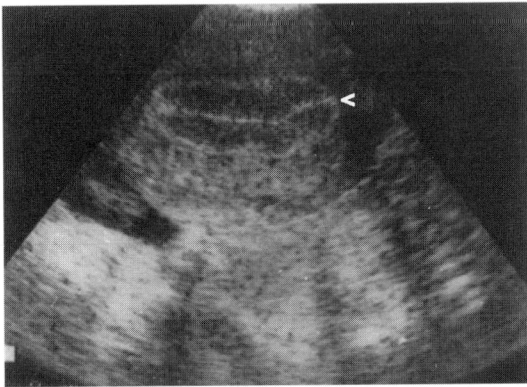

Figure 14 Transvaginal sonography of triple line endometrium

myometrium, and is common in the mid-follicular phase. In grade B patterns, the reflectivity of the endometrium and myometrium are similar in the late follicular phase, close to the estrogen peak. In grade A patterns the endometrium is brighter than the myometrium. Gonen and Casper[40] studied endometrial texture and thickness during ovulation induction for *in vitro* fertilization (IVF) and described three different types of pattern. Type A consists of an entirely homogenous, hyperechogenic endometrium (Figure 12). Type B is an intermediate type characterized by the same reflectivity as myometrium, with a nonprominent or absent central echogenic line (Figure 13). Type C consists of a multilayered endometrium with a 'triple line' appearance, consisting of prominent outer and midline hyperechogenic lines and inner hypoechogenic regions (Figure 14). The authors found that the endometrial pattern and thickness on the day of oocyte retrieval could predict the likelihood of pregnancy. Pattern C and endometrial thickness above 6 mm were associated with a 39.1% pregnancy rate per embryo transfer. There were no pregnancies if the thickness was less than 6 mm. When type A or B endometrium was seen the negative predictive value for the occurrence of pregnancy was 90.5%[40]. The endometrial thickness is measured through the central longitudinal axis of the uterine body, on both sides of the midline. Increased thickness of the endometrium is associated with higher levels of estrogen, with an increased number of preovulatory follicles and with higher rates of fertilization and conception in IVF and ovulation induction cycles[41]. An endometrial thickness of less than 5 mm is usually seen in the early to mid-follicular phase. At the time of ovulation usually a thickness of 10–14 mm is apparent. After ovulation the triple line appearance of the follicular phase disappears and a hyperechogenic endometrium wider than 13 mm can be detected, representative of secretory endometrium[39], similar to the appearance of decidual changes in the early pregnant uterus. The luteal phase endometrial appearance may be out of phase with timing of ovulation, indicating a luteal phase defect. This can be supported by hormonal assay or endometrial biopsy[22].

Sonography has also been used during intra-uterine insemination, enabling verification of the deposition of sperm within the uterine cavity. Insemination is performed when ovulation is apparent and when endometrial thickness is satisfactory. The sperm suspension appears as hyperechogenic spots accentuating the linear uterine cavity[42]. The width of the cervical canal can also be estimated as it may alter on different days of the menstrual cycle, indicating the amount of mucous secretion, secondary to changes in estrogen concentration[43].

Tubal factor infertility

Tubal factors are the cause of 25–40% of infertility cases, mainly due to pelvic inflammatory disease (PID), endometriosis or surgery causing peritubal adhesions, tubal damage and occlusion. Uterine myomas, congenital malformations and torsion can also impair tubal patency.

HSG is an important diagnostic tool which provides information about internal tubal architecture and tubal patency (Figure 15). Tubal obstruction is noted when contrast material does not reach the peritoneal cavity. Peritubal disease may cause distal tubal occlusion or sactosalpinx, namely dilatation of the ampullary portion of the tubes, which does not allow passage of contrast material. Selective salpingography can be used to deliver contrast material directly to the Fallopian tube in some cases where proximal obstruction is suspected, allowing visualization of distal anatomy[44,45]. Tubal spasm, which may be caused by uterine distention during the examination, should be suspected when proximal tubal occlusion is observed. False-positive diagnosis of tubal blockage due to spasm can be prevented by using a gentle technique and obtaining later films[22]. When a history of pelvic inflammatory disease is obtained, the 3% risk of serious infection following HSG should be considered[46,47].

Other techniques have been used to evaluate tubal patency. Observation of fluid in the

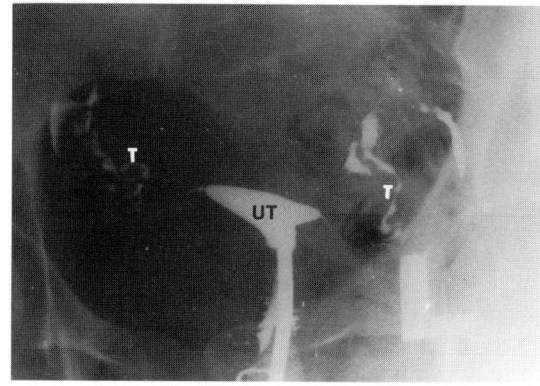

Figure 15 Hysterosalpingograph of normal uterine cavity (UT) and patent tubes (T)

cul-de-sac after transcervical injection of fluid during sonographic examination[48], and detection of radionuclide in the peritoneal cavity after placing it in the vaginal fornix (radionuclide hysterogram) are examples[49]. The disadvantage of these methods is that neither can be used to show intratubal anatomy. Furthermore, there is no way of knowing if both tubes are patent or only one and on which side. In the past, definitive diagnosis and treatment of tubal occlusion required laparoscopy or laparotomy. Laparoscopy is widely used, as it enables direct visualization of the pelvis, as well as surgical intervention for the removal of endometriosis, adhesions, and for tuboplasty, when these are required[16]. Tubal patency is determined by flushing methylene blue dye through the cervix into the uterus and consequently the tubes. With patent tubes the dye flows through the fimbria into the abdominal cavity. When an obstruction exists, the tube may dilate behind the point of obstruction, which often may be difficult to identify with precision. The main disadvantage of laparoscopy is that it is an invasive procedure, and carries the risks of anesthesia and intra-abdominal intervention.

TVS may detect hydrosalpinx or sacto-salpinx as an irregular elongated mass filled with transonic fluid. On transverse sections the dilated tube appears as a cystic structure with internal indentations, which can be differentiated from an ovarian tumor by its elongated structure on longitudinal sections. A tubo-ovarian abscess appears as a dilated, round, thick-walled structure, filled with fluid and frequently with gas bubbles[50]. Cross sections may show different sizes, but the continuity of the tortuous lumen of the thickened tube can be seen. The tube usually embraces the ovary, but some of the ovarian follicles may still be recognized. Pelvic pain will distinguish this lesion from chronic illness. When PID is suspected, pelvic adhesions may be found, appearing as the 'sliding organs sign', namely absence of movement of the ovary or uterus in relation to each other or to the pelvic wall[50].

A relatively recent alternative for tubal assessment is contrast hysterosalpingo-sonography, utilizing an ultrasound contrast medium such as Echovist® and high-resolution TVS[21,51]. Echovist consists of a microbubble-containing microparticle suspension of the water-soluble monosaccharide galactose. The suspension is prepared immediately before the examination, resulting in a white echogenic substance which is stable for 10–15 min. With the patient in the lithotomy position, pelvic examination is performed to rule out infection, and a catheter is inserted through the cervical canal into the uterine cavity and a balloon at its tip is inflated. A small volume (2–3 ml) of contrast material is first instilled. Simple B-mode imaging is used, with a 5–7.5-MHz transvaginal probe. The uterus is scanned in the longitudinal and transverse positions. Additional fluid is instilled for visualization of the tubes in transverse or oblique projections. In our ultrasound service, after positioning the uterine catheter, we first inject normal saline for the evaluation of the uterine cavity, followed by injection of Echovist for tubal patency assessment. When the tubes are patent, the echogenic fluid forms a narrow white line within the tube and the flow can be seen in real time, resulting in spillage into the peritoneal cavity. Tubal occlusion is visualized as an abrupt interruption of the band-shaped course of the Echovist suspension in the case of isthmal occlusion, and a dragging pain may appear on the corresponding side. Ampullar occlusion usually causes fluid collection in the lumen,

simulating a hydrosalpinx. In many cases the ampulla can accommodate up to 20–25 ml of fluid without causing pain. In the case of a pre-existing sactosalpinx the suspension may persist in the occluded portion causing an inflammatory reaction.

Ideally, contrast hysterosalpingo-sonography should be performed between days 8 and 13 of the menstrual cycle, and should not be performed in women with galactosemia. Echovist is reported as being superior to saline in the assessment of tubal patency[52–54]. A high diagnostic reliability for tubal patency has been reported, with concordance values of 80–90% when compared with HSG and with laparoscopy with dye insufflation[55,56]. These values are superior to concordance values between HSG and laparoscopy with dye[57]. However, the diagnosis of tubal occlusion is less reliable than the diagnosis of tubal patency and requires control by a second method. Recent reports advocate the use of contrast hysterosalpingo-sonography as a first-line office procedure, which can be performed by one person with or without an assistant[21,51]. A further advantage of this procedure is that it can include a sonographic assessment of the endometrium and myometrium, as well as the diagnosis of ovarian pathology. Pelvic discomfort is the most commonly reported adverse effect, lasting for several hours and requiring simple analgesia at most[21]. When severe pain is reported, it is often associated with unilateral or bilateral occluded tubes. Injecting Echovist in small boluses and keeping the total volume injected to a minimum appears to reduce the likelihood of pelvic discomfort[21]. Vasovagal reactions may occur, but allergic reactions are rare. An important pre-requisite is adequate training and experience in performing TVS. In some cases the tube may be difficult to assess, in which case color Doppler sonography may be added[58,59]. False-negative findings for tubal patency, namely an occluded tube in the presence of an anatomically patent tube, may occur in the presence of tubal spasm, different resistance between the tubes, poor catheter positioning, and insufficient injection of contrast material. False-positive findings for tubal patency may occur with extravasation of contrast material, tubal fistula or misinterpretation. The pregnancy rate following the procedure is reported to be 35–40% within 1 year, comparable to that reported for HSG and for laparoscopy with dye[51].

Contrast hysterosalpingo-sonography can also be used to diagnose uterine abnormalities. Absence of distention of the uterine cavity suggests the presence of intrauterine adhesions. Polyps may be seen as hypo-intense spherical structures surrounded by Echovist. Myomas are recognized by their moderate echogenicity and a non-homogenic internal structure, surrounded by echogenic fluid. An arcuate uterus can be visualized in longitudinal and transverse projections, as a concave protrusion of the fundus. A bicornuate uterus can be seen as a break in the anticipated transverse oval endometrial structure after instillation of Echovist. For the evaluation of a double uterus, separate balloon catheters should be positioned in each cavity and each filled with contrast fluid simultaneously for comparison and for visualization of a separating wall. Laparoscopy and hysteroscopy are indicated if a major uterine deformity is found.

Contrast hysterosalpingo-sonography is advantageous as an early fertility screen, enabling the identification of those patients who would benefit from further assessment by laparoscopy, hysteroscopy, or HSG. It can replace some of the invasive diagnostic procedures and prevent radiation exposure in patients with normal tubes, and it is cost-effective.

Peritoneal factor infertility

The peritoneal factor generally refers to pelvic adhesions or disruption caused by previous infection, endometriosis or surgery. These may interfere with tubal motility, thus disturbing oocyte pick-up by altering the relationship between the ovary and tube, by preventing oocyte extrusion, or by causing tubal occlusion. Peritubal adhesions may appear on HSG as loculated spillage of contrast material in the peritoneal cavity, ampullary dilatation, or as a convoluted or vertical Fallopian tube. These persist unchanged on delayed views[44,60].

Peritubal loculation is frequently difficult to distinguish from a hydrosalpinx. TVS may in some cases allow the detection of adhesions, causing an aggregate movement of the organs under investigation when pressure is applied simultaneously to the abdomen and by the transvaginal probe[22]. The presence of fluid collection, whether spontaneously or after hydrosonography with saline or Echovist, is also highly suggestive of peritoneal adhesions.

Endometriosis

Typically, endometrial implants are scattered in various extrauterine locations, mainly on the peritoneal surfaces in the pelvis, but also inside the ovaries with the formation of 'chocolate cysts' containing hemolytic blood. Frequently the presence of endometriosis is accompanied by the formation of pelvic and peri-adnexal adhesions, which interfere with ovulation and oocyte transport by the tubes. Impaired fertilization due to endometriosis-related peritoneal factors has also been observed. Diagnosis is based on direct laparoscopic definition of the presence and extent of the endometriotic implants. Although several studies have tried to determine whether ultrasound can be applied for this purpose[61], a common specific echo pattern could not be found[62]. Sandler and Karo[62] defined three categories of lesions according to their sonographic appearance: cystic, mixed and solid. Cystic lesions are characterized by a shaggy, irregular cystic wall with some evidence of septation. Mixed lesions appear similar to pelvic inflammatory disease, while solid lesions suggest ovarian malignancy[61]. The incidence of cystic lesions was reported to be 31–62%, that of mixed lesions 16–47%, and that of solid lesions 10–30%. Ultrasound was found to be accurate in determining the size, shape, and location of endometriomas, enabling the diagnosis of pelvic masses not assessable clinically[63,64]. Friedman and colleagues[65] compared routine ultrasound and laparoscopy in the detection of endometriosis. They found that routine ultrasound does not have a role in the diagnosis of endometriosis in women without a suspected pelvic abnormality[65], although it may support a clinical suspicion of endometriosis[66]. The classical chocolate cyst may appear as a non-echogenic cyst with a semisolid content. The cyst may appear homogenic, or partially solid and partially cystic, and may be difficult to differentiate from other hemorrhagic ovarian masses, such as corpus luteum cysts, from complex cystic neoplasms, or from tubo-ovarian abscesses[66]. A hemorrhagic corpus luteum cyst has a pattern which changes over time, which may aid in distinguishing it from endometriosis. Endometriomas and chocolate cysts usually remain of constant parenchymatous texture, representing the paste-like content, while a hemorrhagic corpus luteum cyst changes in pattern due to fibrinolysis of the hemolytic content of the cyst, and thus the proportion of cystic and solid elements changes. These criteria may aid in the correct sonographic diagnosis of endometriotic lesions[66].

On MRI, the presence of endometriosis is suggested by multiple complex hemorrhagic multiloculated masses[34]. The MRI appearance of endometriosis varies according to the form of the disease. Endometrial implants have the same signal intensity characteristics as normal endometrium. Endometriomas are generally multiloculated with low signal-intensity walls, while the signal intensity characteristics vary with the state of the blood breakdown products (Figure 16). An endometrioma may appear heterogeneous and may have posterior shading. Indistinct borders with adjacent organs can suggest adhesions, and invasion into bowel or bladder can be noted. Although MRI is currently the best imaging modality for detection of endometriosis, neither sonography nor MRI are sensitive enough for the diagnosis of small endometriotic lesions or intraperitoneal implants[17]. Thus, laparoscopy remains the gold standard for diagnosis and staging[17,60], while MRI or TVS can be used to follow response to hormonal therapy[67].

OVULATION INDUCTION AND *IN VITRO* FERTILIZATION

Ovulatory problems are present in 10–20% of infertile couples. However, induction of ovulation is applied much more frequently, since it

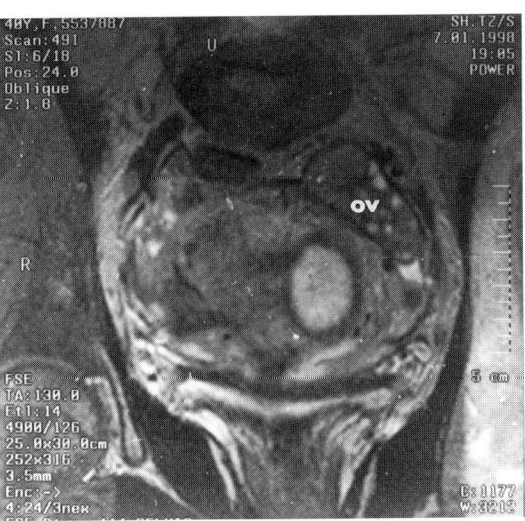

Figure 16 Magnetic resonance imaging of ovarian structure (OV)

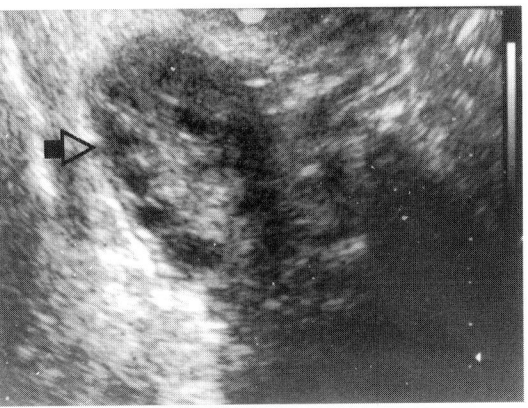

Figure 17 Transvaginal sonography of polycystic ovary. Note necklace appearance of peripheral cysts (arrow)

increases conception rates in other causes of infertility as well, for example male factor and unexplained infertility. The main goal of sonography in this context is in monitoring follicular growth and timing of ovulation, but it is also valuable in the correct diagnosis of disorders of ovulation, such as polycystic ovaries and luteinized unruptured follicle syndrome (LUFS). Polycystic ovaries, which are seen in 5% of women, may be suggested by characteristic sonographic features (Figure 17). Ovarian enlargement with spherical ovaries greater than 6 cm in diameter may be seen in approximately two-thirds of patients[68]. Peripheral cysts less than 1 cm in diameter, representing immature atretic follicles, may appear in about 50% of patients with polycystic ovaries. LUFS should be suspected when a dominant follicle is still apparent 48 h after the luteinizing hormone (LH) surge[69]. An atretic ovary that does not contain follicles may be visualized in women with Turner's syndrome.

Sonography is a vital tool for monitoring women undergoing ovulation induction and IVF. Ultrasound is used to follow follicular size, to aid in aspiration of oocytes from the mature follicles, to follow endometrial thickness, and to aid in the transfer of embryos into the uterine cavity. For ovulation induction, typically clomiphene citrate, human menopausal gonadotropin (hMG) or follicle-stimulating hormone (FSH) are used. In IVF, usually concomitant treatment with gonadotropin-releasing hormone agonists (GnRH-a) with hMG/FSH is used in order to avoid a spontaneous LH surge. TVS is preferably used, as it provides a higher resolution and less interference from surrounding bowel loops. An initial scan of the pelvis is mandatory to rule out any ovarian or uterine pathology. Sonography can simultaneously monitor follicular and endometrial growth, and is usually initiated on the 5th day of gonadotropin administration, by which time the developing follicles are around 10 mm in diameter. Follicular measurement determines maximum diameter longitudinally and transversely and then uses the mean as the index number[31]. Normal follicles increase by 1–4 mm per day until the size of a mature follicle is reached, averaging at 15–24 mm[31,39]. In a natural cycle, ovulation occurs within a narrow range of follicular diameters of 20 to 25 mm[70] (Figure 18), but this may vary considerably in induced cycles. In an induced cycle, when the largest follicle, used as a guide for oocyte maturity, has reached a size of 18–20 mm (Figure 19), ovulation is initiated by the administration of human chorionic gonadotropin (hCG). Sonography is important in assessing timing and dosage of the ovulation induction protocol. Visualization of the cumulus oophorus indicates follicular maturity,

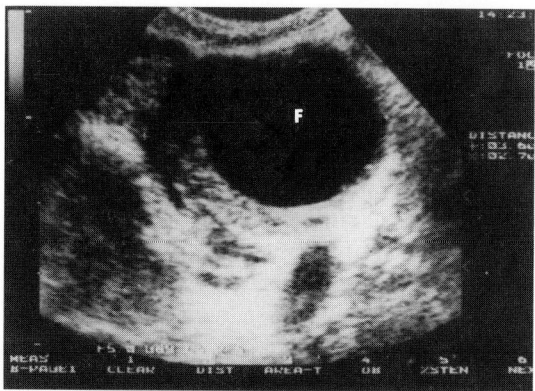

Figure 18 Transvaginal sonography of mature ovarian follicle (F)

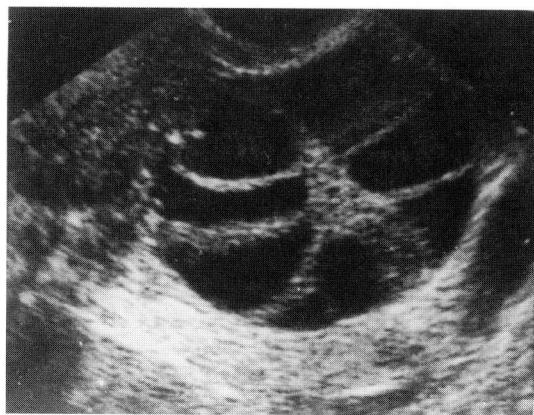

Figure 19 Transvaginal sonography of ovary with multiple mature follicles following induction of ovulation with menotropins

meaning that ovulation will occur within 36 h[66]. Although other signs of follicular maturity and impending ovulation have been documented, such as double contour and changes in ovarian and uterine blood flow, none has been reliably shown to predict imminent ovulation[31,71,72].

Normal follicular growth correlates with estradiol measurements. A mature follicle secretes about 250–300 pg/ml of estradiol[39,73]. Although follicular size is more accurate than estradiol measurements in predicting ovulation, using both parameters may achieve better timing[39]. In induced cycles the correlation between follicular size and estradiol levels is lower, as estradiol levels also represent the cohort of small follicles. Thus, the correlation with total follicular volume is better, as the rate of individual follicular growth may alter during the cycle[39]. A satisfactory estradiol level may be produced by a few mature follicles or by many small immature follicles. HCG is usually administered when estradiol has reached at least 500 pg/ml or when sonography shows at least one follicle 17 mm in diameter or greater. As the estradiol level rises, there is an increased frequency of ovarian hyperstimulation syndrome (OHSS)[74]. Thus, in induced cycles, sonography is extremely valuable in withholding hCG administration when estradiol levels are apparently ovulatory, but result from the development of multiple small follicles[70]. Premature administration of hCG at a follicular diameter smaller than 14 mm may result in follicular atresia and a short luteal phase[39]. When hCG is administered too late the oocytes may be overmature. Correct follicular monitoring is also important in ovulation induction protocols which do not include GnRH-a administration, which carry the risk of ovulation occurring prior to oocyte pick-up, due to a spontaneous LH surge.

For accurate monitoring, it is necessary to differentiate ovarian follicles from other anatomical structures with similar appearance. Blood vessels can be differentiated by changing the position of the transducer by 90° and by the presence of pulsatility and color Doppler. Bowel shows peristaltic movements and an echogenic content. Other structures such as a hydrosalpinx or an ovarian cyst will appear constant on serial scans in contrast with the changing size of the growing follicle[66].

Recent studies by Van Blerkom and colleagues[75] suggest that oocytes that reside in follicles experiencing severe hypoxia prior to ovulation may suffer changes in cellular physiology of fundamental developmental significance, with the occurrence of such follicles increasing with maternal age. The application of color pulsed Doppler provides an indirect indication of perifollicular vascularity that correlates well with the level of follicular oxygenation. These findings indicate differences

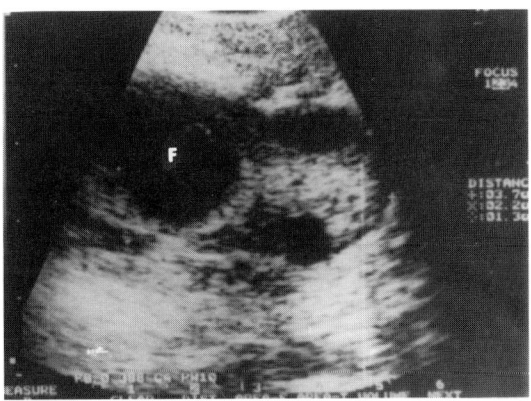

Figure 20 Transvaginal sonography of preovulatory follicle (F) in low responder IVF patient

in follicle-specific perifollicular blood flow characteristics that may reflect differential angiogenesis in the perifollicular capillary bed. Severe intrafollicular hypoxia may influence the normality of chromosomal organization and segregation in the oocyte. Thus, Doppler analysis of individual preovulatory follicles may provide an indirect indication of follicular quality and possibly the competence of the corresponding oocyte[75] (Figure 20).

Sonographic indicators of ovulation include a sudden collapse of the growing follicle, central echoes within the follicle, crenation of the follicular wall, decreased follicular size, and appearance of fluid in the cul-de-sac. With the formation of the corpus luteum, the internal follicular area fills and becomes isoechoic with respect to the surrounding ovary[76]. This series of events, which may take no more than a few hours, is considered compatible with ovulation[66]. Some fluid may appear in the cul-de-sac prior to ovulation, resulting from transudate from the growing dominant follicle[39].

Monitoring complications of ovulation induction

Ovarian hyperstimulation, characterized by cystic enlargement of the ovaries after ovulation, is not a rare occurrence in ovulation induction protocols[69] (Figure 19). Ovarian hyperstimulation syndrome (OHSS), however, is a less common complication, characterized by massive cystic enlargement of the ovaries,

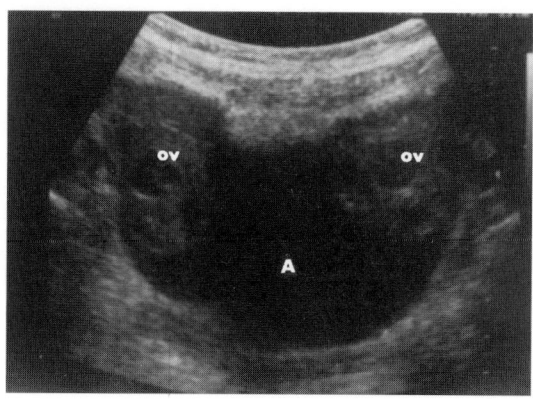

Figure 21 Ovarian hyperstimulation syndrome following induction of ovulation and oocyte pick-up; Transvaginal sonography monitoring of enlarged ovaries (OV) and massive ascites (A)

ascites, edema, pleural effusion, and hemoconcentration (Figure 21). Steering a pathway between desired ovarian hyperstimulation and full OHSS requires continuous ultrasonic monitoring along with estradiol measurements. The development of this syndrome can be suggested by the appearance of multiple follicles (more than 35) correlated with an estradiol level above 4000 pg/ml[77]. When these appear it is advisable to withhold or limit hCG administration or to administer GnRH-a. The symptoms and signs start developing soon after ovulation and reach a peak at 8–10 days after ovulation. When pregnancy fails to occur, the symptoms diminish within 10 days, while in the presence of pregnancy these may persist for several weeks. The degree of severity is determined by the presence of the clinical signs mentioned above and ultrasonic parameters, such as ovarian size or the presence of fluid in the peritoneal or pleural cavities. Ultrasound is a vital tool in monitoring the course of OHSS and determining treatment measures.

Persistent cysts, which may appear during ovulation induction, can be followed ultrasonically. Response to treatment by oral contraceptive drugs or by GnRH-a can be monitored.

Multiple pregnancies are a common complication of ovulation induction, occurring in 7% with clomiphene citrate, in 18% with gonadotropins and in over 25% in IVF protocols. The rate of multiple gestation can be decreased by limiting the number of embryos transferred in IVF cycles[78]. Ultrasound can be used to monitor and decrease the rate of multiple pregnancy, by limiting the number of follicles in ovulation induction. Furthermore, ultrasound-guided reduction of multiple gestation has been shown to improve pregnancy and newborn outcome[79–81]. The transvaginal and transabdominal approaches are comparable for this application[82].

The prevalence of ectopic pregnancy is increased in the population undergoing IVF, possibly due to the increased rate of endometriosis and pelvic inflammatory disease in this group. Monitoring of patients includes serial β-hCG measurements correlated with sonographic appearances. A intrauterine gestational sac should be visible by transabdominal sonography (TAS) when the hCG level is greater than 4000 mIU/ml or by TVS at 1000 mIU/ml[69,83]. Failure to demonstrate an intrauterine sac at these levels strongly suggests an ectopic gestation. Demonstrating a fetal pole or a yolk sac within the uterus by week 6 from the last menstrual period using TAS or by day 32 to 35 using TVS excludes ectopic gestation in most cases, although heterotopic pregnancy may occur, at an incidence of 1 : 300 in induced/IVF cycles[84].

Follicular aspiration and embryo transfer

Sonographically guided oocyte pick-up is today the almost exclusive method for oocyte recovery in IVF and for monitoring embryo transfers[39,85]. Early studies have reported the use of a transabdominal-transvesical approach[86,87], replacing laparoscopic oocyte retrieval. During the last 12 years the transvaginal approach has prevailed[88] by offering a shorter distance between the probe and the ovary, enabling the use of probes with higher frequency and higher resolution, achieving a better yield in terms of number of oocytes aspirated and consequently higher pregnancy rates. Furthermore, with this method, the aspiration needle inserted into the vaginal fornix traverses a shorter intra-abdominal distance, thus reducing the danger of injury to bowel or blood vessels. Because of all these advantages and because it is better tolerated by the patients, the transvaginal approach is usually performed as an outpatient procedure, becoming the method of choice for oocyte pick-up[69]. Rarely, a transabdominal approach may be necessary if the ovaries are situated very high, outside the pelvis[78]. One difficulty of ultrasonically guided oocyte retrieval is spatial orientation. When the retrieval needle is not in the plane of the sound beam it is not visible and can be difficult to control. This is mostly overcome by the use of a biopsy guide attached to the probe, which couples the path of the needle to the plane of the ultrasound beam. Inadvertent introduction of the needle into blood vessels and bowel is a rare event and can be prevented in most cases by a thorough examination of all pelvic structures in both the long and short axis, prior to initiation of oocyte pick-up.

Embryo transfer necessitates adequate positioning of the embryos in the uterine cavity. With the use of TAS with a full bladder, it is possible to measure the distance from the external os of the cervix to the desired location within the uterus. Uterine straightening is achieved, allowing a smooth passage of the transfer catheter into the uterine cavity, thus improving pregnancy rates[89]. Furthermore, once the embryos have been transferred it is possible to view the echogenicity of the air bubbles transferred with the medium at the point of their deposition.

ASSESSMENT OF THE MALE PARTNER

Male factor infertility is present in approximately 40% of infertile couples. The pathogenesis of most male factor-related disturbances is unclear. The function of the male genital system is dependent on the central nervous system (namely, the hypothalamus and hypophysis), the adrenal gland, the testes, the epididymis, the seminal vesicles and the prostate gland. As all these participate in sperm production and transport, any malfunction may affect the male reproductive capacity. Spermatogenesis takes place in the germinal epithelium of the seminiferous tubules (sertoli cells) in the testis and requires approximately 74 days. Sperm transport through the epididymis and vas deferens varies in duration, averaging 12 days, during which time the spermatozoon acquires its oocyte penetration ability.

When male factor infertility is suspected, imaging of the ejaculatory apparatus is necessary, in order to rule out structural abnormalities. Lesions which are associated with excretory male infertility include congenital (Wolffian and Mullerian duct anomalies), acquired (Cowper duct and peripheral-zone prostatic cysts), infectious (prostatitis) and hormonal (seminal vesicle atrophy) entities. Vasography is the traditional method for evaluation of the excretory tract. It is an invasive procedure which carries the risk of post-procedure stricture of the vas deferens.

Recent advances have enabled the application of ultrasonography in the assessment of male infertility. Scrotal and transrectal ultrasonography (TRUS) are used in the evaluation of reproductive tract disorders. Color flow Doppler ultrasonography is used for the assessment of varicocele. TRUS combined with seminal vesiculography is used for the evaluation of distal ejaculatory duct obstruction. Other methods include computed tomography (CT) and endorectal MRI.

Scrotal sonography

Ultrasonography is the primary imaging modality for scrotal abnormalities, used to confirm findings of physical examination, such as varicocele and parenchymal irregularities in the testicle or epididymis. Examination is performed on a supine patient using 7.5- or 10-MHz transducers, so that abnormalities as small as 0.5 mm may be identified.

The normal adult testis measures 3 to 5 cm in length, 2 to 3 cm in width, and 2 to 3 cm in anteroposterior depth, with a volume of 15 to 20 ml. The sonographic appearance is homogenous of low to medium echogenicity.

Occasionally, the septa that extend from the mediastinum testis and divide the testis into the lobuli testis may produce a characteristic echogenic linear pattern. The posterolateral epididymis, which consists of a head, a body and a tail, is generally 6–8 mm in diameter. Small amounts of fluid in the tunica vaginalis are considered normal[69]. Sonography is accurate within 10% of the actual volume and is better than physical examination in detecting testicular asymmetry[90]. Two-thirds of men with male factor infertility have an abnormality in testicular size, manifested by testes of less than 3 cm in length and less than 2 cm in diameter[91]. Conditions associated with atrophy and non-obstructive azoospermia or severe oligoteratoasthenospermia (OTA) include varicocele, cryptorchidism, post-pubertal mumps, tuberculosis, syphilis, Klinefelter's syndrome, and hepatic cirrhosis. Ultrasound is the first approach used for the detection and localization of an undescended testis. Infertility is common in this population[92], and in later years there is an increased risk of testicular cancer. Testicular irregularities on physical examination require prompt ultrasound evaluation. Testicular tumors are most common in the age group presenting with fertility problems, as there is an association between testicular tumors and infertility[93]. Ultrasound is extraordinarily sensitive, capable of revealing even small tumors which are not clinically palpable. However, it is not specific, as orchitis, hemorrhage, infarction and abscesses may be of similar appearance[69]. Most testicular tumors appear as a focal hypoechoic lesion within the normally homogenous texture of the testis. Seminoma, the most common germ cell tumor, is also the most common tumor associated with cryptorchidism, which clearly predisposes to male infertility. Cystic degeneration, fibrosis, local hemorrhage and necrosis are more commonly seen with non-seminoma germ cell tumors. Most intratesticular lesions in this age group are malignant. Benign lesions such as microlithiasis, intratesticular cysts and old hematomas may occasionally occur[94], but their relation to infertility is not clear[95].

Adult varicocele is present in approximately 40% of infertile men, and its occurrence in healthy young men reaches 13.4%[96]. Most common are left-sided varicoceles, but bilateral lesions occur in 40% of infertile patients with varicocele. Scrotal sonography may be used for the screening of varicocele when physical examination is uncertain. Ultrasound examination reveals serpiginous tubular structures within the epididymis, which may be further distended when the patient stands or performs a Valsalva maneuver[69]. Although venography is still considered the gold standard for diagnosis, it is an invasive procedure and therefore not favored[97]. This has led to the pursuit of alternative diagnostic measures, including radionuclide angiography, which has a high false-negative rate, and scrotal thermography, which has widely variable results.

Ultrasonic applications used in the diagnosis of varicocele include Doppler stethoscope, real-time ultrasonography and color flow Doppler imaging[95]. The Doppler stethoscope has a significantly high false-positive rate compared to venography[98]. The presence of a prolonged venous flow augmentation or reflux, usually detected as a venous rush during the Valsalva maneuver, is considered diagnostic. False-positive results may occur in normal men when a transient flow augmentation appears during the Valsalva maneuver, and secondary to active cremasteric contractions[95]. High resolution, real-time scrotal sonography using 7- to 10-MHz probes defines varicocele as a hollow tubular structure that increases in size with the Valsalva maneuver. A vein 3 mm in diameter or larger in a resting patient is considered to be a varicocele[95,99]. Bidirectional Doppler ultrasound can be used to classify varicoceles as stop-type, having a retrograde flow alone, or shunt-type, having both retrograde and orthograde venous blood flow. The stop-type pattern is more common with subclinical mild varicoceles[100]. Reversal of flow characteristics of varicocele may be confirmed by color flow Doppler. The appearance is of prolonged flow augmentation within a colored flow area which reverses with real-time imaging (color change). Inguinal sonography can also be performed accurately in a longitudinal alignment[95,101].

Ultrasound examination of the epididymis is helpful for the diagnosis of epididymal cysts or spermatocele, both of which are asymptomatic conditions which may be associated with infertility, but are usually not the cause of it. Rarely, an epididymal cyst may become obstructive and result in oligo- or azoospermia. The appearance of an epididymal cyst is hypoechoic and circumscribed with good transmission and with posterior wall enhancement. Ultrasound is not helpful in the evaluation of suspected epididymal obstruction[95].

A hydrocele is characterized by a hypoechoic, fluid-filled tunica vaginalis sac surrounding the testis. The presence of a testicular tumor should be ruled out in the infertile male with a hydrocele[95].

Transrectal ultrasonography

TRUS is an excellent approach for visualizing the seminal vesicles, prostate, and ejaculatory ducts. TRUS can assess obstructions, and determine the absence or hypoplasia of the seminal vesicle and ejaculatory ducts. Combined with seminal vesiculography, TRUS can assess distal ejaculatory duct obstruction, which reduces the need for more invasive procedures. Ejaculatory duct obstruction manifests itself as primary or secondary infertility with oligo- or azoospermia, depending on the etiology and time of occurrence of the obstruction. Perineal discomfort, pain with ejaculation, and epididymal pain may occur. Absolute indications for performing TRUS are low-volume azoospermia or severe oligospermia without testicular atrophy and without the presence of retrograde ejaculation. However, normal volume does not exclude an ejaculatory duct obstruction[102]. Other indications include midline cysts or asymmetry on rectal examination[95]. A midline cyst may be of Mullerian (utricular, may contain sperm), Wolffian (diverticulae, contains sperm), or prostatic (retention cyst, does not contain sperm) origin. The Mullerian cysts are the most common in infertile men[103].

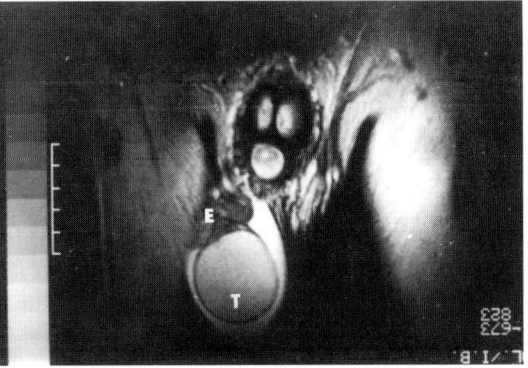

Figure 22 Magnetic resonance imaging of normal testis (T) and epididymis (E)

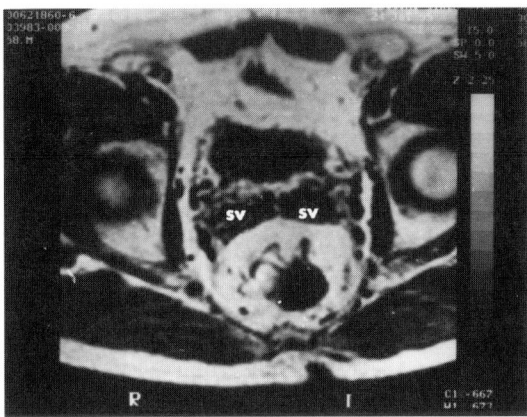

Figure 23 Magnetic resonance imaging of normal seminal vesicles (SV)

TRUS is the best screening test for ejaculatory duct obstruction. Ejaculatory duct cysts, calcification or dilation, and seminal vesicle dilation on TRUS are all consistent with ejaculatory duct obstruction[95]. TRUS is also indicated in men with severe oligospermia and a low-volume ejaculate, because a partial obstruction may be present[104]. Intraoperative use of TRUS is helpful in localizing the obstructing cysts and in determining the depth of resection of the obstructed ejaculatory duct[105]. A disadvantage of TRUS is that it cannot exclude obstructions proximal to the prostate and seminal vesicles. TRUS-guided seminal vesiculography is a recent development which can effectively diagnose ejaculatory duct obstruction without the risk of vasal scarring associated with vasography[95].

The seminal vesicles have a typical bow-tie appearance, and they are homogenous with few internal echoes. Ejaculatory duct obstruction can be associated with seminal vesicle dilation above 1.5 cm[102], or with asymmetry. Men with congenital absence of the vas deferens (CAVD) should undergo TRUS, as up to 90% of men with unilateral CAVD have aplasia of the ipsilateral seminal vesicle, and 20% have aplasia of the controlateral seminal vesicle[106]. Men with bilateral CAVD may have coexisting aplasia or hypoplasia (decrease in size of 30% or more) of the seminal vesicles, and should be tested for cystic fibrosis. Renal ultrasound is warranted, due to coexisting renal malformations[95].

MRI has multiplanar capability and provides high-resolution images of the prostate gland and adjacent structures, but it cannot replace ultrasound in the initial evaluation of patients with infertility. MRI should be reserved for selected patients in whom TRUS is not conclusive, as it is more expensive and not as widely available[107] (Figures 22 and 23).

References

1. Mishell, D. R. Jr. and Davajan, V. (1991). Evaluation of the infertile couple. In Mishell, D. R. Jr, Davajan, V. and Lobo, R. A. (eds.) *Infertility, Contraception and Reproductive Endocrinology*, 3rd edn., pp. 557–70. (Cambridge, MA: Blackwell Scientific Publications)

2. Hull, M. G. R., Glazener, C. M. A., Kelly, N. J., Conway, D. I., Forster, P. A., Hinton, R.A., Coulson, C., Lambert, P. A., Watt, E. M. and Desai, K. M. (1985). Population study of causes, treatment, and outcome of infertility. *Br. Med. J.*, **291**, 1693–7

3. Congressional Board of the 100th Congress, Office of Technology Assessment (1988). *Infertility: Medical and Social Choices*, Publication no. 20510–8025. (Washington, DC: Government Printing Office)

4. Jones, H. W. and Toner, J. P. (1993). The infertile couple. *N. Engl. J. Med.*, **329**, 1710–15

5. Belsey, M. A. and Ware, A. (1986). Epidemiological, social and psychosocial aspects of infertility. In Insler, V. and Lunenfeld, B. (eds.) *Infertility: Male and Female*, pp. 631–47. (New York: Churchill Livingstone)

6. Menken, J., Trussell, J. and Larsen, U. (1986). Age and infertility. *Science*, **233**, 1389–94

7. Howe, G., Westhoff, C., Vessey, M. and Yeates, D. (1985). Effects of age, cigarette smoking, and other factors on fertility: findings in a large prospective study. *Br. Med. J. Clin. Res. Ed.*, **290**, 1697–1700

8. Wilcox, A., Weinberg, C. and Baird, D. (1988). Caffeinated beverages and decreased fertility. *Lancet*, **2**, 1453–6

9. Hull, M. G., Savage, P. E., Bromham, D. R., Ismail, A. A. and Morris, A. F. (1982). The value of a single serum progesterone measurement in the midluteal phase as a criterion of a potentially fertile cycle ('ovulation') derived from treated and untreated conception cycles. *Fertil. Steril.*, **37**, 355–60

10. Alper, M. M., Garner, P. R., Spence, J. E. and Quarrington, A. M. (1986). Pregnancy rates after hysterosalpingography with oil- and water-soluble contrast media. *Obstet. Gynecol.*, **68**, 6–9

11. Schenker, J. G. and Margalioth, E. J. (1982). Intrauterine adhesions: an updated appraisal. *Fertil. Steril.*, **37**, 593–610

12. Fayez, J. A., Mutie, G. and Schneider, P. J. (1987). The diagnostic value of hysterosalpingography and hysteroscopy in infertility investigation. *Am. J. Obstet. Gynecol.*, **156**, 558–60

13. Howards, S. S. (1995). Treatment of male infertility. *N. Engl. J. Med.*, **332**, 312–17

14. Kruger, T. F., Menkveld, R., Stander, F. S. H., Lombard, C. J., Van der Merwe, J. P., Vanzyl, J. A. and Smith, K. (1986). Sperm morphologic features as a prognostic factor in *in vitro* fertilization. *Fertil. Steril.*, **46**, 1118–23

15. American Institute of Ultrasound in Medicine (1985). *Safety Considerations for Diagnostic Ultrasound Equipment*. (Bethesda: AIUM)

16. Mehta, A. C. (1989). Evaluation of tubal factor for infertility. In Belfort, P., Pinotti, J. A. and Eskes, T. K. A. B. (eds.) *Advances in Gynecology and Obstetrics*, Series Vol. 1. (Carnforth, UK: Parthenon Publishing)

17. Woodward, P. J., Wagner, B. J. and Farley, T. E. (1993). Magnetic resonance imaging in the evaluation of female infertility. *Radiographics*, **13**, 293–310

18. Blumenfeld, Z., Dirnfeld, M. and Beck, H. (1990). Comparison of treatment of uterine leiomyomata with three GnRH agonistic analogues – efficacy and side-effects. In Vickery, B. and Lunenfeld, B. (eds.) *GnRH Analogues in Cancer and Human Reproduction*, Vol. 3, p. 45. (Boston: Kluwer Academic Publishers)

19. Goldberg, B. B., Liu, J. B., Kuhlman, K., Merton, D. A. and Kurtz, A. B. (1991). Endoluminal gynecologic ultrasound: preliminary results. *J. Ultrasound Med.*, **10**, 583–90

20. Cullinan, J. A., Fleischer, A. C., Kepple, D. M. and Arnold, A. L. (1995). Sonohysterography: a technique for endometrial evaluation. *Radiographics*, **15**, 501–16

21. Ayida, G., Harris, P., Kennedy, S., Seif, M., Barlow, D. and Chamberlain, P. (1996). Hysterosalpingo-contrast sonography (HyCoSy) using Echovist-200 in the outpatient investigation of infertility patients. *Br. J. Radiol.*, **69**, 910–13

22. Krysiewicz, S. (1992). Infertility in women: diagnostic evaluation with hysterosalpingography and other imaging techniques. *Am. J. Roentgenol.*, **159**, 253–61

23. Hamilton, C. J. C. M., Evers, J. L. H. and de Haan, J. (1986). Ultrasound increases the prognostic value of the postcoital test. *Gynecol. Obstet. Invest.*, **21**, 80–8

24. Daly, D. C., Reuter, K., Cohen, S. and Mastroianni, J. (1989). Follicle size by ultrasound versus cervical mucus quality: normal and abnormal patterns in spontaneous cycles. *Fertil. Steril.*, **51**, 598–603

25. Daly, D. C. (1992). Hysteroscopy and infertility. In Sciarra, J. J. (ed.) *Gynecology and Obstetrics*, Vol. 5 (Philadelphia: JB Lippincott Company)

26. Dudiak, C. M., Turner, D. A., Patel, S. K., Archie, J. T., Silver, B. and Norusis, M. (1988). Uterine leiomyomas in the infertile patient: preoperative localization with magnetic resonance imaging versus ultrasound and hysterosalpingography. *Radiology*, **167**, 627–30

27. Carrington, B. M. and Hricak, H. (1992). The uterus and vagina. In Hricak, H. and Carrington, B. M. (eds.) *MRI of the Pelvis: a Text Atlas*, pp. 93–184. (London: Dunitz)

28. Golan, A., Langer, R., Bukovsky, I. and Caspi, E. (1989). Congenital anomalies of the mullerian system. *Fertil. Steril.*, **51**, 747–55

29. Harger, J. H., Archer, D. F., Marchese, S. G., Muracca-Clemens, M. and Garver, K. L. (1983). Etiology of recurrent pregnancy losses and outcome of subsequent pregnancies. *Obstet. Gynecol.*, **62**, 574–81

30. Clark, R. L. and Keefe, B. (1989). Infertility: imaging of the female. *Urol. Radiol.*, **11**, 233–7

31. Winfield, A. C. and Wentz, A. C. (1987). *Diagnostic Imaging of Infertility*. (Baltimore: Williams and Wilkins)

32. Reuter, K. L., Daly, D. C. and Cohen, S. M. (1989). Septate versus bicornuate uteri: errors in imaging diagnosis. *Radiology*, **172**, 749–52

33. Mintz, M. C. and Grumbach, K. (1988). Imaging of congenital uterine anomalies. *Semin. Ultrasound Comput. Tomogr. Magn. Reson.*, **9**, 167–74

34. McCarthy, S. (1990). Magnetic resonance imaging in the evaluation of infertile women. *Magn. Reson. Q.*, **6**, 239–49

35. Parsons, A. K. and Lense, J. J. (1993). Sonohysterography for endometrial abnormalities: preliminary results. *J. Clin. Ultrasound*, **21**, 87–95

36. Keltz, M. D., Olive, D. L., Kim, A. H. and Arici, A. (1997). Sonohysterography for screening in recurrent pregnancy loss. *Fertil. Steril.*, **67**, 670–4

37. Gaucherand, P., Piacenza, J. M., Salle, B. and Rudigoz, R. C. (1995). Sonohysterography of the uterine cavity: preliminary investigations. *J. Clin. Ultrasound*, **23**, 339–48

38. Smith, B., Porter, R., Ahuja, K. and Craft, I. (1984). Ultrasonic assessment of endometrial changes in stimulated cycles in an *in vitro* fertilization and embryo transfer program. *J. In Vitro Fertil. Embryo Transfer*, **1**, 233–8

39. Drugan, A., Blumenfeld, Z., Erlik, Y., Timor-Tritsch, I. and Brandes, J. M. (1988). The use of trasvaginal sonography in infertility. In Timor-Tritsch, I. E. and Rottem, S. (eds.) *Transvaginal Sonography*, pp. 143–58. (New York: Elsevier Science Publishing Company, Inc.)

40. Gonen, Y. and Casper, R. F. (1990). Prediction of implantation by the sonographic appearance of the endometrium during controlled ovarian stimulation for *in vitro* fertilization (IVF). *J. In Vitro Fertil. Embryo Transfer*, **7**, 146–52

41. Rabinowitz, R., Laufer, N., Lewin, A. *et al.* (1986). The value of ultrasonographic endometrial measurement in the prediction of pregnancy following IVF. *Fertil. Steril.*, **45**, 824–8

42. Blumenfeld, Z. and Nahhas, F. (1989). Pretreatment of sperm with human follicular fluid for borderline male infertility. *Fertil. Steril.*, **51**, 863–8

43. Timor-Tritsch, I. E., Rottem, S. and Boldes, R. (1988). Scanning the uterus. In Timor-Tritsch, I. E. and Rottem, S. (eds.) *Transvaginal Sonography*, p. 27. (New York: Elsevier Science Publishing Company, Inc.)

44. Yoder, I. C. (1988). *Hysterosalpingography and Pelvic Ultrasound: Imaging in Infertility and Gynecology*. (Boston: Little Brown)

45. Thurmond, A. S. (1991). Selective salpingography and fallopian tube recanalization. *Am. J. Roentgenol.*, **156**, 33–8

46. Speroff, L., Glass, R. H. and Kase, N. G. (1989). Investigation of the infertile couple. In *Clinical Gynecologic Endocrinology and Infertility*, 4th edn, p. 513. (Baltimore: Williams and Wilkins)

47. Stumpf, P. G. and March, C. M. (1980). Febrile morbidity following hysterosalpingography: identification of risk factors and recommendation for prophylaxis. *Fertil. Steril.*, **33**, 487–92

48. Rasmussen, F., Larsen, C. and Justesen, P. (1986). Fallopian tube patency demonstrated at ultrasonography. *Acta Radiol.*, **27**, 61–3

49. Angtuaco, T. L., Boyd, C. M., London, S. N., Powell, L. G., Diner, W. C., Vandergrift, J. F., Bersey, M. L., Bass, B. M. and Donovan, S. A. (1989). Technetium-99m hysterosalpingography in infertility: an accurate alternative to contrast hysterosalpingography. *Radiographics*, **9**, 115–28

50. Timor-Tritsch, I. E., Rottem, S. and Levron, Y. (1988). The fallopian tubes. In Timor-Tritsch, I. E. and Rottem, S. (eds.) *Transvaginal Sonography*, p. 45. (New York: Elsevier Science Publishing Company, Inc.)

51. Degenhardt, F., Jibril, S. and Eisenhauer, B. (1996). Hysterosalpingo-contrast sonography (HyCoSy) for determining tubal patency. *Clin. Radiol.*, **51**, S15–18

52. Randolph, J., Ying, Y., Maier, D., Schmidt, C. L., Riddick, D. H. and Randolph, J. F., Jr. (1986). Comparison of real-time ultrasonography, hysterosalpingography and laparoscopy/hysteroscopy in the evaluation of uterine abnormalities and tubal patency. *Fertil. Steril.*, **46**, 828–32

53. Bonilla-Musoles, F., Simon, C., Serra, V., Sampaio, M. and Pellicer, A. (1992). An assessment of hysterosalpingography (HSSG) as a diagnostic tool for uterine cavity defects and tubal patency. *J. Clin. Ultrasound*, **20**, 175–81

54. Balen, F., Allen, C., Siddle, N. and Lees, W. (1993). Ultrasound contrast hysterosalpingography – evaluation as an outpatient procedure. *Br. J. Radiol.*, **66**, 592–9

55. Deichart, U., Schlief, R., Van de Sandt, M. and Juhnke, I. (1989). Transvaginal hystero-contrast-sonography (HyCoSy) compared with conventional tubal diagnostics. *Hum. Reprod.*, **4**, 418–24

56. Schlief, R. and Deichart, U. (1991). Hysterosalpingo-contrast sonography of the uterus and fallopian tubes: results of a clinical trial of a new contrast medium in 120 patients. *Radiology*, **178**, 213–15

57. Gabos, P. (1976). A comparison of hysterosalpingography and endoscopy in evaluation of tubal function in infertile women. *Fertil. Steril.*, **27**, 238–42

58. Deichart, U., Schlief, R., Van de Sandt, M. and Daume, E. (1992). Transvaginal hysterosalpingo-contrast-sonography for the assessment of tubal patency with gray-scale imaging and additional use of pulsed wave Doppler. *Fertil. Steril.*, **57**, 62–7

59. Yarali, H., Gurgan, T., Erden, A. and Kisnisci, H. (1994). Color Doppler hysterosalpingosonography: a simple and potentially useful method to evaluate fallopian tubal patency. *Hum. Reprod.*, **9**, 64–6

60. Karasick, S. and Goldfarb, A. F. (1989). Peritubal adhesions in infertile women: diagnosis with hysterosalpingography. *Am. J. Roentgenol.*, **152**, 777–9

61. Galle, P. C. (1989). Clinical presentation and diagnosis of endometriosis. *Obstet. Gynecol. Clin. North. Am.*, **16**, 29–42

62. Sandler, M. A. and Karo, J. J. (1978). The spectrum of ultrasonic findings in endometriosis. *Radiology*, **127**, 229–31

63. Coleman, B. G., Arger, P. H. and Mulhern, C. B. Jr. (1979). Endometriosis: clinical and ultrasonic correlation. *Am. J. Roentgenol.*, **132**, 747–9

64. Goldman, S. M. and Minkin, S. I. (1980). Diagnosing endometriosis with ultrasound. *J. Reprod. Med.*, **25**, 178–82

65. Friedman, H., Vogelzang, R. L., Mendelson, E. B., Neiman, H. L. and Cohen, M. (1985). Endometriosis detection by ultrasound with laparoscopic correlation. *Radiology*, **157**, 217–20

66. Blumenfeld, Z., Yoffe, N. and Brohnstein, M. (1990). Transvaginal sonography in infertility and assisted reproduction. *Obstet. Gynecol. Surv.*, **46**, 36–49

67. Zawin, M., McCarthy, S., Scoutt, L. *et al.* (1990). Monitoring therapy with a gonadotropin-releasing hormone analog: utility of MRI imaging. *Radiology*, **175**, 503–6

68. Hann, L. E., Hall, D. A., McArdle, C. R. and Seibel, M. M. (1984). Polycystic ovarian disease: sonographic spectrum. *Radiology*, **150**, 531–4

69. McArdle, C. K. (1990). Ultrasound in infertility. In Seibel, M. M. (ed.) *Infertility: A Comprehensive Text*, pp. 285–302. (Norwalk, CT: Appleton and Lange)

70. DeCherney, A. H. and Laufer, N. (1984). The monitoring of ovulation induction using ultrasound and estrogen. *Clin. Obstet. Gynecol.*, **27**, 993–1002

71. Steer, C. V., Campbell, S., Pampiglione, J. S., Kingsland, C. R., Mason, B. A. and Collins, W. P.

(1990). Transvaginal colour flow imaging of the uterine arteries during the ovarian and menstrual cycles. *Hum. Reprod.*, **5**, 391–5

72. Sterzik, K., Grab, D., Sasse, V., Hutler, W., Rosenbusch, B. and Terinde, R. (1989). Doppler sonographic findings and their correlation with implantation in an *in vitro* fertilization program. *Fertil. Steril.*, **52**, 825–8

73. Hackeloer, B. J., Fleming, R. and Robinson, H. P. (1979). Correlation of ultrasonic and endocrinologic assessment of human follicular development. *Am. J. Obstet. Gynecol.*, **135**, 122–8

74. Schenker, J. G. and Weinstein, D. (1978). Ovarian hyperstimulation syndrome: a current survey. *Fertil. Steril.*, **30**, 255–68

75. Van Blerkom, J., Antzak, M. and Schrader, R. (1997). The developmental potential of the human oocyte is related to the dissolved oxygen content of follicular fluid: association with vascular endothelial growth factor levels and perifollicular blood flow characteristics. *Hum. Reprod.*, **12**, 1047–55

76. Picker, R. H., Smith, D. H., Tucker, M. M. and Saunders, D. M. (1983). Ultrasonic signs of imminent ovulation. *J Clin. Ultrasound*, **11**, 1–2

77. Blankstein, J., Shalev, J., Saadon, T. *et al.* (1987). Ovarian hyperstimulation syndrome: prediction by number and size of preovulatory follicles. *Fertil. Steril.*, **47**, 597–602

78. Laufer, N., Grunfeld, L. and Garrisi, J. (1990). *In vitro* fertilization. In Seibel, M. M. (ed.) *Infertility: A Comprehensive Text*. (Norwalk, CT: Appleton and Lange)

79. Lipitz, S., Reichman, B., Uval, J., Shaler, J., Achiron, R., Barkai, B., Lasky, A. and Mashiach, S. (1994). A prospective comparison of the outcome of triplet pregnancies managed expectantly or by multifetal reduction to twins. *Am. J. Obstet. Gynecol.*, **170**, 874–9

80. Lipitz, S., Uval, J., Achiron, R., Sehiff, E., Lusky, A. and Reichman, B. (1996). Outcome of twin pregnancies reduced from triplets compared with nonreduced twin gestations. *Obstet. Gynecol.*, **87**, 511–14

81. Berkowitz, R. L., Lynch, L., Stone, J. and Alvarez, M. (1996). The current status of multifetal pregnancy reduction. *Am. J. Obstet. Gynecol.*, **174**, 1265–74

82. Lipitz, S., Yaron, Y., Shalev, J., Achiron, R., Zolti, M. and Mashiach, S. (1994). Improved results in multifetal pregnancy reduction: a report of 72 cases. *Fertil. Steril.*, **61**, 59–61

83. Nyberg, D. A., Filly, R. A., Mahoney, B. S., Monroe, S., Laing, F. C. and Jeffrey, R. B., Jr. (1985). Early gestation: correlation of hCG levels and sonographic identification. *Am. J. Roentgenol.*, **144**, 951–4

84. Risk, B., Tan, S. L., Morcos, S., Riddle, A., Brinsden, P., Mason, B. A. and Edwards, R. G. (1991). Heterotopic pregnancies after *in vitro* fertilization and embryo transfer. *Am. J. Obstet. Gynecol.*, **164**, 161–4

85. Lenz, S., Lauritsen, J. G. and Kjellow, M. (1981). Collection of human oocytes for *in vitro* fertilization by ultrasonically guided follicular puncture. *Lancet*, **1**, 1163–4

86. Lenz, S. and Lauritsen, J. G. (1982). Ultrasonically guided percutaneous aspiration of human follicles under local anesthesia: a new method of collecting oocytes for *in vitro* fertilization. *Fertil. Steril.*, **38**, 673–7

87. Lewin, A., Laufer, N., Rabinowitz, R. and Schenker, J. G. (1986). Ultrasonically guided oocyte collection under local anesthesia: the first choice method for *in vitro* fertilization – a comparative study with laparoscopy. *Fertil. Steril.*, **46**, 257–61

88. Dellenbach, P., Nisand, I., Moreau, L., Feger, B., Plumere, C., Gerlinger, P., Brun, B. and Rumpler, Y. (1984). Transvaginal sonographically controlled ovarian follicle puncture for egg retrieval. *Lancet*, **1**, 1467

89. Lewin, A., Schenker, J. G., Avrech, O., Shapira, S., Safran, A. and Friedler, S. (1997). The role of uterine straightening by passive bladder distention before embryo transfer in IVF cycles. *J. Assist. Reprod. Genet.*, **14**, 32–4

90. Costabile, R. A., Skoog, S. and Radowich, M. (1992). Testicular volume assessment in the adolescent with varicocele. *J. Urol.*, **147**, 1348–50

91. McClure, R. D. and Hricak, H. (1986). Scrotal ultrasound in the infertile man: detection of subclinical unilateral and bilateral varicoceles. *J. Urol.*, **135**, 711–15

92. Lipshultz, L. I. and Greenberg, S. H. (1981). Varicocele and male subfertility. In Sciarra, J. (ed.) *Gynecology and Obstetrics*, Vol. 5 pp. 1–9. (Hagerstown: Harper and Row)

93. Foster, R. S. and Donohue, J. P. (1995). Fertility in testicular cancer patients. *AUA Update Series XIV*, **19**, 153–60

94. Krone, K. D. and Carroll, B. A. (1985). Scrotal ultrasound. *Radiol. Clin. North. Am.*, **23**, 123–9

95. Kim, E. D. and Lipshultz, L. I. (1996). Role of ultrasound in the assessment of male infertility. *J. Clin. Ultrasound*, **24**, 437–53

96. Cockett, A. T. K., Takihara, H. and Cosentino, M. J. (1984). The varicocele. *Fertil. Steril.*, **41**, 5–11

97. Hirsh, A. V., Kellett, M. J., Robertson, G. *et al.* (1980). Doppler flow studies, venography and thermography in the evaluation of varicoceles of fertile and subfertile men. *Br. J. Urol.*, **52**, 560–5

98. Hirsh, A. V., Cameron, K. M., Tyler, J. P. *et al.* (1980). The Doppler assessment of varicoceles and internal spermatic vein reflux in infertile men. *Br. J. Urol.*, **52**, 50–6

99. Gonda, R., Karo, J., Forte, R. *et al.* (1987). Diagnosis of subclinical varicocele in infertility. *Am. J. Roentgenol.*, **148**, 71–5

100. Sigmund, G., Gall, H. and Bahren, W. (1987). Stop-type and shunt-type varicoceles: venographic findings. *Radiology*, **163**, 105–10

101. Orda, R., Sayfan, J., Manor, H., Witz, E. and Sofer, Y. (1987). Diagnosis of varicocele and postoperative evaluation using inguinal ultrasonography. *Ann. Surg.*, **296**, 99–101

102. Carter, S. S. C., Shinohara, K. and Lipshultz, L. I. (1989). Transrectal ultrasonography in disorders of the seminal vesicles and ejaculatory ducts. *Urol. Clin. North. Am.*, **16**, 787–99

103. Jarow, J. P. (1993). Transrectal ultrasonography of infertile men. *Fertil. Steril.*, **60**, 1035–9

104. Ruiz Rubio, J. L., Fernandez Gonzales, I., Quijano Barosa, P., Hervero Payo, J. A., Berenger Sanchez, A. (1995). The value of transrectal ultrasonography in the diagnosis and treatment of partial obstruction of the seminal duct system. *J. Urol.*, **153**, 435–6

105. Goldwasser, B. Z., Weinerth, J. L. and Carson, C. C. (1985). Ejaculatory duct obstruction: the case for aggressive diagnosis and treatment. *J. Urol.*, **134**, 964–6

106. Hall, S. and Oates, R. D. (1993). Unilateral absence of the scrotal vas deferens associated with contralateral mesonephric duct anomalies resulting in infertility: laboratory, physical, and radiographic findings, and therapeutic alternatives. *J. Urol.*, **15**, 1161–4

107. Parsons, R. B., Fisher, A. M., Bar-Chama, N. and Mitty, H. A. (1997). Magnetic resonance imaging in male infertility. *Radiographics*, **17**, 627–37

Ultrasound and the ovary

2

D. Nugent, J. Smith and A. H. Balen

THE OVARY AND ASSISTED REPRODUCTION

Some of the most important advances in assisted conception therapies have resulted from developments in ultrasonography. The development of this technology has simplified oocyte retrieval techniques, enabling transvaginal ultrasound-directed procedures to be performed under sedation, thereby superceding laparoscopic oocyte collection under general anesthesia. It is also now the preferred method for monitoring follicular growth, and such is its accuracy that many centers have largely abandoned endocrine monitoring of ovarian stimulation by gonadotropins[1,2]. *In vitro* fertilization (IVF) is a relatively successful therapy with cumulative conception rates that compare favorably with spontaneous conception in women of the same age[3,4]. In a recent analysis of 36 961 IVF cycles performed in the UK, the livebirth rate after a single cycle was 13.9% for women under the age of 35 years[5]. Ovulation induction therapies for anovulatory infertility also produce very favorable success rates. In a recent series of 200 women who underwent 1227 cycles of ovulation induction, the overall cumulative conception and livebirth rates were 80% and 65%, respectively, after 12 cycles of treatment[2].

This chapter outlines the usefulness of ultrasound in monitoring both the normal ovarian cycle and the artificially stimulated ovary, as well as in aiding oocyte retrieval procedures. The importance of identifying ovarian morphology correctly will be discussed. The complications that may arise during treatment, such as ovarian cysts and the ovarian hyperstimulation syndrome (OHSS), will also be outlined. Finally, some areas of ongoing research and development will be touched upon.

Transvaginal ultrasound examination of the pelvic organs is preferred to the transabdominal approach, as it not only obviates the need for a full bladder with its associated discomfort, but also allows higher frequencies to be used due to the close proximity of the probe to the organs under examination. This improved resolution provides greater precision in measurements of pelvic structures, including endometrial thickness and follicle diameters[6]. It is especially advantageous in those patients with lower abdominal scars, as scar tissue may impair the penetration of ultrasound. Furthermore, adhesions tend to immobilize the ovaries deep within the pelvis and limit their elevation when the bladder is filled for a transabdominal scan. Andreotti and colleagues[7], in a comparison of transabdominal with transvaginal scanning, showed that the margins of the follicles were more sharply defined in 90% of cases when the transvaginal approach was used compared with only 41% with a transabdominal approach. The same study found that the numbers and sizes of the dominant follicle(s) correlated better with the serum estradiol concentrations with transvaginal scanning.

OVARIAN MORPHOLOGY

Three distinct morphological appearances are recognizable within the ovary on ultrasound examination: normal, polycystic and multicystic (Figures 1–3). Multicystic ovaries are characteristically observed in pubertal girls and women with weight loss-related amenorrhea[8]. These multicystic (or multifollicular) ovaries are normal in size or slightly enlarged and contain six or more cysts that are 4–10 mm in diameter. Importantly, and in contrast to women with polycystic ovaries, the stroma is normal. The multicystic ovary appears to

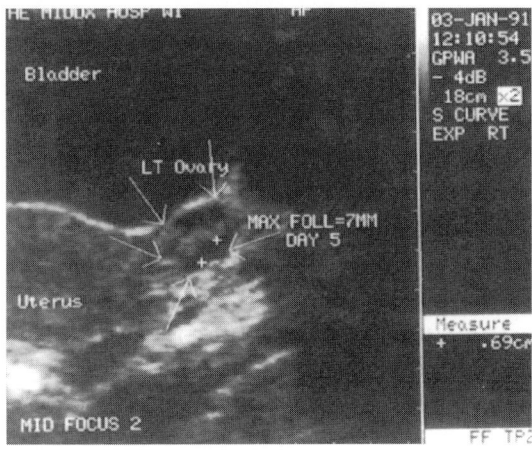

Figure 1 Transabdominal ultrasound scan of a normal ovary in the early follicular phase of the cycle. Arrows outline the ovary

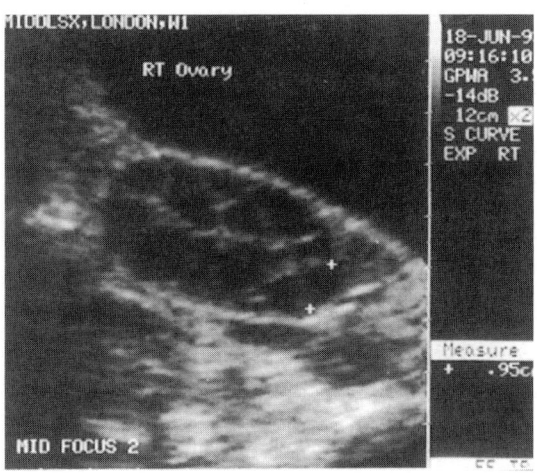

Figure 3 Transabdominal ultrasound scan of an unstimulated multicystic ovary. Note the absence of a thickened stroma, in contrast to the polycystic ovary

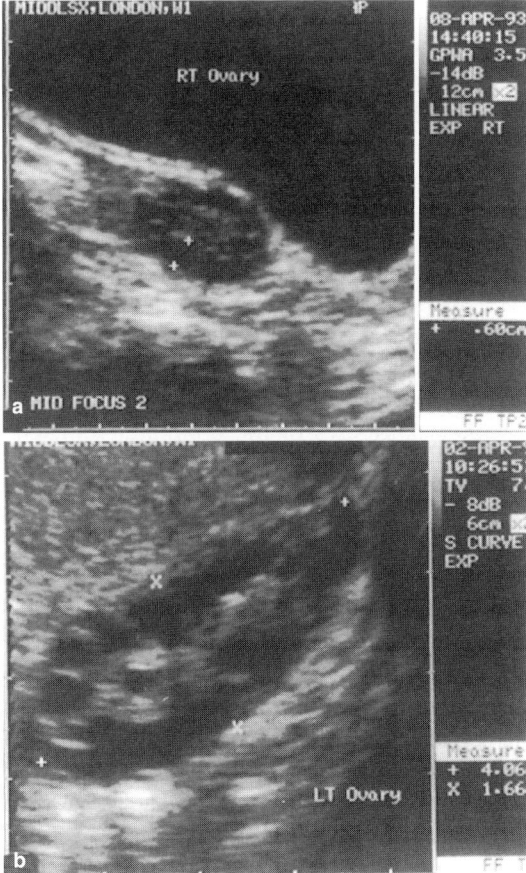

Figure 2 (a) Transabdominal and (b) transvaginal ultrasound scans of a polycystic ovary

develop as a consequence of reduced hypothalamic secretion of gonadotropin-releasing hormone (GnRH), which results in subnormal stimulation of the ovaries by the gonadotropins. As one might anticipate, the multicystic ovary exhibits a normal response to exogenous stimulation, by either pulsatile GnRH or gonadotropins, after which the ultrasound appearance of the ovary usually reverts to normal[8].

Polycystic ovaries are recognized separately, both in their appearance on ultrasound and in their response to ovulation induction and ovarian stimulation for *in vitro* fertilization. In 1935 Stein and Leventhal[9] first described the association between enlarged, sclerocystic ovaries and amenorrhea, infertility and hirsutism, now known as the polycystic ovary syndrome (PCOS). Since then it has become clear that polycystic ovaries may be present in women who are non-hirsute and who have regular menstrual cycles. Thus, a clinical spectrum exists between the symptomless patient with polycystic ovaries and the typical features of PCOS described by Stein and Leventhal[9]. While the diagnosis of polycystic ovaries simply describes the morphological appearance of the ovary, the diagnosis of PCOS should be reserved for polycystic ovaries in association with menstrual disturbance (amenorrhea or, more commonly, oligomenorrhea) and/or complications of hyperandrogenization (seborrhea, acne and hirsutism) and/or obesity. Furthermore, patients with PCOS exhibit considerable heterogeneity in terms of the number and severity of their symptoms[10].

PCOS is also associated with endocrinological abnormalities, in particular with elevated serum concentrations of luteinizing hormone (LH), prolactin, estrogens and androgens. In about 40% of cases, plasma concentrations of LH are raised and there is an increased ratio of LH to follicle-stimulating hormone (FSH)[10]. As with the clinical spectrum, these changes are variable and patients with PCOS may have normal endocrine concentrations.

Such variations in the clinical and biochemical manifestations of polycystic ovaries mean that the diagnosis is most reliably based on ovarian morphology. Fortunately, the advent of high-resolution ultrasound has made the identification of polycystic ovaries simple, and ovarian biopsy, which is invasive and possibly damaging to future fertility, is now obsolete. While the definition varies between authors, ovaries may be described as polycystic if there are 10 or more cysts of 2–8 mm in diameter, arranged around a dense stroma or scattered throughout an increased amount of stroma[10].

The prevalence of polycystic ovaries in women with ovulatory disorders is well documented. Franks and associates[11] described a prevalence of more than 50% in patients presenting with oligo- or amenorrhea. Using high-resolution ultrasound, it is apparent that as many as 87% of patients with oligomenorrhea and 26% with amenorrhea have polycystic ovaries[12]. Polycystic ovaries have also been identified in women with hypogonadotropic hypogonadism attending for ovulation induction[13], and while these patients had no endogenous production of gonadotropins, they responded to stimulation in a characteristically 'polycystic' fashion, with a sudden growth of multiple follicles[13,14]. Polson and colleagues[15] found the prevalence of polycystic ovaries to be 22% in a volunteer 'normal' population. While the prevalence of polycystic ovaries in patients referred for IVF has rarely been studied, a series of over 500 patients who underwent IVF showed that 34% had the appearance of polycystic ovaries on ultrasound scanning[16].

Clearly, polycystic ovaries with or without clinical symptoms are a common finding in patients referred for ovulation induction or IVF. Indeed, the primary diagnosis is often not PCOS but rather another cause of subfertility that necessitates assisted conception therapy[16]. It is of the utmost importance to make a careful assessment of the morphological appearance of the ovary prior to commencing ovarian stimulation, as the presence of polycystic ovaries should alert one to the risks and complications that might occur (particularly the ovarian hyperstimulation syndrome). This allows time for appropriate tailoring and monitoring of the cycle.

Future improvements in both sonographic equipment technology and computer-guided image analysis offer the prospect of a more precise and quantitative approach to the diagnosis of polycystic ovaries. The quality of the images produced by the use of three-dimensional imaging is an obvious example of the advantages of recent technological advances[17]. With the use of appropriate computer software it is possible to make use of the three-dimensional reconstructions to judge more accurately the number and location of individual follicles. This invites the possibility of examining in greater detail than previously the dynamics of spontaneous or induced follicular growth in women with polycystic ovaries[18].

OVARIAN CYSTS

Since the widespread use of GnRH agonists (GnRH-a), functional ovarian cysts have been commonly encountered during IVF cycles, with the initial surge of FSH when a GnRH-a is commenced being the accepted trigger of functional cyst formation[19]. While the reported incidence of ovarian cysts during IVF cycles varies considerably, a review of the larger series reveals an incidence of at least 5%, with a higher incidence if the GnRH-a is commenced during the follicular phase compared with the luteal phase of the cycle[20]. Thus, in addition to noting the underlying ovarian morphology, the prestimulation baseline ultrasound scan is used to examine for the presence of ovarian cysts[21]. While there is conflicting evidence about the influence of such cysts on IVF outcome, the majority viewpoint suggests that there is a detrimental effect only if the cysts are functionally active[22,23]. The first priority in management of cysts should be prevention of development, which may be achievable in several ways. As mentioned above, commencing the GnRH-a during the luteal phase of the cycle reduces the incidence, as may the concomitant administration of a progestogen[24].

Once a functional cyst has developed, a conservative approach has been shown to be effective, in which the GnRH-a is continued until the serum estradiol concentrations fall, although occasionally this may take several weeks[25,26]. Thus, an alternative, effective and simple approach to persistent functional ovarian cysts is aspiration prior to ovarian stimulation[27–29], which does not appear to adversely affect the pregnancy rate[29]. It has also been proposed, but not fully investigated, that if a functional ovarian cyst represents a dysfunctional ovarian follicle, then a single injection of human chorionic gonadotropin (hCG) may successfully rupture the follicle[20].

If cyst aspiration is performed, potential complications may arise. These include infection within or bleeding from any pelvic structure traversed by the needle, such as the ovaries, uterus, iliac vessels or even the bowel. Fortunately, ovarian abscesses after follicular aspiration for IVF and embryo transfer are rare events but have been reported[30,31]. If the patient is known to have endometriosis in particular it is important to avoid aspirating the cyst at any stage during treatment because of the greater risk of infection. An endometrioma has a characteristic hazy and relatively echodense appearance when compared with a fluid-filled cyst on ultrasound scanning, and inadvertent or unavoidable aspiration necessitates full antibiotic cover (Figure 4).

Another rare complication that may arise is pelvic hematoma formation from accidental introduction of the needle into a pelvic vessel[32]. The application of transvaginal ultrasound

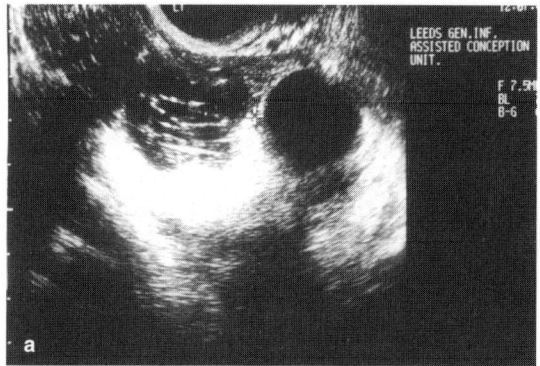

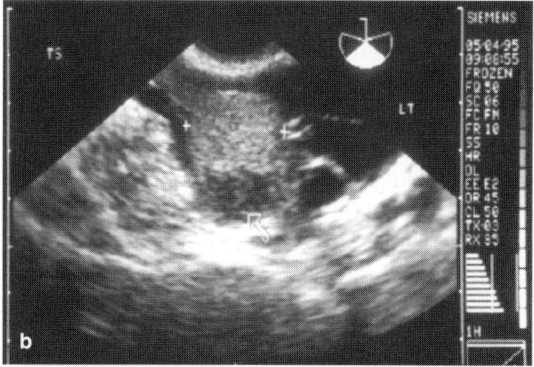

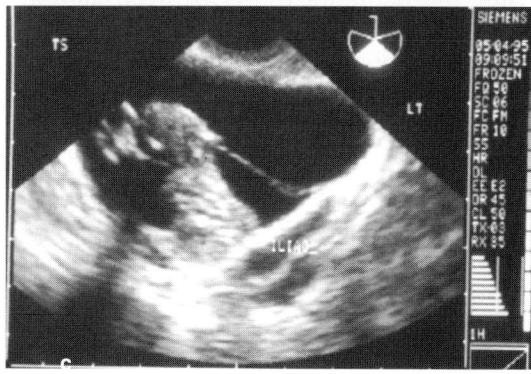

Figure 4 Three different complex cysts seen on baseline scans of women about to undergo assisted conception treatments. These should be managed by laparoscopic surgery (ideally) prior to commencing ovarian stimulation. All cysts should be investigated because of the potential risk of malignancy and the putative association between ovarian stimulation and ovarian cancer. (a) Dermoid cyst; (b) endometrioma; (c) complex serous cystadenoma

can help to prevent this if the operator carefully visualizes all round structures in both the long and the short axis to delineate a vessel from a follicle before advancing the needle. Ultrasound guidance also allows visualization

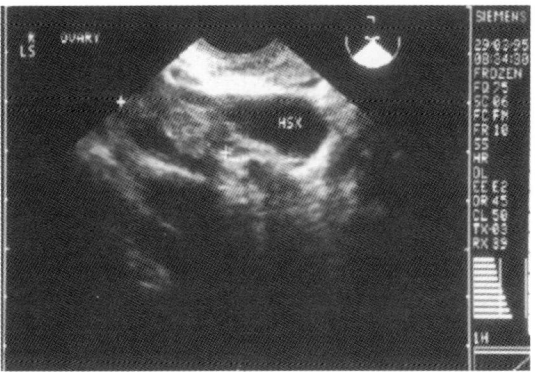

Figure 5 Hydrosalpinx (HSX) adjacent to the ovary; there is a trend towards removing hydrosalpinges prior to *in vitro* fertilization because of their putative adverse effect on implantation

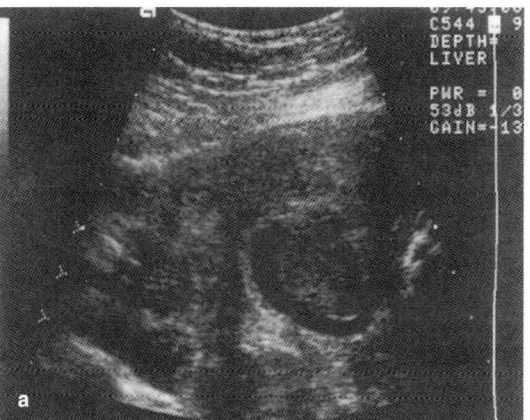

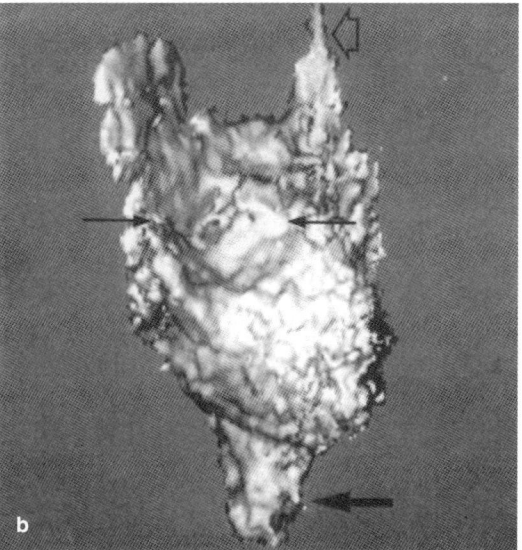

Figure 6 Submucous fibroid. (a) Plain transabdominal ultrasound after introduction of normal saline into the uterine cavity. The hypoechoic saline is shown surrounding the submucosal fibroid. (b) Three-dimensional reconstruction of the saline-filled uterine cavity, illustrating the fundal filling defect (small arrows) caused by the submucosal fibroid. The cervical canal is delineated by the large arrow and the left cornu by the open arrow. Reproduced with permission from Balen, F.G., Allen, C.M., Gardener, J.E., Siddal, N. and Lees, W.R. (1993). Three dimensional reconstruction of ultrasound images of the uterine cavity. *Br. J. Radiol.*, **66**, 588–91

of the peristaltic bowel, again differentiating it from follicular structure. Fortunately inadvertent puncture of the bowel is rare. There is one report of a case of appendicitis after transvaginal oocyte retrieval with the finding of puncture holes in the appendix at surgery, strongly suggesting a causal relationship[33].

The situation is slightly different in patients who are undergoing ovulation induction for anovulatory infertility. In such patients cysts are usually functional and secrete estrogens and progesterone. If a cyst is seen in these patients on a baseline ultrasound scan, the usual policy is to commence ovarian stimulation only after the patient has had a spontaneous menstrual bleed, which indicates that the endogenous secretion of ovarian hormones has reached baseline levels[2]. Further confirmation of this is provided by a thin ($\leqslant 5$ mm) endometrium.

The baseline ultrasound scan also permits inspection of the other pelvic structures and might reveal the presence of hydrosalpinges (Figure 5), submucous fibroids (Figure 6) endometrial polyps or even an elusive intrauterine contraceptive device.

NATURAL CYCLE MONITORING AND IVF

Ultrasound has been widely used to monitor the menstrual cycle, providing information on ovarian morphology, endometrial thickness and co-existent pelvic masses. The spatial resolution of transvaginal and transabdominal scans is 2–3 mm and 3–5 mm, respectively, so small follicles can be visualized easily as echo-free structures and usually lie towards the periphery of the more echogenic ovarian tissue. The internal diameter of the follicle should be measured in three planes and the mean value calculated. The intra-observer standard deviation of transabdominal follicular measurement was reported in one study to be 0.6 mm, and the interobserver standard deviation 1.2 mm, irrespective of the follicular diameter[34]. Thus, the 95% confidence limits for any particular measurement should be ± 2.4 mm[34], and one would expect transvaginal measurements to confer even greater accuracy[35]. In spontaneous cycles the small antral follicles should be visible about 10 days before the day of ovulation (day −10). By day −5 there is usually a dominant follicle which grows at a rate of approximately 2–3 mm daily until ovulation[36,37], while the other follicles undergo atresia or developmental arrest[38]. Bakos and colleagues[39] and Randall and Templeton[40] have also used ultrasound to monitor the menstrual cycle in healthy ovulatory women. Bakos and colleagues found that the size of the dominant follicle increased throughout the follicular phase to a mean diameter of 21.5 mm at ovulation[39]. They also found variability in the size of the follicle at ovulation; the mean diameters ranged from 17.4 to 27.0 mm (Figure 7). The plasma estradiol concentrations correlate well with follicular diameter in natural cycles[36], although not in superovulated cycles[2]. The mean levels in the natural cycle have been found to be 1012 pmol/l, with a range of 490 to 1710 pmol/l[39]. The increase in circulating estrogen levels results in an increase in the overall uterine size and a thickening of the endometrium[41], which serves as a useful clinical bioassay for estrogen production.

Historically, the natural cycle was used in the first successful IVF pregnancies, which were achieved in spontaneous, unstimulated cycles[42]. However, the limitations of natural cycle IVF soon became evident. These include the development of only a single follicle, the high possibility of not retrieving an oocyte on the collection day, and the necessity for intensive monitoring to detect a spontaneous pre-ovulatory LH surge. The pregnancy rates are higher with the transfer of several embryos and superovulation strategies have now become routine to increase the total number

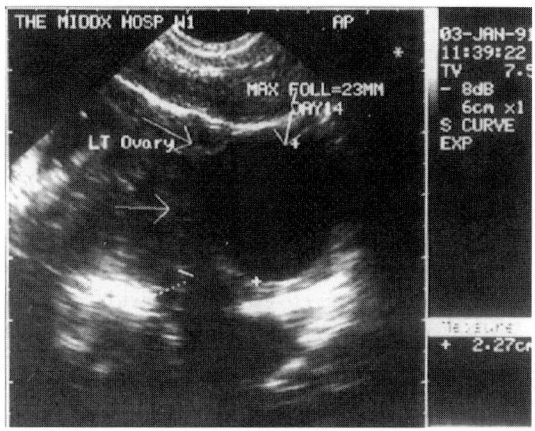

Figure 7 Transvaginal ultrasound scan of unifollicular development on day 14 of ovulation induction in a normal ovary, with a single 23-mm follicle. Arrows outline the edge of the ovary

of oocytes available[43]. Nevertheless, there has been a slight resurgence of interest in natural cycle IVF in recent years[44,45], to avoid some of the known complications of superovulation such as multiple pregnancy and the ovarian hyperstimulation syndrome (OHSS), as well as putative risks such as the possible increased risk of ovarian neoplasia[46]. Some centers have been remarkably successful with this approach, which probably relates in part to careful patient selection. Foulot and colleagues[45] reported a 22.5% pregnancy rate per cycle of natural cycle IVF. They monitored the patients with daily ultrasound scans from day 9 or 10, depending on the length of the menstrual cycle. Human chorionic gonadotropin (hCG) was administered when the dominant follicle was > 18 mm in diameter, unless the daily assays of serum LH indicated the onset of a spontaneous surge, in which case the oocyte retrieval operation was brought forward[45]. More recently, Fahy and associates[47] suggested that natural cycle IVF should be reserved for patients with tubal or unexplained infertility, in whom they achieved an overall fertilization rate of 80% and an implantation rate of 14%.

OVULATION INDUCTION CYCLES

In ovulation induction cycles for *in vivo* fertilization (either timed intercourse, donor insemination, or intrauterine insemination using either husband or donor semen) the first ultrasound scan is scheduled for day 8 of ovarian stimulation, i.e. 1 week after the baseline scan[2]. The result of this scan determines both whether the dose of stimulatory drugs should be increased and the timing of the next scan. If clomiphene citrate or pulsatile GnRH are being used it should only be necessary to scan a patient every 2–4 days[2].

If gonadotropins are used, hCG is administered when the dominant follicle is 17–18 mm in diameter, and the patient is advised when best to have intercourse. Even when a spontaneous LH surge occurs it should be augmented with hCG, as the surge in superovulated cycles is often attenuated[48] and might be insufficient to trigger ovulation. If there are more than three follicles greater than 16 mm in diameter, or more than six follicles greater than 14 mm in diameter, hCG should be withheld and intercourse avoided because of the risks of multiple pregnancy and OHSS[2]. An endometrial thickness of greater than 7–8 mm on the day of administration of hCG is suitable for implantation, although pregnancies are more likely to occur if the endometrial thickness is at least 9 mm[2].

CONTROLLED OVARIAN STIMULATION IN IVF CYCLES

The initial attempts at ovarian stimulation for IVF treatment used human menopausal gonadotropin (hMG), with or without clomiphene citrate[49]. While good results are possible with such an approach, close monitoring of follicular growth is necessary, and despite this 15–30% of cases will have a spontaneous LH surge. Pituitary desensitization with a gonadotropin-releasing hormone agonist[50] has thus become increasingly practiced in most assisted conception clinics. The reversible hypogonadotropic hypogonadism so produced permits unimpeded control over follicular development[51] and leads to improved pregnancy rates in IVF programs[52,53], although there have been relatively few prospective, randomized studies comparing the use of

GnRH-a with conventional stimulation regimens in patients who do not have a specific indication for GnRH-a use[54]. A meta-analysis of randomized and quasi-randomized studies was reported by Hughes and associates in 1992[55]. They found that the routine use of GnRH-a reduced cancellation rates, increased the number of oocytes recovered, and improved clinical pregnancy rates per cycle commenced and per embryo transfer, compared with conventional stimulation regimens. When GnRH-a is used in the long protocol there is virtually no risk of an LH surge occurring and so ovarian stimulation may be continued until the optimal number of follicles have developed[56]. Indeed, once the largest follicle has attained a diameter of at least 18 mm there is a window of at least 3 days during which hCG can be given without affecting the rates of fertilization and pregnancy[56].

The regimen we use most commonly involves administration of nafarelin acetate 600 µg daily by nasal spray, commencing in the mid-luteal phase of the menstrual cycle. Once pituitary suppression has been confirmed, with a thin endometrium and quiescent ovaries on ultrasound examination, the dose of nafarelin is decreased to 400 µg daily and ovarian stimulation commenced. The initial daily dose of FSH is based upon age; 150 IU for women < 35 years and 225 IU for those ≥ 35 years. This standard dose is adjusted upwards in older women and in previous poor responders, and downwards in patients with polycystic ovaries because of the increased risk of OHSS[57]. The next ultrasound scan is after 8 days of ovarian stimulation, while the subsequent frequency of ultrasound monitoring depends on both the individual clinic's policy and the treatment regimen that is being used. At each scan, the number and size of the follicles are documented and plotted graphically so that one can see at a glance the rate of follicular growth in each ovary. When multiple folliculogenesis occurs the follicles are rarely spherical and it is therefore important to measure three orthogonal diameters for each follicle and then calculate the mean diameter (Figure 8). For reasons given

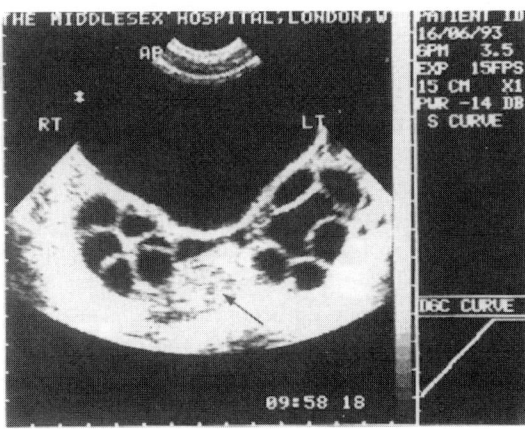

Figure 8 Transabdominal ultrasound scan of multifollicular development during superovulation induction for *in vitro* fertilization. Axial scan through uterine fundus (arrow) and both ovaries

above, regimens that involve clomiphene citrate or gonadotropins alone require more frequent monitoring than those in which a GnRH-a is used, and daily ovarian scans are necessary once a dominant follicle has formed.

Hormonal monitoring may be performed by means of an estradiol assay at the time of each scan, although increasingly this is deemed unnecessary with the use of high-resolution transvaginal ultrasound scanning[58,59]. Follicles of different sizes secrete estradiol at widely differing rates, and there is a wide range of estradiol levels for any given ultrasound picture[2]. Ultrasonography also demonstrates the location of the follicles for aspiration during oocyte retrieval and it has been found that follicular dimensions, based on the volume of aspirated fluid, correlate well with the ultrasonic measurements[60]. This study also found no correlation between the diameter of the largest follicle and the serum concentration of estradiol. Moreover, Golan and colleagues[58], using transvaginal ultrasound monitoring, found no difference in the number of days of stimulation, oocytes obtained, fertilization rates, pregnancy rates or complications with or without concomitant estradiol estimation.

In the main, ultrasound monitoring should now be regarded as sufficiently accurate for it to be used alone in monitoring gonadotropin

therapy for both *in vivo*[2,61] and *in vitro* fertilization[60], particularly when GnRH agonists are used in IVF cycles[56]. However, estradiol measurements may provide additional information which is of particular relevance when it comes to predicting the likelihood of a patient developing OHSS. Also, at the other end of ovarian response, if there are only one or two follicles, the serum estradiol concentration may provide an additional guide as to whether the cycle should be cancelled. Traditionally, the serum estradiol concentration on the day of hCG administration should be at least 2500 pmol/l, although with wider use of recombinant FSH products, deficient in LH, the mean estradiol level per follicle is reduced[62].

In GnRH-a cycles, because the spontaneous LH surge is abolished, the timing of hCG administration is not as critical and a number of assisted conception programs have used this approach to simplify cycle programming to avoid weekend oocyte retrievals[63,64], or even to schedule oocyte retrievals on as few as 3 working days each week[65]. It has been found that when the short protocol of GnRH-a is used, accurate timing of hCG remains critical. In a prospective randomized study by Clark and co-workers[66], looking at the timing of hCG when the short protocol of GnRH-a is used, it was found that prolonging follicular stimulation by 1 day significantly reduced pregnancy rates. In the case of long protocol GnRH-a administration there have been a number of retrospective studies that have demonstrated that the day of hCG administration can be safely delayed for 1 or 2 days beyond the standard time of administration[67,68]. In addition, there is a recently performed prospective study in which 247 patients, all of whom were on the long protocol with buserelin, were randomized into three groups[56]. Patients in Group 1 (*n* = 79) had hCG administered when the mean diameter of the largest follicle had reached 18 mm and at least two other follicles were greater than 14 mm in diameter. Patients in Groups 2 (*n* = 84) and 3 (*n* = 84) had hCG administered 1 day and 2 days, respectively, after the above criteria had been reached. Whilst there was a significantly progressive increase in the mean diameter of the largest follicle and the mean serum estradiol concentration among the three groups, there were no differences in the mean number of preovulatory or medium-sized follicles, the number of oocytes collected or the number of embryos transferred. There were also no significant differences in the oocyte recovery, fertilization or cleavage rates, and the pregnancy rates were similar in the three groups. Thus there is no significant advantage in the precise timing of hCG administration when GnRH agonists are used to desensitize the pituitary during IVF cycles, and this enables greater flexibility and simplicity in programming the workload of the clinic.

OVARIAN STIMULATION IN POLYCYSTIC OVARIES

The response of the polycystic ovary to stimulation in the context of ovulation induction aimed at unifollicular ovulation is well documented and differs significantly from that of the normal ovary. The response tends to be slow initially, followed by a significant risk of ovarian hyperstimulation and/or cyst formation. The therapies that are used aim for unifollicular development (Figure 9) in order to achieve a singleton pregnancy by either timed intercourse, donor insemination or intrauterine insemination.

The simplest methods of ovulation induction involve short courses of an anti-estrogen (clomiphene citrate, cyclofenil or tamoxifen) administered in the early follicular phase. The cumulative conception rate in anovulatory PCOS is about 80% by 12 months[69]. Women with PCOS who do not respond to oral therapy may succeed in having ovulation induced by gonadotropins, either hMG or FSH alone[2]. Again the possibility of OHSS exists, although regimens have been developed which, by a gradual stepwise increase in dose, reduce this risk[70]. One proposed scheme is to commence on one ampule of hMG daily for up to 14 days, until a response is seen with ultrasound monitoring. If no response is obtained after this time the daily dose is increased by

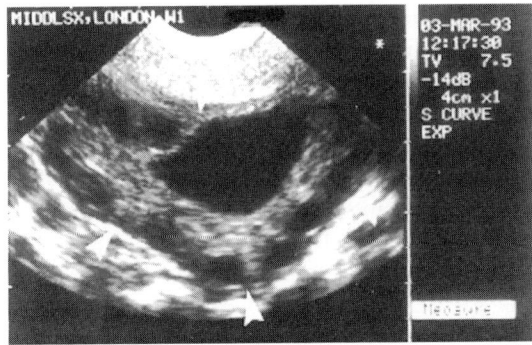

Figure 9 Transvaginal scan of unifollicular development in a polycystic ovary, with the edges of the ovary delineated by arrows

half an ampule every 7 days until a response is seen[71].

Stimulated IVF nowadays most commonly depends on inducing multifollicular recruitment using long protocol regimens. As might be predicted from the response of the polycystic ovary to ovulation induction regimens the response to multifollicular drug regimens also differs from the normal ovary. Jacobs and colleagues[72] described an increase in follicular production in patients with polycystic ovaries and others refer to the 'explosive' nature of the ovarian response[73]. There are several possible explanations for this 'explosive' response. There are numerous partially developed follicles present in the polycystic ovary and these are readily stimulated to give rise to the typical multifollicular response. The thecal hyperplasia present in polycystic ovaries provides large amounts of androstenedione and testosterone, which act as substrates for estrogen production. Granulosa cell aromatase, while deficient in the 'resting' polycystic ovary, is readily stimulated by FSH. Thus, normal quantities of FSH can act on large amounts of substrate (testosterone and androstenedione) to produce large amounts of intra-ovarian estrogen. Ovarian follicles, present in excess, are increasingly sensitive to FSH (receptors for which are up-regulated by high local concentrations of estrogen) and as a result there is multiple follicular development associated with very high levels of circulating estrogen. In a comparison of 76 patients with polycystic ovaries and 76 consecutive controls (matched for age, diagnosis and stimulation regimen) undergoing IVF therapy, the number of follicles (14.9 ± 0.7 vs. 9.8 ± 0.6 in the controls, $p < 0.001$) and peak serum estrogen levels (5940 ± 255 vs. 4370 ± 240 pmol/l, $p < 0.001$) were significantly increased in the polycystic ovary group[57]. Both groups of patients received similar total amounts of hMG. Again the greater sensitivity to exogenous stimulation of polycystic ovaries compared with normal ovaries means that this group is particularly susceptible to OHSS[57,74].

Two recent studies have suggested that the use of GnRH-a may reduce miscarriage rates in patients with PCOS. Homburg and colleagues[75] looked at 239 women with PCOS who were clomiphene treatment failures treated by GnRH-a and hMG ($n = 110$) or hMG only ($n = 128$) for ovulation induction ($n = 138$) or IVF ($n = 101$). The miscarriage rate in those undergoing ovulation induction who had GnRH-a plus hMG was 16.7% compared with 39.4% in those who had hMG alone. For patients undergoing IVF, the comparable figures were 18.2 and 38.5%. In a study by Balen and associates[16] the miscarriage rate was 23.6% in women with normal ovaries compared with 35.8% in those with polycystic ovaries. Women with normal ovaries on ultrasound were just as likely to miscarry if they were treated with gonadotropins and clomiphene citrate or with the long buserelin protocol. Those with polycystic ovaries, however, had a significant reduction in the rate of miscarriage when treated with the long buserelin protocol (20.3%) compared with gonadotropins and clomiphene citrate (47.2%). There was no difference found in miscarriage rates between those who received the short or ultrashort buserelin regimens and those who received gonadotropins and clomiphene citrate. These observations are consistent with the concept of an adverse effect of LH hypersecretion, which is known to be a feature of PCOS[76]. The long protocol regimens widely used in IVF treatment cycles may thus provide additional benefit to this group of patients.

THE OVARIAN HYPERSTIMULATION SYNDROME

The ovarian hyperstimulation syndrome (OHSS) is a well-recognized complication of ovulation induction (Figure 10). It is caused by symptomatic ovarian enlargement resulting from luteinization of multiple follicles and stromal edema. It may result in fluid retention, ascites, oliguria and weight gain, and may progress to electrolyte disturbances, thromboembolism, pleural effusions and hydrothorax[77,78]. While relatively common with gonadotropin treatment[79], severe OHSS is rarely associated with clomiphene usage alone[78]. If the severe form arises during IVF it is the only life-threatening condition associated with ovarian stimulation in IVF[73,77,80]. When GnRH agonists were initially incorporated into ovarian stimulation protocols it was hoped that their use might reduce the incidence of OHSS, since it is known that it is rare in patients with hypogonadotropic hypogonadism. Unfortunately, however, the use of GnRH-a does not reduce the incidence of OHSS, and in fact several studies have suggested that there may be an increased incidence when GnRH-a is used[81,82]. More recently, MacDougall and colleagues[57,80] studied the association of OHSS with IVF and found that pre-treatment with GnRH-a significantly increased the prevalence of severe OHSS (1.1% compared with 0.2%, $p < 0.05$).

Patients with anovulatory PCOS are at higher risk of developing OHSS, whether undergoing ovulation induction[74,76] or IVF[57,73]. In a total population of 1302 patients, MacDougall and colleagues[80] identified 15 patients who underwent ovarian stimulation for IVF or other assisted conception techniques and developed OHSS of sufficient severity to merit hospital admission (prevalence of 1.2%, with 0.6% having severe OHSS). Of these patients, 15% had ultrasonographically diagnosed polycystic ovaries and 87% were undergoing their first attempt at IVF. All had received luteal support in the form of hCG. Although the pregnancy rate in this group was very high (93.3%), the multiple pregnancy

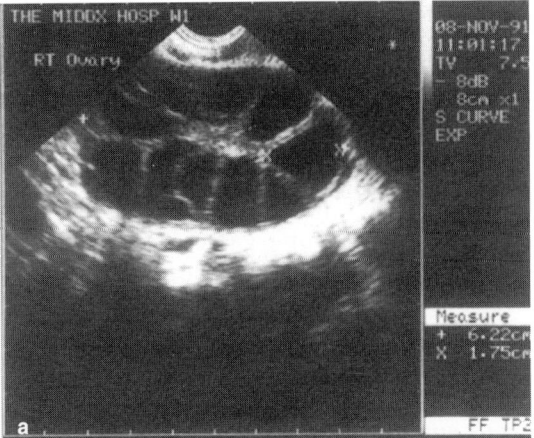

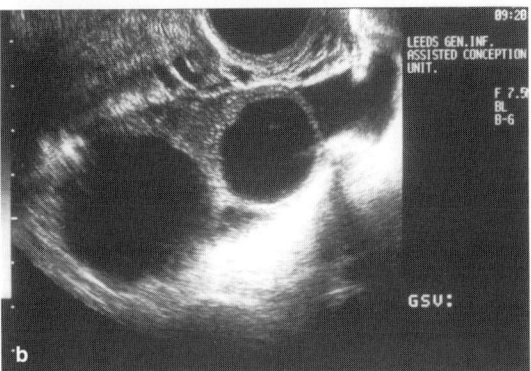

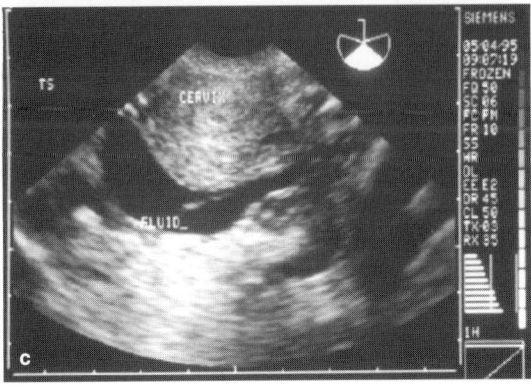

Figure 10 (a) Transvaginal scan of an overstimulated ovary. (b) Closer view of an overstimulated ovary with ascites adjacent to ovarian cysts. (c) Free ascitic fluid in the pouch of Douglas, behind the cervix

rate was 57% with a miscarriage rate of 14.3%[80]. As a result of such evidence, many centers now recommend that the dose of gonadotropins be reduced if polycystic ovaries are identified on the baseline ultrasound scan.

Prevention remains the most successful therapy for OHSS, because management is mostly palliative when the symptoms are progressing, and this may necessitate hospitalization in the more severe cases. One group has demonstrated a correlation between OHSS and multiple intermediate-sized preovulatory-sized follicles[83], while another has found an increased risk for the disease when serum estradiol levels are > 4000 pg/ml on the day of hCG administration[84]. A combination of serial follicular monitoring with transvaginal ultrasound and serum estradiol measurements is still used by many for the monitoring of ovulation induction cycles. In particular, the judicious use of transvaginal ultrasound scanning for follicular monitoring while inducing ovulation with gonadotropins remains critical for the prevention of OHSS. Multiple intermediate-sized follicles serve as predictive tools. When this pattern is seen a number of options can be considered. These include cycle cancellation by withholding hCG administration and commencing a new cycle 1 or 2 months later. This is the safest option but may be costly in emotional and financial terms and may result in cancellation of a high proportion of cycles which would not have progressed to clinical hyperstimulation. Second, the hCG can be withheld and the GnRH-a continued until estradiol levels fall, at which point the gonadotropins are recommenced at a lower dose. However, it may take between 24 and 56 days before it is possible to restart stimulation[81]. Third, one may proceed with the oocyte retrieval but freeze all pre-embryos for transfer in a subsequent cycle[85]. However, a study by Wada and associates[86] showed that although elective cryopreservation of all embryos from women with high estradiol levels reduced the severity of symptomatic OHSS, it did not reduce the incidence. If an oocyte recovery is performed then every follicle, including small and medium-sized ones, should be emptied because these contribute significantly to the risk of developing OHSS[83].

A further strategy is to administer glucocorticoids after oocyte recovery and reduce the dose slowly over 10 days. However, the only prospective randomized study that has addressed this issue has shown no benefit of glucocorticoid administration[87]. The use of intravenous albumin in patients at high risk of developing OHSS has been suggested[88], but some recent studies have questioned its usefulness[89]. If a fresh embryo transfer is performed in those patients at risk, the transfer of a maximum of two embryos will reduce the multiple pregnancy rate where the hCG levels would be higher. In addition, luteal phase support in the form of progesterone should be administered rather than hCG. When the disease is in progress, management requires careful attention to fluid and electrolyte balance and prevention of thromboembolic events. The use of transvaginal ultrasound scanning can be used to monitor the ovarian volume and keep a record of the number of follicles and their size, and can also be helpful in diagnosing ascites. Although paracentesis is rarely needed and is reserved for those patients with severe respiratory compromise, skilled ultrasonographic guidance helps avoid ovarian trauma[90]. Clearly at present there is no ideal way of preventing OHSS. If polycystic ovaries are noted on ultrasound the dose of gonadotropins should be lowered. If despite this there are many preovulatory follicles and high serum estradiol levels noted then the choice of strategies will need to be carefully considered for each individual patient.

OOCYTE RETRIEVAL

Concurrent with the evolution of assisted conception therapies has been an advancement in the methods for collecting oocytes. The pioneers of IVF, Steptoe and Edwards, first described the technique of oocyte collection via laparoscopy[91]. However, the disadvantages of this method were soon apparent, such as the need for general anesthesia and the invasiveness of the technique. These considerations are made more important when repeated attempts are required by some patients before conceiving[3]. Some patients who undergo IVF will also have severe pelvic adhesions, which in 5–10% of cases make

laparoscopic oocyte collection impossible[92]. In general, laparoscopic oocyte retrieval is now confined to gamete intrafallopian transfer (GIFT) procedures, since laparoscopy remains the preferred approach for transfer of the gametes into the Fallopian tubes, although many perform a transvaginal oocyte retrieval before the laparoscopic gamete transfer.

Ultrasound-directed follicle aspiration for oocyte recovery was first described by Lenz and colleagues in 1981 using the transcutaneous, transvesical route[93]. Subsequently, a number of other transabdominally visualized routes have been employed, including the transvaginal transvesical[94] and perurethral approaches[95]. However, these techniques were difficult to learn and it was not until the advent of the direct transvaginal approach[96] that ultrasound-directed follicle aspiration superceded laparoscopic methods. Direct transvaginal oocyte collection permits easy access to the ovaries, usually takes less than 30 min and can be performed under sedation (e.g. intravenous midazolam and fentanyl). What is more, the oocyte retrieval rate is comparable to that of the laparoscopic technique[32], and patient satisfaction is high[97]. It is also preferable for patients with pelvic adhesions because laparoscopic or transabdominal access may be limited[98].

An ultrasound machine that provides a clear image is essential for follicular aspiration, and high ultrasound frequencies are utilized (5–7.5 MHz). The biopsy probe should lie flush with the transducer and be securely attached so that the needle is stable and in the center of the image throughout the procedure. With the patient in the lithotomy position, the vagina is first cleansed and the needle then introduced into the ovary via the lateral fornix of the vagina. When the bevel of the needle is in the center of a follicle, suction is applied and the needle is then gently rotated while the follicle is seen to collapse on ultrasound imaging (Figure 11). The follicular fluid is examined by an embryologist for the presence of an oocyte surrounded by its expanded cumulus mass. It is usual practice to flush the follicle only once with culture medium. The oocytes that are collected in the initial aspirate and

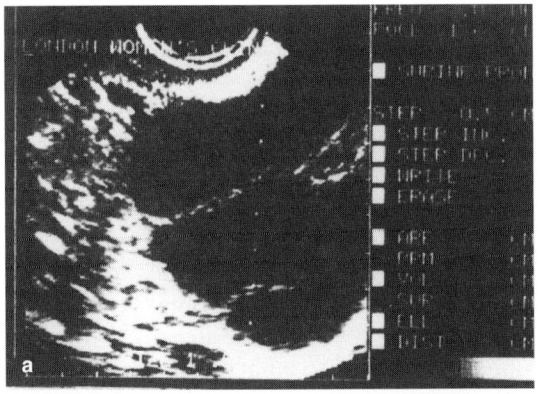

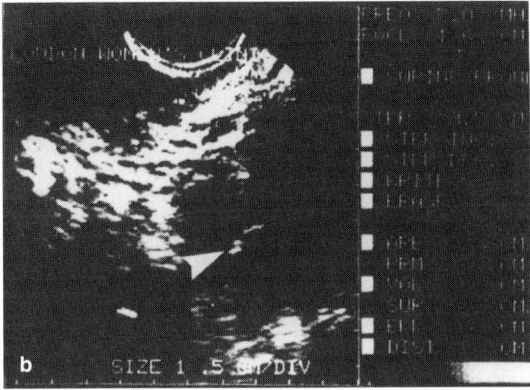

Figure 11 Transvaginal ultrasound-guided oocyte retrieval. (a) Dotted line indicates guideline for passage of the needle into a stimulated ovary. (b) After follicular aspiration, the needle can be seen (arrow) in a collapsed follicle

the myometrium and even the endometrium to reach a posteriorly fixed ovary, or to use the transabdominal route for ovaries that are fixed high above the pelvis. These cases increase the risk of hemorrhage and if the endometrium is traversed may lead to intrauterine infection and reduced implantation rates[100]. In difficult cases the uterus may be avoided by placing a tenaculum on the cervix to manipulate a clear path for the needle to the ovary[101]. The combination of transvaginal ultrasound with uterine manipulation by the cervical tenaculum can also be used to stabilize the ovary that moves out of the needle path as attempts are made to enter the ovary with the transvaginally applied needle[101].

Vaginal bleeding remains the commonest intra-operative complication and, fortunately, almost always responds to firm pressure on the bleeding point. This complication can be minimized by carefully visualizing vessels before advancing the collection needle and avoiding movement of the needle in the vaginal wall, particularly laterally, which can cause vaginal tearing. It should be regarded as mandatory to have easy access to resuscitation equipment in case of a vasovagal faint, an apneic attack or other analgesic complications.

THE LUTEAL PHASE

It is important to perform an ultrasound scan in the mid-luteal phase of both natural and stimulated cycles for *in vivo* fertilization. The corpus luteum may have a number of appearances, being either ovoid or irregular in outline with either a cystic, echo-free interior or a hazy, echogenic appearance because of the presence of cellular debris and blood[102] (Figure 12). Ovulation occurs 36–38 h after the serum peak LH surge[103], and is associated with shrinkage or disappearance of the follicle in most instances[39,40]. Fluid is seen in the cul-de-sac in 50% of cases, and when present it is maximal 4–5 days post-ovulation[40]. While Bakos and colleagues[39] found no correlation between corpus luteum size and progesterone levels, the combination of a corpus luteum visualized on ultrasound and an elevated

first flush, compared with those from subsequent flushes, have better fertilization and cleavage rates and form the embryos that are most likely to achieve pregnancies[99]. When the follicle has been completely emptied, often shown by the presence of a little blood-stained fluid in the collection tubing, the needle is moved to the adjacent follicle. Generally, the needle is not withdrawn from the ovary until every follicle has been emptied, and the procedure is then repeated for the contralateral ovary. The pelvis should be inspected before withdrawing the ultrasound probe to ensure that there is no excessive collection of fluid or blood in the pouch of Douglas.

Occasionally the ovaries are inaccessible through the lateral fornices and it becomes necessary to pass the needle directly through

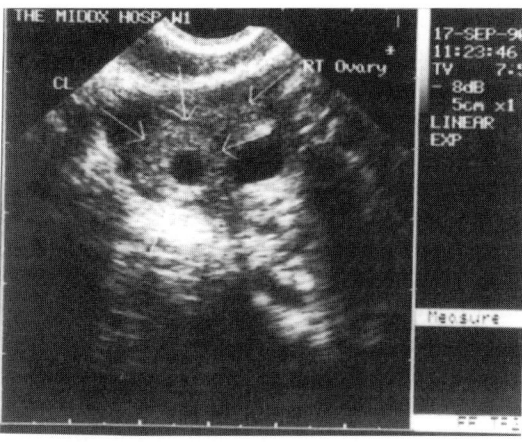

Figure 12 Transvaginal scan of a corpus luteum (arrowed)

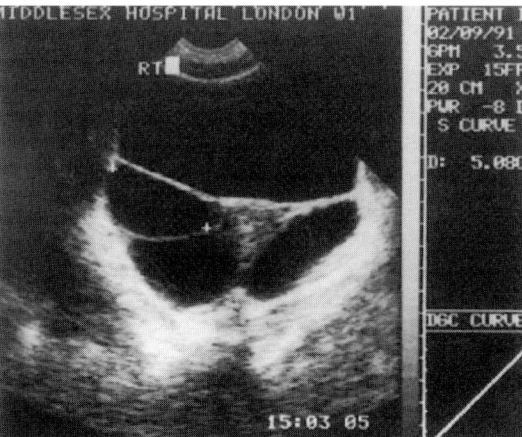

Figure 13 Several large corpus luteal cysts

serum progesterone concentration confirms ovulation[39]. Occasionally, no follicular rupture occurs and a cystic structure persists in the luteal phase of the cycle associated with elevated serum progesterone concentrations otherwise consistent with ovulation[104,105] (Figure 13). This is referred to as a 'luteinized unruptured follicle', the exact incidence of which is unknown.

DOPPLER ULTRASOUND IN ASSISTED CONCEPTION

The combination of transvaginal ultrasound with color Doppler flow measurements may provide details of follicular events around the time of ovulation[106], as well as allowing assessment of the uterine blood flow to predict endometrial receptivity[107,108]. The probability of a pregnancy occurring during assisted conception procedures depends both on the embryo quality and uterine receptivity. In order to improve the chance of conception it has become customary to transfer two, three or four pre-embryos, and in some centers even more. In the UK it is now illegal to transfer more than three pre-embryos in any one cycle and many centers are turning to the routine transfer of two pre-embryos, particularly in women under the age of 35 years who have a higher chance of a multiple pregnancy and a reduced rate of miscarriage[16,109,110]. It is possible that improved assessment of endometrial receptivity for implantation might help prevent the transfer of precious pre-embryos in cycles that are virtually doomed to failure. The embryos could then be frozen and transferred later, in a cycle that is judged to be optimal for implantation – perhaps following hormonal manipulation of the endometrial response. Alternatively, in cycles where endometrial receptivity is deemed good, the numbers of embryos could be minimized to reduce the chances of multiple pregnancy. Until recently, the only way to assess endometrial receptivity was via a biopsy, but now Doppler ultrasound is proving to be a valuable, non-invasive alternative which provides an instantaneous picture of uterine blood flow (Figure 14).

Blood flow through the uterine and ovarian arteries has been extensively investigated in both spontaneous[107,108] and stimulated cycles[111]. Steer and colleagues[108] were the first to use transvaginal color Doppler to study the uterine arteries in 23 normally cycling women, and they found that the lowest pulsatility index (PI) occurred 9 days after the LH peak. This indicates that the maximum uterine perfusion occurs at about the time of expected implantation. Another index of blood flow, the resistance index, was measured on the day of embryo transfer in a series of women undergoing IVF[111], and it was found to be lower in those who subsequently became pregnant.

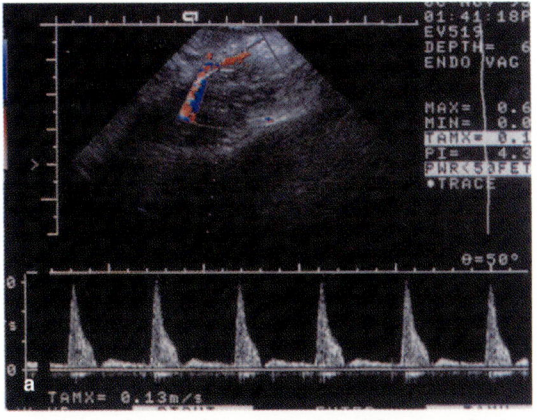

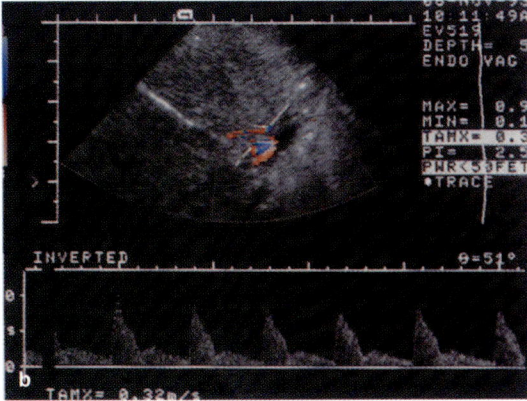

Figure 14 Doppler studies of uterine blood flow in a frozen embryo replacement cycle, during which a regimen of estrogen and progesterone is administered. (a) the pulsatility index (1.39) indicates resistance to flow and so estrogen therapy is continued for 2 more days until (b) the pulsatility index is more favorable

A similar study was performed by Steer and associates in 82 patients undergoing IVF[112]. The authors measured the PI on the day of embryo transfer, classified it as being low (1–1.99; $n = 27$), medium (2–2.99; $n = 36$) or high ($\geqslant 3$; $n = 19$), and related pregnancy rates to the PI. There were no pregnancies in the high PI group. The pregnancy rate, implantation rate and multiple pregnancy rate in the low PI group were 41%, 15.5% and 27.3%, respectively, compared with 47%, 22.2% and 47.1% in the medium PI group. The authors suggested that the PI on the day of embryo transfer could be used to alter the

management, such that a high value (> 3) would lead to elective freezing of the embryos for transfer at a later date in a more favorable cycle. If the PI is normal, the number of embryos transferred could be reduced to minimize the risk of a multiple pregnancy.

Doppler studies of the ovarian circulation are still very much at the research stage. It has been reported in one study in natural cycles that resistance to arterial flow is lower on the side containing the dominant follicle[113], and in gonadotropin-stimulated cycles it has been reported that ovarian impedance is inversely proportional to the number of follicles greater than 15 mm in diameter[114]. It has also been reported that, in IVF cycles, there is a lower ovarian impedance 3 days after embryo transfer in those patients who conceive, compared with those who do not[115]. Bourne and colleagues[106] found that the first signs of perifollicular blood flow could only be detected after the mid-cycle LH surge. They found that there was a rapid increase in the number of small vessels around the preovulatory follicle in the few hours preceding ovulation, which was accompanied by an increase in the blood flow velocity. Immediately after follicular rupture the blood flow velocity to the corpus luteum rose even further, suggesting a process of rapid angiogenesis at this time. The significance of these findings and possible clinical applications remain to be seen. The future might hold the possibility of timing the administration of hCG to coincide with optimal ovarian blood flow for either the release or collection of the highest quality oocytes.

IN VITRO MATURATION

In the future, other possibilities may be available to reduce the length of *in vitro* fertilization treatment cycles. One strategy which may reduce the amount of stimulation used in IVF is the clinical development of *in vitro* maturation (IVM) of oocytes. This involves minimal or no ovarian stimulation, collection of a cohort of immature oocytes (germinal vesicle) and their maturation to metaphase II oocytes in *in vitro* culture, usually over a 48-h period. While enjoying significant success in animal breeding, this remains an experimental tool in humans[116]. Nevertheless, significant progress is being made and some human pregnancies have been achieved[116]. While the largest published series in humans quotes a pregnancy rate of less than 2%[117], a more recent report gives a pregnancy rate of 25.5% in 47 cycles involving PCOS patients[118]. To collect immature oocytes from small antral follicles (range 4–10 mm) requires the use of modified oocyte retrieval needles and lower vacuum pressures than for existing oocyte retrieval. To allow visualization of such small follicles the utilization of high-resolution transvaginal ultrasound is again important.

CONCLUSIONS

Ultrasound assessment of the ovaries and other pelvic structures is a vital adjunct to the successful management of the subfertile patient. It not only provides invaluable information about the ovarian morphology and natural menstrual cycle but also improves the chances of safe and effective treatment, whether it be via ovulation induction for anovulatory infertility or superovulation regimens for assisted conception procedures. It is important to diagnose polycystic ovaries at the time of the baseline scan so that appropriate stimulation regimens are administered and the patient and clinician are alerted to the possibilities of OHSS and multiple pregnancy.

Ultrasound monitoring of follicular growth provides a reliable assessment of ovulation induction therapy and enables appropriate scheduling of the administration of the preovulatory injection of hCG. In assisted conception cycles, when GnRH agonists are used to achieve pituitary desensitization, there is at least a 3-day window for the effective administration of hCG once the largest follicle has reached a diameter of 18 mm. Thus assisted conception procedures can be simplified and made to be more cost effective, with expensive endocrine monitoring being reserved for difficult cases only – for example, those patients thought to be at particular risk of developing OHSS. New techniques, such as color Doppler flow imaging, are providing interesting insights into ovarian and uterine blood flow and might have a future clinical role in optimizing the timing of hCG administration and embryo transfer. The use of three-dimensional ultrasound may provide more detailed analysis of the ovary, particularly in conditions such as polycystic ovaries. Ultrasound-guided follicular aspiration has replaced laparoscopy as the optimal method for collecting oocytes as it is a quick, safe and efficient procedure. In the future this may be extended to the retrieval of immature oocytes for *in vitro* maturation. An ultrasound scan in the luteal phase helps to confirm that ovulation has occurred and, hopefully, a few weeks later, can be used to visualize the gestational sac of an early pregnancy.

References

1. Tan, S. L. (1994). Simplifying *in vitro* fertilization therapy. *Curr. Opin. Obstet. Gynecol.*, **6**, 111–14
2. Balen, A. H., Braat, D. D. M., West, C., Patel, A. and Jacobs, H. S. (1994). Cumulative conception and livebirth rates after the treatment of anovulatory infertility. An analysis of the safety and efficacy of ovulation induction in 200 patients. *Hum. Reprod.*, **9**, 1563–70
3. Tan, S. L., Royston, P., Campbell, S., Jacobs, H. S., Betts, J., Mason, B. and Edwards, R. G. (1992). Cumulative conception and livebirth rates after *in vitro* fertilization. *Lancet*, **339**, 1390–4
4. Hull, M. G. R., Eddowes, H. A., Fahy, U., Abuzeid, M. I., Mills, M. S., Cahill, D. J., Fleming, C. F., Wardle, P. G., Ford, W. C. L. and McDermott, A. (1992). Expectations of

assisted conception for infertility. *Br. Med. J.*, **304**, 1465–9

5. Templeton, A., Morris, J. K. and Parslow, W. (1996). Factors that affect outcome of *in vitro* fertilization treatment. *Lancet*, **348**, 1402–6

6. Yee, B., Barnes, R. B., Vargyas, J. M. and Marrs, R. P. (1987). Correlation of transabdominal and transvaginal ultrasound measurements of follicle size and number with laparoscopic findings for *in vitro* fertilization. *Fertil. Steril.*, **47**, 828–32

7. Andreotti, R. F., Thompson, G. H., Janowitz, W., Shapiro, A. G. and Zusmer, N. R. (1989). Endovaginal and transabdominal sonography of ovarian follicles. *J. Ultrasound Med.*, **8**, 555–60

8. Adams, J., Polson, D., Abdulwahid, N., Morris, D. V., Franks, S., Mason, H. D., Tucker, M., Price, J. and Jacobs, H. S. (1985). Multifollicular ovaries: clinical and endo-crine features and response to pulsatile gonadotrophin-releasing hormone. *Lancet*, **2**, 1375–9

9. Stein, I. F. and Leventhal, M. L. (1935). Amenorrhea associated with bilateral polycystic ovaries. *Am. J. Obstet. Gynecol.*, **29**, 181–91

10. Conway, G. S., Honour, J. W. and Jacobs, H. S. (1989). Heterogeneity of the polycystic ovary syndrome: clinical, endocrine and ultrasound features in 556 patients. *Clin. Endocrinol.*, **30**, 459–70

11. Franks, S. Adams, J., Mason, H. and Polson, D. (1985). Ovulatory disorders in women with polycystic ovary syndrome. In Jacobs, H. S. (ed.) *Clinical Obstetrics and Gynaecology*, Vol. 12, pp. 605–32. (Philadelphia: W.B. Saunders)

12. Adams, J., Polson, D. W. and Franks, S. (1986). Prevalence of polycystic ovaries in women with anovulation and idiopathic hirsutism. *Br. Med. J.*, **293**, 355–8

13. Shoham, Z., Conway, G. S., Patel, A. and Jacobs, H. S. (1992). Polycystic ovaries in patients with hypogonadotrophic hypogonadism: similarity of ovarian response to gonadotrophin stimulation in patients with polycystic ovary syndrome, *Fertil. Steril.*, **58**, 37–45

14. Schachter, M., Balen, A. H., Patel, A. and Jacobs, H. S. (1996). Hypogonadotrophic patients with ultrasonographically diagnosed polycystic ovaries: endocrine response to pulsatile gonadotrophin-releasing hormone. *Gynecol. Endocrinol.*, **10(5)**, 327–35

15. Polson, D. W., Wadsworth, J., Adams, J. and Franks, S. (1988). Polycystic ovaries: a common finding in normal women. *Lancet*, **1**, 870–2

16. Balen, A. H., Tan, S. L., MacDougall, J. and Jacobs, H. S. (1992). Miscarriage rates following *in vitro* fertilization are increased in women with polycystic ovaries and reduced by

pituitary desensitisation with buserelin. *Hum. Reprod.*, **8**, 959–64

17. Kyei-Mensah, A., Zaidi, J. and Campbell, S. (1996). Ultrasound diagnosis of polycystic ovary syndrome. *Balliéres Clin. Endocrinol. Metab.*, **10**, 249–62

18. Franks, S. (1997). Polycystic ovary syndrome: approaching the millenium. *Hum. Reprod.*, **12**, 43–5

19. Jenkins, J. M., Anthony, F. W., Wood, P., Rushen, D., Masson, G. M. and Thomas, E. (1993). The development of functional ovarian cysts during pituitary down-regulation. *Hum. Reprod.*, **8**, 1623–7

20. Jenkins, J. M. (1996). The influence, development and management of functional ovarian cysts during IVF cycles. *Hum. Reprod.*, **11**, 132–6

21. Hornstein, M. D., Barbieri, R. L., Ravnikar, V. A. and McShane, P. M. (1989). The effects of baseline ovarian cysts on the clinical response to controlled ovarian stimulation in an *in vitro* fertilization program. *Fertil. Steril.*, **52**, 437–40

22. Thatcher, S. S., Jones, E. and DeCherney, A. H. (1989). Ovarian cysts decrease the success of controlled ovarian stimulation and *in vitro* fertilization. *Fertil. Steril.*, **52**, 812–16

23. Karande, V. C., Scott, R. T., Jones. G. S. and Muasher, S. J. (1990). Non-functional ovarian cysts do not affect ipsilateral or contralateral ovarian performance during *in vitro* fertilization. *Hum. Reprod.*, **5**, 431–3

24. Aston, K., Arthur, I., Masson, G. M. and Jenkins, J. M. (1995). Progestogen therapy may prevent the development of functional ovarian cysts during pituitary down-regulation with GnRH agonists. *Br. J. Obstet. Gynaecol.*, **102**, 835–7

25. Ron-El, R., Raziel, A., Herman, A., Soffer, Y., Golan, A. and Caspi, E. (1989). Follicle cyst formation following long-acting gonadotrophin-releasing hormone analogue administration. *Fertil. Steril.*, **52**, 1063–6

26. Sampaio, M., Serra, V., Miro, F., Calatayud, C., Castellvi, R. M. and Pellicer, A. (1991). Development of ovarian cysts during gonadotrophin-releasing hormone agonist (GnRHa) administration. *Hum. Reprod.*, **6**, 194–7

27. Rizk, B., Tan, S. L., Kingsland, C., Steer, C., Mason, B. A. and Campbell, S. (1990). Ovarian cyst aspiration and the outcome of *in vitro* fertilization. *Fertil. Steril.*, **54**, 661–4

28. Jenkins, J. M., Davies, D. W., Anthony, F. W., Wood, P., Gadd, S., Watson, R. H. and Masson, G. M. (1992). The management of functional ovarian cysts during IVF cycles. *J. Obstet. Gynecol.*, **12**, 64–5

29. Silverberg, K. M., Olive, D. L, and Schenken, R. S. (1990). Ovarian cyst aspiration prior to initiating ovarian hyperstimulation for *in vitro* fertilization. *J. In Vitro Fertil. Embryo Transfer*, **7**, 153–6

30. Padilla, S. L. (1993). Ovarian abscess following puncture of an endometrioma during ultrasound-guided oocyte retrieval. *Hum. Reprod.*, **8**, 1282–3

31. Howe, R. S., Blasco, L., Wheeler, C., Tureck, R., and Mastroianni, L. (1988). Pelvic infection after transvaginal ultrasound-guided ovum retrieval. *Fertil. Steril.*, **49**, 726–8

32. Feldberg, D., Goldman, J. A., Ashkenazi, J., Shelef, M., Dicker, D. and Samuel, N. (1988). Transvaginal oocyte retrieval controlled by vaginal probe for *in vitro* fertilization: a comparative study. *J. Ultrasound Med.*, **7**, 339–43

33. Van Hoorde, G. J., Verhoeff, A, and Zeilmaker, G. H. (1992). Perforated appendicitis following transvaginal oocyte retrieval for *in vitro* fertilization and embryo transfer. *Hum. Reprod.*, **7**, 850–1

34. Eissa, M. K., Hudson, K., Docker, M. F., Sawers, R. S. and Newton, J. R. (1985). Ultrasound follicle diameter measurement: an assessment of inter-observer and intra-observer variation. *Fertil. Steril.*, **44**, 751–4

35. Gonzalez, C. J., Curson, R. and Parsons, J. (1988). Transabdominal versus transvaginal ultrasound screening of ovarian follicles: are they comparable? *Fertil. Steril.*, **50**, 657

36. Hackeloer, B. J., Fleming, R., Robinson, H. P., Adam, A. H. and Coutts, J. R. T. (1979). Correlation of ultrasonic and endocrinologic assessment of human follicular development. *Am. J. Obstet. Gynecol.*, **135**, 122–8

37. DeCherney, A. H., Romero, R. and Polan, M. L. (1982). Ultrasound in reproductive endocrinology. *Fertil. Steril.*, **37**, 323

38. Speroff, L., Glass, R. and Kase, N. (1994). *Clinical Gynecological Endocrinology and Infertility*, 5th edn. (Baltimore: Williams and Wilkins)

39. Bakos, O., Lundkvist, O., Wide, L. and Bergh, T. (1994). Ultrasonographic and hormonal description of the normal ovulatory menstrual cycle. *Acta Obstet. Gynecol. Scand.*, **73**, 790–6

40. Randall, J. M. and Templeton, A. (1991). Transvaginal sonographic assessment of follicular and endometrial growth in spontaneous and clomiphene citrate cycles. *Fertil. Steril.*, **56**, 208–12

41. Adams, J., Tan, S. L., Wheeler, M. J., Morris, D. V., Jacobs, H. S. and Franks, S. (1988). Uterine growth in the follicular phase of spontaneous ovulatory cycles and during luteinizing hormone-releasing hormone-induced cycles in women with normal or polycystic ovaries. *Fertil. Steril.*, **49**, 52–5

42. Edwards, R. G., Steptoe, R. G. and Purdy, J. M. (1980). Establishing full-term human pregnancies using cleaving embryos grown *in vitro*. *Br. J. Obstet. Gynaecol.*, **87**, 737–56

43. Tan, S. L., Doyle, P., Campbell, S., Beral, V., Risk, P., Brinsden, P., Mason, B. A. and Edwards, R. G. (1992). Obstetric outcome of pregnancies resulting from *in vitro* fertilization compared with normally occurring pregnancies. *Am. J. Obstet. Gynecol.*, **167**, 778–84

44. Paulson, R. J., Sauer, M. V. and Lobo, R. A. (1989). *In vitro* fertilization in unstimulated cycles: a new application. *Fertil. Steril.*, **51**, 1059–60

45. Foulot, H., Ranoux, C., Dubuisson, J.-B., Rambaud, D., Aubriot, F.-X. and Poirot, C. (1989). *In vitro* fertilization without ovarian stimulation: a simplified protocol applied to 80 cycles. *Fertil. Steril.*, **52**, 617–21

46. Nugent, D., Salha, O., Balen, A. H. and Rutherford, A. J. (1998). Ovarian neoplasia and subfertility treatments. *Br. J. Obstet. Gynaecol.*, **105**, 584–91

47. Fahy, U. M., Cahill, D. J., Wardle, P. G. and Hull, M. G. (1995). *In vitro* fertilization in completely natural cycles. *Hum. Reprod.*, **10**, 572–5

48. Balen, A. H. and Jacobs, H. S. (1991). Gonadotrophin surge attenuating factor – a missing link in the control of LH secretion? *Clin. Endocrinol.*, **35**, 399–402

49. Fleming, R. and Coutts, J. R. T. (1990). Induction of multiple follicular development for *in vitro* fertilization. In Edwards, R. G. (ed.) *Assisted Human Conception. Br. Med. Bull.*, **46**, 596–615. (Edinburgh: Churchill Livingstone)

50. Porter, R. N., Smith, W., Craft, I. L., Abdulwahid, N. A. and Jacobs, H. S. (1984). Induction of ovulation for *in vitro* fertilization using buserelin and gonadotrophins. *Lancet*, **2**, 1284–5

51. Fleming, R., Haxton, M. J., Hamilton, M. P. R., McCune, G. S., Black, W. P., McNaughton, M. C. and Coutts, J. R. T. (1985). Successful treatment of infertile women with oligomenorrhoea using a combination of a luteinizing hormone-releasing hormone agonist and exogenous gonadotrophins. *Br. J. Obstet. Gynaecol.*, **92**, 369–74

52. Rutherford, A. J., Subak-Sharpe, R. J., Dawson, K. J., Margara, R. A., Franks, S. and Winston, R. M. L. (1988). Improvement of *in vitro* fertilization after treatment with buserelin, an agonist of luteinizing hormone-releasing hormone. *Br. Med. J.*, **296**, 1765–8

53. Frydman, R., Fries, N., Testart, J., Belaisch Allart, J. C., Forman, R., Hazout, A. and

Testart, J. (1988). Luteinizing hormone-releasing hormone agonists in *in vitro* fertilization: different methods of utilization and comparison with previous ovulation stimulation treatments. *Hum. Reprod.*, **3**, 559–61

54. Tan, S. L. (1996). Gonadotrophin-releasing hormone agonists in assisted reproductive therapy. *Hum. Reprod.*, **11**, 137–42

55. Hughes, E. G., Federkow, D. M., Daya, S. Sagle, M., de Koppel, P. and Collins, J. (1992). The routine use of gonadotrophin-releasing hormone agonists prior to *in vitro* fertilization and gamete intrafallopain transfer: a meta-analysis of randomised controlled trials. *Fertil. Steril.*, **58**, 888–96

56. Tan, S. L., Balen, A. H., el Hussein, E., Mills, C., Campbell, S., Yovich, J. and Jacobs, H. S. (1992). A prospective randomised study of the optimum timing of human chorionic gonadotrophin administration after pituitary desensitisation in *in vitro* fertilization. *Fertil. Steril.*, **57**, 1259–64

57. MacDougall, M. J., Tan, S. L., Balen, A. H. and Jacobs, H. S. (1993). A controlled study comparing patients with and without polycystic ovaries undergoing *in vitro* fertilization. *Hum. Reprod.*, **8**, 233–7

58. Golan, A., Herman, A., Soffer, Y., Burkowsky, I. and Ron-El, R. (1994). Ultrasonic control without hormonal determination for ovulation induction in *in vitro* fertilization/embryo transfer with gonadotrophin-releasing hormone analogue and human menopausal gonadotrophin. *Hum. Reprod.*, **9**, 1631–3

59. Haning, R. V., Austin, C. W., Kuzma, D. L., Shapiro, S. S. and Zweibel, W. J. (1982). Ultrasound evaluation of estrogen monitoring for induction of ovulation with menotropins. *Fertil. Steril.*, **37**, 627–32

60. Montzavinos, T., Garcia, J. E. and Jones, H. W. (1983). Ultrasound measurement of ovarian follicles stimulated by human gonadotrophins for oocyte recovery and *in vitro* fertilization. *Fertil. Steril.*, **40**, 461–5

61. Bordt, J., Hander, J. P. and Schneider, H. P. G. (1986). Ultrasound controlled gonadotrophin therapy of anovulatory infertility. *Fertil. Steril.*, **46**, 818–22

62. Out, H. J., Mannaerts, B. M. J. L., Driessen, S. G. A. J. and Celingh Bennink, H. J. T. (1996). Recombinant follicle-stimulating hormone in assisted reproduction: more oocytes, more pregnancies. Results from five comparative studies. *Hum. Reprod. Update*, **2**, 162–71

63. Zorn, J. R., Boyer, P. and Guichard, A. (1987). Never on a Sunday: programming for IVF-ET and GIFT. *Lancet*, **1**, 385–6

64. Vauthier, D. and Lefebvre, G. (1989). The use of gonadotrophin-releasing hormone analogs for *in vitro* fertilization: comparison between the standard form and long-acting formulation of D-Trp-6-luteinizing hormone-releasing hormone. *Fertil. Steril.*, **51**, 100–4

65. Dimitry, E. S., Bates, S. A., Oskarsson, T., Margara, R. and Winston, R. M. L. (1991). Programming *in vitro* fertilization for a 5- or 3-day week. *Fertil. Steril.*, **55**, 934–8

66. Clark, L., Stanger, J. and Brinsmead, M. (1991). Prolonged follicle stimulation decreases pregnancy rates after *in vitro* fertilization. *Fertil. Steril.*, **55**, 1192–4

67. Conaghan, J., Dimitry, E. S., Mills, M., Margara, R. A. and Winston, R. M. L. (1989). Delayed human chorionic gonadotrophin administration for *in vitro* fertilization. *Lancet*, **1**, 1323–4

68. Abdalla, H., Baber, R., Leonard, T., Kirkland, A., Power, M., Mitchell, A., Owen, E. and Studd, J. (1989). Timed oocyte collection in an assisted conception programme using GnRH analogue. *Hum. Reprod.*, **4**, 927–30

69. Hull, M. G. R., Savage, P. E. and Bromham, D. R. (1982). Anovulatory and ovulatory infertility: results with simplified management. *Br. Med. J.*, **284**, 1681–5

70. Franks, S., Mason, S., Polson, D. W., Winston, R. M. L., Margara, R. and Reed, M. J. (1988). Mechanism and management of ovulatory failure in women with polycystic ovary syndrome. *Hum. Reprod.*, **3**, 531–4

71. Hamilton-Fairley, D. and Franks, S. (1990). Common problems in induction of ovulation. *Bailliére's Clin. Obstet. Gynaecol.*, **4**, 609–26

72. Jacobs, H. S., Porter, R., Eshel, A. and Craft, I. (1987). Profertility uses of luteinizing hormone-releasing hormone agonist anologs. In Vickery, B. H. and Nestor, J. J. (eds.) *LHRH and its Analogs*, pp. 303–22. (Lancaster, UK: MTP Press Ltd.)

73. Smitz, J., Camus, M., Devroey, P., Evard, P., Wisanto, A. and Van Steirteghen, A. C. (1991). Incidence of severe ovarian hyperstimulation syndrome after gonadotrophin-releasing hormone agonist/hMG superovulation for *in vitro* fertilization. *Hum. Reprod.*, **6**, 933–7

74. Salat-Baroux, J. and Antoine, J. M. (1990). Accidental hyperstimulation during ovulation induction. *Balliére's Clin. Obstet. Gynaecol.*, **4**, 627–37

75. Homburg, R., Levy, T., Berkovitz, D., Farhi, J., Feldberg, D., Ashkenazi, J. and Ben-Rafael, Z. (1993). Gonadotrophin-releasing hormone agonist reduces the miscarriage rate for pregnancies achieved in women with polycystic ovary syndrome. *Fertil. Steril.*, **59**, 527–31

76. Schenker, J. G. and Weinstein, D. (1978). Ovarian hyperstimulation syndrome: a current survey. *Fertil. Steril.*, **30**, 255

77. Golan, A., Ron-El, R., Herman, A., Weinraub, Z., Soffer, Y. and Caspi, E. (1989). Ovarian hyperstimulation syndrome: an update review. *Obstet. Gynecol. Surv.*, **44**, 430–40

78. Polishuk, W. and Schenker, J. (1969). Ovarian overstimulation syndrome. *Fertil. Steril.*, **20**, 443–50

79. Raj, S., Berger, M., Grimes, E. and Taymor, M. (1977). The use of gonadotrophins for the induction of ovulation in women with polycystic ovarian disease. *Fertil. Steril.*, **28**, 1280–4

80. MacDougall, M. J., Tan, S. L. and Jacobs, H. S. (1992). *In vitro* fertilization and the ovarian hyperstimulation syndrome. *Hum. Reprod.*, **7**, 597–600

81. Forman, R. G., Frydman, R., Egan, D., Ross, C. and Barlow, D. H. (1990). Severe ovarian hyperstimulation syndrome using agonists of gonadotrophin-releasing hormone for *in vitro* fertilization: a European series and a proposal for prevention. *Fertil. Steril.*, **53**, 502–9

82. Tanbo, T., Dale, P. O., Kjekhus, E. and Abyholm, T. (1990). Stimulation with human menopausal gonadotrophin versus follicle-stimulating hormone after pituitary suppression in polycystic ovarian syndrome. *Fertil. Steril.*, **53**, 798–803

83. Blankstein, J., Shalev, J., Saadon, T., Kukia, E.E., Rubinovici, J., Pariente, C., LunenField, B., Serr, D.M. and Mashiach, S. (1987). Ovarian hyperstimulation syndrome: prediction by numbers and size of preovulatory ovarian follicles. *Fertil. Steril.*, **47**, 597–602

84. Haning, R. V. Jr, Austin, C. W., Carlson, I. H., Kuzma, D. L., Shapiro, S. S. and Zweibel, W. J. (1983). Plasma estradiol is superior to ultrasound and urinary estriol glucuronide as a predictor of ovarian hyperstimulation during induction of ovulation with menotropins. *Fertil. Steril.*, **40**, 31–6

85. Amso, N. N., Ahuja, K. K., Morris, N. and Shaw, R. W. (1990). The management of predicted ovarian hyperstimulation syndrome involving gonadotrophin-releasing hormone analog with effective cryopreservation of all pre-embryos. *Fertil. Steril.*, **53**, 1087–90

86. Wada, I., Matson, P. L., Troup, S. A., Morroll, D. R., Hunt, L. and Lieberman, B. A. (1993). Does elective cryopreservation of all embryos from women at risk of ovarian hyperstimulation syndrome reduce the incidence of the condition. *Br. J. Obstet. Gynaecol.*, **100**, 265–96

87. Tan, S. L., Balen, A. H., Hussein, E., Campbell, S. and Jacobs, H. S. (1992). The administration of glucocorticoids for the prevention of ovarian hyperstimulation syndrome in *in vitro* fertilization. A prospective randomized study. *Fertil. Steril.*, **57**, 378–83

88. Asch, R. H., Ivery, G., Goldsamn, M., Frederick, J. L., Stone, S. C. and Balmaceda, J. P. (1993). The use of intravenous albumin in patients at risk of severe ovarian hyperstimulation syndrome. *Hum. Reprod.*, **8**, 1015–20

89. Shaker, A., Zosmer, A., Dean, N., Bekir, J. S., Jacobs, H. S. and Tan, S. L. (1996). Comparison of intravenous albumin and transfer of fresh embryos with cryopreservation of all embryos for subsequent transfer in prevention of ovarian hyperstimulation syndrome. *Fertil. Steril.*, **65**, 992–6

90. Padilla, S., Zamaria, S., Baramki, T. and Garcia, J. (1990). Abdominal paracentesis for the ovarian hyperstimulation syndrome with severe respiratory compromise. *Fertil. Steril.*, **53**, 365–7

91. Steptoe, P. and Edwards, R. G. (1970). Laparoscopic recovery of preovulatory human oocytes after priming of ovaries with gonadotrophins. *Lancet*, **2**, 683–9

92. Daniell, F., Pittway, D. E. and Maxton, W. S. (1983). The role of laparoscopic adhesiolysis in an *in vitro* fertilization program. *Fertil. Steril.*, **40**, 49–52

93. Lenz, S., Lauritsen, J. G. and Kjellow, M. (1981). Collection of human oocytes for *in vitro* fertilization by ultrasonically guided follicular puncture. *Lancet*, **1**, 1163–4

94. Dellenbach, P., Nisand, I., Moreau, L., Feger, B., Plumere, C. and Gerlinger, P. (1985). Transvaginal sonographically controlled follicle puncture for oocyte retrieval. *Fertil. Steril.*, **44**, 656–62

95. Parsons, J., Riddles, A. and Booker, M. (1985). Oocyte retrieval for *in vitro* fertilization by ultrasonically guided needle aspiration via the urethra. *Lancet*, **1**, 1076

96. Wikland, M., Lennart, E. and Hamberger, L. (1985). Transvesical and transvaginal approaches for the aspiration of follicles by the use of ultrasound. *Ann. NY Acad. Sci. USA*, **442**, 184–92

97. Hammarberg, K., Enk, L., Nilsson, L. and Wikland, M. (1987). Oocyte retrieval under the guidance of a vaginal transducer: evaluation of patient acceptance. *Hum. Reprod.*, **2**, 487–90

98. Taylor, P. J., Wiseman, D., Mahadevan, M. and Leader, A. (1986). 'Ultrasound rescue': a successful alternative form of oocyte recovery in patients with periovarian adhesions. *Am. J. Obstet. Gynecol.*, **154**, 240–4

99. Hussein, E. E., Balen, A. H. and Tan, S. L. (1992). A prospective study comparing the outcome of eggs retrieved in the aspirate to those retrieved in the flush during transvaginal ultrasound-directed oocyte recovery for *in vitro* fertilization. *Br. J. Obstet. Gynaecol.*, **99**, 841–4

100. Ashkenazi, J., Farhi, J., Dicker, D., Feldberg, D., Halev, J. and Ben Rafael, Z. (1994). Acute pelvic inflammatory disease after oocyte retrieval: adverse effects on the results of implantation. *Fertil. Steril.*, **61**, 526–8

101. Licciardi, F. L., Schwartz, L. B. and Schmidt-Sarosi, C. (1995). A tenaculum improves the ovarian accessibility during difficult transvaginal follicular aspiration: a novel but simple technique. *Fertil. Steril.*, **63**, 677–9

102. Deichert, U., Hackelöer, B. J. and Daume, E. (1986). The sonographic and endocrinologic evaluation of the endometrium in the luteal phase. *Hum. Reprod.*, **1**, 219–22

103. Ritchie, W. G. (1985). Ultrasound in the evaluation of normal and induced ovulation. *Fertil. Steril.*, **43**, 167–81

104. Marik, J. and Hulka, J. (1978). Luteinized unruptured follicle syndrome: a subtle cause of infertility. *Fertil. Steril.*, **29**, 270–4

105. Daly, D. C., Soto-Albors, C., Walters, C., Ying, Y. K. and Riddick, D. H. (1985). Ultrasonographic assessment of luteinized unruptured follicle syndrome in unexplained infertility. *Fertil. Steril.*, **43**, 62–5

106. Bourne, T. H., Jurkovic, D., Waterstone, J., Campbell, S. and Collins, W. P. (1991). Intrafollicular blood flow during human ovulation. *Ultrasound Obstet. Gynecol.*, **1**, 53–9

107. Scholtes, M. C. W., Wladimiroff, J. W., van Rijen, H. J. M. and Hop, W. C. (1989). Uterine and ovarian flow velocity waveforms in the normal menstrual cycle: a transvaginal Doppler study. *Fertil. Steril.*, **52**, 981–5

108. Steer, C., Campbell, S., Pampiglione, J., Kingsland, C., Mason, B. A. and Collins, W. (1990). Transvaginal color flow imaging of the uterine arteries during ovarian and menstrual cycles. *Hum. Reprod.*, **5**, 391–5

109. Balen, A. H., MacDougall, J. and Tan, S. L. (1993). The influence of the number of embryos transferred during *in vitro* fertilization on pregnancy outcome. *Hum. Reprod.*, **8**, 1324–8

110. Tan, S. L., Maconochie, N., Doyle, P., Campbell, S., Balen, A. H., Bekir, J., Brinsden, P., Edwards, R. G. and Jacobs, H. S. (1994). Cumulative conception and livebirth rates after *in vitro* fertilization, with and without pituitary desensitization with the gonadotropin-releasing hormone agonist buserelin. *Am. J. Obstet. Gynecol.*, **171**, 513–20

111. Sterzik, K., Grab, D., Sasse, S., Hutter, H., Rosenbusch, B. and Torinde, R. (1989). Doppler sonographic findings and their correlation with implantation in an *in vitro* fertilization program. *Fertil. Steril.*, **52**, 825–8

112. Steer, C. V., Campbell, S., Tan, S. L., Crayford, T., Mills, C., Mason, B. A. and Collins, W. P. (1992). The use of transvaginal color flow imaging after *in vitro* fertilization to identify optimum uterine conditions before embryo transfer. *Fertil. Steril.*, **57**, 372–6

113. Taylor, K., Burns, P., Wells, P., Conway, D. and Hull, M. (1985). Ultrasound Doppler flow studies of the ovarian and uterine arteries. *Br. J. Obstet. Gynaecol.*, **92**, 240–6

114. Deutinger, J., Reinthaller, A. and Bernaschek, G. (1989). Transvaginal pulsed Doppler measurement of blood flow velocity in the ovarian arteries during cycle stimulation and after follicle puncture. *Fertil. Steril.*, **51**, 466–70

115. Baber, R. J., McSweeney, M. B., Gill, R. W., Porter, R. N., Picker, R. H., Warren, P. S., Kossof, G. and Saunders, D. M. (1988). Transvaginal pulsed Doppler ultrasound assessment of blood flow to the corpus luteum in IVF patients following embryo transfer. *Br. J. Obstet. Gynaecol.*, **95**, 1226–30

116. Gosden, R. G., Wynn, P., Krapez, J., Rutherford, A. J., Sharma, V. and Rutherford, A. J. (1998). *In vitro* maturation of oocytes. In O'Brien, P. M. S. (ed.) *The Yearbook of Obstetrics and Gynaecology*, Vol. 6, pp. 330–8. (London: RCOG Press)

117. Trounson, A. O., Bongso, A., Szell, A. and Barnes, F. L. (1996). Maturation of human and bovine primary oocytes in *in vitro* fertilization and embryo production. *Singapore J. Obstet. Gynecol.*, **27**, 78–84

118. Cha, K. Y. (1997). *In vitro* maturation of follicles and oocytes: oocytes from unstimulated follicles. In Porcu, E. and Flamigni, C. (eds.) *Human Oocytes: From Physiology to IVF*, Bologna, Italy: pp. 157–61 Monduzzi Editore

Ovarian circulation

3

S. Kupesic and A. Kurjak

Over the last 5 years there has been a large increase in the number of studies on normal and abnormal ovarian vascularity. Transvaginal color Doppler has opened up exciting new possibilities for a better understanding of the physiology and pathophysiology of ovarian blood flow, resulting in a number of completely new diagnostic parameters.

OVARIAN VASCULAR ANATOMY

For adequate application of Doppler technology in studies of hemodynamics, it is important to be familiar with the vascular anatomy of the ovary, which consists of an arterial, venous and lymphatic system. Although in the near future, Doppler assessment of the lymphatic system may be possible, it is not so at the moment. Similarly, evaluation of the venous flow is feasible, but the technique has not been standardized. Therefore, the first objective of our research is to study arterial anatomy and blood flow changes, which reflect functional activity and pathological circumstances in the most intensive form.

The ovarian vascular system can be divided into extrinsic and intrinsic vascular systems. The extrinsic vascular system consists of arteries that start from big abdominal trunks before they enter into the ovary and the homologous venous system. The intrinsic vascular system is formed by vessels which enter the ovary from the ovarian hilus, giving rise to the microcirculation and posteriorly causing venous drainage[1]. Although we are dealing with a topographical division, as the adjacent systems together constitute one vascular system, it is interesting from a functional point of view. The cyclic changes of ovarian vascularization are manifest most intensively in the intrinsic vascular system.

Extrinsic vascular system

The pattern of the ovarian blood supply is similar in all mammals, although it grows more complex closer to the top of the phylogenetic scale[1].

Arteries

The ovary receives its arterial vascularization from two sources: the ovarian artery and the utero-ovarian branch of the uterine artery[2]. These arteries anastomose, forming an arch parallel to the ovarian hilus, and constitute the vascular genital arcade. The ovarian artery emerges from the abdominal aorta beneath the renal arteries. From there, it descends obliquely and, crossing the ureter and iliac vessels, enters into the infundibulopelvic ligament. The artery approaches the ovary at its upper pole. At this level, the external tubarian artery, which does not participate in the vascularization of the ovary, branches off. The other artery involved in blood perfusion of the ovary is the utero-ovarian artery. This artery begins from the uterine artery at the altitude of the uterine horn and goes to the lower pole of the ovary. Both arteries anastomose directly or through branches which enter into the ovary by the front or the ovarian hilus. Although embryological evolution apparently demonstrates that the principal share of blood in the ovary originates from the ovarian artery, the importance of supply by the utero-ovarian artery seems to be related to the type of anastomosis. Topographically, between two arteries, four types of anastomosis are observed, with equal participation or with one dominant anastomosis.

Veins

Ovarian veins leave the ovary at the level of the hilus, giving rise to the pampiniform plexus, with its many characteristic interconnections. Anastomosing with veins coming from the uterus, it forms a utero-ovarian vein, consisting of two canals, interconnected by numerous anastomoses[3]. Both canals ascend to the abdomen and end by joining together into a single utero-ovarian vein, opening on the left to the renal vein, and on the right to the vena cava.

Intrinsic vascular system (microcirculation)

The ovary has an arterial supply known for its special pattern and obvious functional changes. From the ovarian hilus, arterial branches penetrate the stroma[1] and acquire a tortuous and helicoid pathway (they roll up around their own axis). For such a special pattern, they are named spiral or helical arteries. Getting further into the ovarian stroma, spiral arteries divide more and more and become progressively smaller in diameter. In the cortical zone the diameter becomes 40–60 μm, and dividing at a right or sharp angle from the principal branch they successively form arterioles of the first capillary system[3]. The abundance of spiral arteries in the ovarian stroma constitutes an authentic medulla at this stage[1]. The arterial system drains by the agency of a venous system rolled up into a ball, with a diameter larger than that of the arteries (80 μm), called the ovarian bulb.

The spiral pattern of the ovarian arteries plays an important role in the hemodynamics of cyclic structural adaptation of the ovary. The helicoid pathway of the arteries enlarges the surface of friction as blood flows through, increasing resistance and lowering blood pressure, which is necessary to contain the elevated pressure at the entrance of the ovarian artery[1]. An arterial pattern of this kind generates a centrifugal force, rather than a blood circulation which has turbulations in the system. Angular bifurcation of the arterioles contributes to the stability of the flow with minimum energetic waste. Finally, such a structure facilitates accommodation to changes in size, due to development of the follicle and the corpus luteum. When they grow, arteries unwind and become larger, returning to the basal state during follicular atresia or luteal regression[4]. This is vitally important for the understanding of changes in intraovarian Doppler velocimetry.

PHYSICAL PRINCIPLES

Ultrasound imaging has provided a unique method for the non-invasive study of ovarian structural changes. The measurement of blood flow velocity by ultrasound is based on the Doppler effect, which is named after the Austrian physicist Christian Johann Doppler (1803–53). The Doppler effect occurs when the frequency of a sound wave emitted from a stationary source and reflected from a moving interface changes according to the velocity and direction of the moving interface[5]. Movements toward the source will increase the frequency of the reflected waves, and movements away from the source will decrease it. The changes of frequency are directly proportional to the velocity of the moving interface. This change of frequency is called the Doppler shift. If the ultrasound beam is sent towards a blood vessel, the moving erythrocytes will act as reflectors and cause a change of the reflected sound frequency. The Doppler shift F_D is described by the standard equation:

$$F_D = \frac{2F_0 \, v \cos \theta}{c}$$

where v is the velocity of the reflector, F_0 is the frequency of the emitted sound, c is the velocity of ultrasound in the medium and θ is the angle between the insonating sound wave and the direction of the moving reflector.

The Doppler effect can be used to measure mean blood velocity across a vessel area. With two-dimensional ultrasound, all necessary information regarding the angle between the vessel direction and the insonating sound, and the diameter of the vessel, can be obtained. Once the standard form of the Doppler equation is used for quantification of blood volume, the total rate of blood flow in the vessel can be calculated easily by multiplying the average velocity by the cross-sectional area of the vessel:

$$Q = vr^2/\cos \theta$$

where Q is the blood-flow volume, v is the mean blood velocity over the vessel cross-sectional area, r is the vessel radius and θ is the angle of approach of the Doppler beam to the vessel. However, quantification of the blood flow can be performed only in the vessels that are demonstrated by ultrasound. The analysis of the blood flow in thin non-visualized vessels can be based on blood flow velocity waveform analysis. The velocity waveform shows the frequency shift vs. time. It represents maximum Doppler shifts throughout the cardiac cycle, thus reflecting the pulsatile nature of blood flow in arterial vessels. Analysis of flow velocity is an alternative method of blood flow assessment. The major advantage of this analysis is angle-independence and there is no need for simultaneous vessel visualization and diameter measurement. More than ten indices have been used for velocity waveform analysis. The A/B ratio, resistance index (RI) and pulsatility index (PI) are predominantly used:

A/B ratio = A/B (peak systole/end diastole)
RI = (A − B)/A ((peak systole − end diastole)/peak systole)
PI = (A − B)/(mean (peak systole − end diastole)/mean frequency)

Doppler ultrasound has the potential to study patterns of ovarian blood flow and hence identify functional changes[6]. Until recently the use of this method for examination of flow in specific deep vessels has been difficult, since conventional continuous waveform meters provide confusing signals from flow or tissue movements occurring anywhere along the entire length of the ultrasound beam. The availability of pulsed Doppler instruments has made it possible to sample the signals at a chosen depth and thus to detect flow in any selected deep vessel. Pulsed Doppler combined with real-time ultrasound imaging, the so-called 'duplex' method, allows the precise localization of a deep vessel and positioning of the Doppler sample volume within it[7]. Furthermore, recent technological advances have resulted in transvaginal color Doppler ultrasonography. The system uses pulsed Doppler, which performs flow analysis at multiple points along each scan line of echo data[8,9]. Flow information is then color-coded and displayed on an entirely corresponding two-dimensional image. The main advantages of the color system are rapid and definitive determination of the position of small and tortuous normal and newly formed vessels, accuracy of the measurement and precise indication of flow direction and velocity. Red indicates flow towards the transducer, and blue away from the transducer. The brightness of the color is proportional to the velocity of flow within the vessel, whilst turbulent flow may appear as various shades of green. After simultaneous visualization of morphological and blood flow information, a pulsed Doppler range gate is placed over the area of interest to provide flow velocity waveforms which may be analyzed in a conventional fashion. This new modality carries many safety advantages when compared to the use of transvaginal pulsed Doppler alone[10]. By reducing the time required to find and sample a vessel, the total exposure of the area of interest to ultrasound should be reduced.

COLOR DOPPLER VELOCIMETRY OF THE OVARY

Ovarian artery

The ovarian artery is a tributary of the upper aorta and reaches the lateral aspect of the ovary through the infundibulopelvic ligament[1]. In some patients, these vessels are not clearly visualized and the sample volume should be moved across the ligament and then through the substance of the ovary until the arterial signal is identified. Signals from the ovarian artery are characterized by the low Doppler shifts of a small vessel with low velocity (Figure 1). The waveform shape varies with the state of activity of the ovary. Studies of ovarian artery blood flow velocity waveforms show the difference in the vascular impedance between the two ovarian arteries depending on the presence of the dominant follicle or corpus luteum[11,12]. A longitudinal study of the ovarian artery over the ovarian cycle performed at the Ultrasonic Institute of the University of Zagreb suggested decreased pulsatility and resistance indices, reflecting vascular impedance and implying increased flow to the ovary containing the dominant follicle or corpus luteum. The ovarian artery of the 'inactive' ovary showed low end-diastolic flow or absence of diastolic flow. A rise in the end-diastolic flow velocity of the 'active' ovary is most obvious on day 21 and this suggests that the corpus luteum acts as a low-impedance shunt (Figure 2). The increased blood supply to the functioning corpus luteum is essential for delivery of precursors involved in steroidogenesis and for removal of progesterone[13–15].

Various invasive and non-invasive techniques of ovarian blood flow measurement in mammals have been used, including micro-

spheres[13], direct blood collection[16], and implantation of Doppler flow meters[17] and electromagnetic flow meters in cows[14]. These techniques have shown that 80–90% of the blood flow to the ovary is supplied to the corpus luteum[18]. A rapid decrease in ovarian blood flow accompanying luteolysis is noticed in animal models[16]. Prostaglandin $F_{2\alpha}$ is reported to be the active luteolysin, and a reduction of 90% in luteal flow has been reported follow-

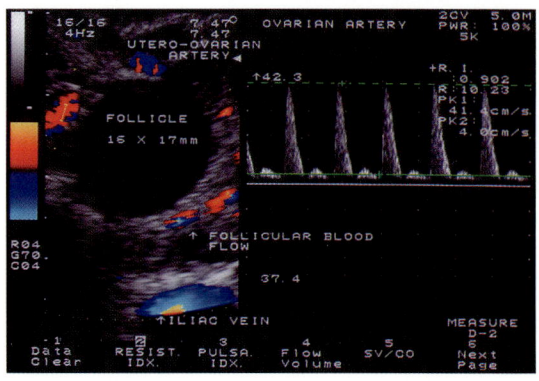

Figure 1 Flow velocity waveforms obtained from the ovarian artery during the periovulatory phase of the menstrual cycle. Notice the continuous diastolic flow and the resistance index (RI) of 0.90

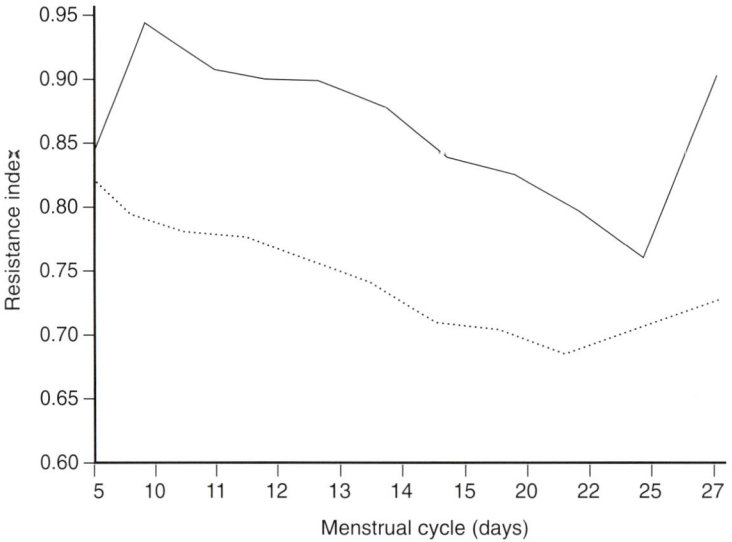

Figure 2 Ovarian artery blood flow changes during the ovulatory menstrual cycle. The resistance indices of the 'active' ovary (solid line) and 'inactive' ovary (dotted line) are shown

ing its local administration[19]. Patients treated with clomiphene citrate and/or human menopausal gonadotropin (hMG) at our institution typically developed multiple follicles bilaterally, and both ovarian arteries showed low pulsatility waveforms typical of low impedance[11].

If pregnancy occurs, the corpus luteum maintains its function for the first trimester of pregnancy and the active waveforms persist during this period. Pregnancy is known to be dependent on a functioning corpus luteum, and Doppler ultrasound is a good means by which to identify this activity.

Intraovarian blood flow

The ovarian artery is a high-pressure system with flow velocity waveforms totally different from intraovarian waveforms. Near the ovarian hilus the penetration vessels are coiled and tortuous. This type of vascularity demonstrates high-resistance blood flow.

The fundamental unit of the ovary is the follicle, which consists of the female germ cell (oocyte) surrounded by a series of specialized cell layers, the granulosa and theca cells. Every month during the woman's reproductive life, one oocyte is released from the single mature follicle that has completed development. A number of biochemical, morphological and vascular changes occur within the cell layers

during this process, and a significant proportion of them can be studied by color Doppler. With this modality, areas of vascularity on the follicular rim can be detected when the dominant follicle reaches 10 mm in diameter (Figure 3). The resistance index (RI) is around 0.54 while ovulation approaches (Figure 4).

A decline begins 2 days before ovulation and reaches its nadir at ovulation (0.44 ± 0.04)[20]. The increase in the peak systolic blood velocity within the follicle in the presence of a relatively constant RI is a particularly interesting finding that might herald impending

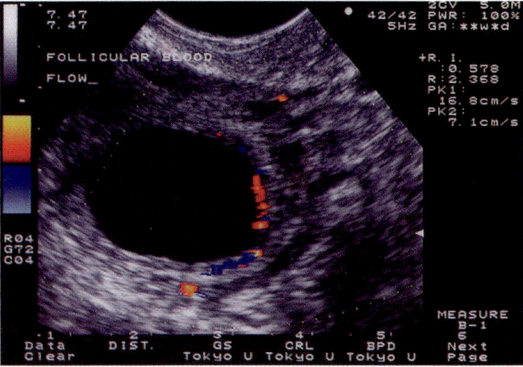

Figure 3 Transvaginal ultrasound scan demonstrating a ring of angiogenesis around the follicle during the moment of presumed ovulation

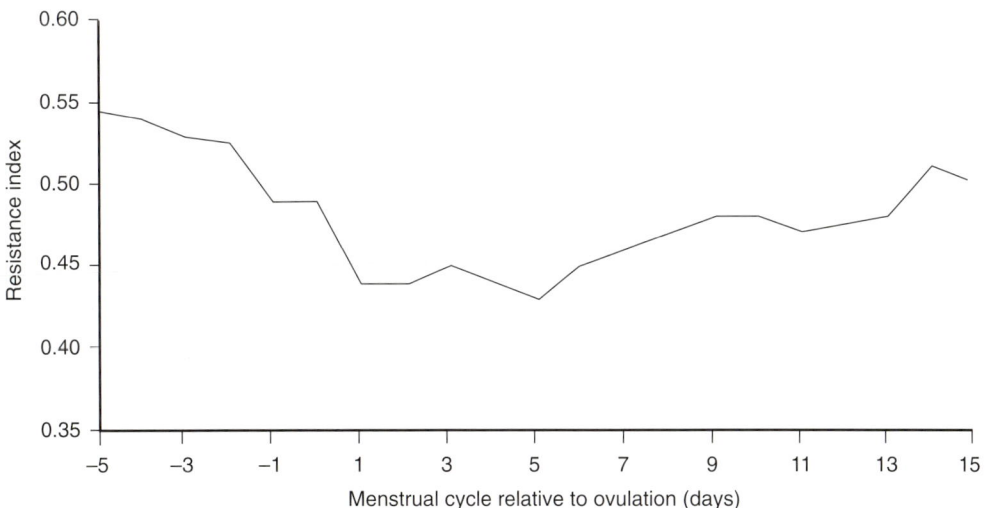

Figure 4 Intraovarian blood flow changes during the ovulatory menstrual cycle

ovulation. Increased vascularity on the innermost rim of the follicle[21] may represent the dilatation of new vessels that have developed between the relatively vascular theca cell layer and the normally hypoxic granulosa cell layer of the follicle. Disruption of these vascular changes has profound effects on the oxygen concentration across the follicular epithelium[22,23]. It is hoped that information on ovarian perfusion may be used both to predict ovulation and to investigate ovulatory dysfunction. We have observed 12 cases of luteinized unruptured follicles with a failure of the peak blood velocity in the preovulatory period. These data support the hypothesis that changes in oxygen tension within the follicular wall are necessary for follicular rupture[21–23]. If the process of oogenesis or ovulation can be inhibited independently from the main pathways of steroidogenesis, then novel methods of avoiding conception may be advised. Steroids that inhibit angiogenesis in the presence of heparin have already been identified[24]. It is apparent that transvaginal sonography with color Doppler facilities can be used to monitor the progress towards these novel contraceptive methods.

The same modality can follow changes of the intraovarian circulatory network in patients with polycystic ovarian syndrome (Figure 5). In a study of 34 oligo- or amenorrheic women with bilaterally increased ovarian volume, thickened ovarian capsule and numerous cystic structures measuring 2–8 mm in diameter, hormonal parameters (luteinizing hormone/follicle-stimulating hormone ratio > 3, increased androgen level) and intraovarian blood flow were measured[20]. We found no changes in resistance indices of the ovarian arteries and intraovarian parenchymal vessels during the menstrual cycle. High diastolic flow patterns were followed continuously from the ovarian stroma, resulting in a mean RI of 0.54 (Figure 6). These vascular changes are the possible effect of local hyperandrogenism and/or luteinizing hormone (LH) stimulus to (vascular) theca cells.

Color flow is more easily obtainable from ovarian tissue in the luteal phase (Figure 7).

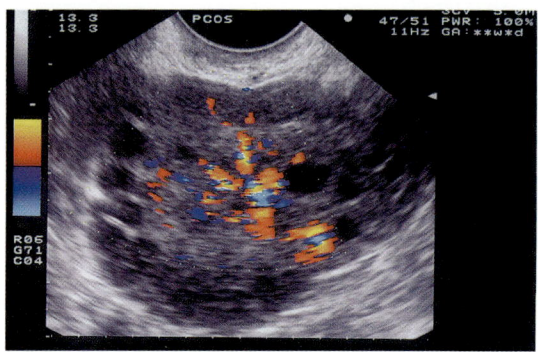

Figure 5 A transvaginal ultrasound scan of a polycystic ovary. A large number of small cystic structures are crowded together and stand out from the surface of the enlarged ovarian stroma

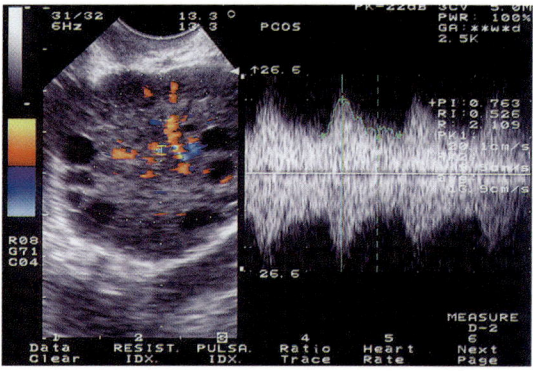

Figure 6 In the same patient as in Figure 5, Doppler waveform analysis obtained from the stroma demonstrates moderate impedance to flow (resistance index 0.53)

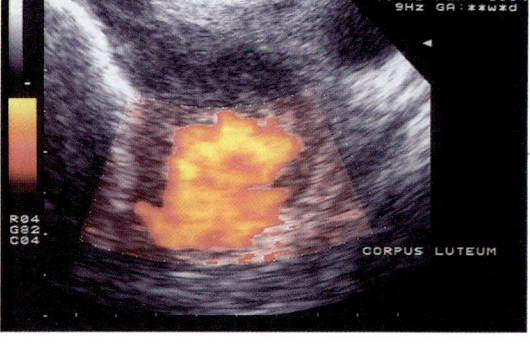

Figure 7 Demonstration of increased vascularity in the corpus luteum as seen using the power Doppler technique

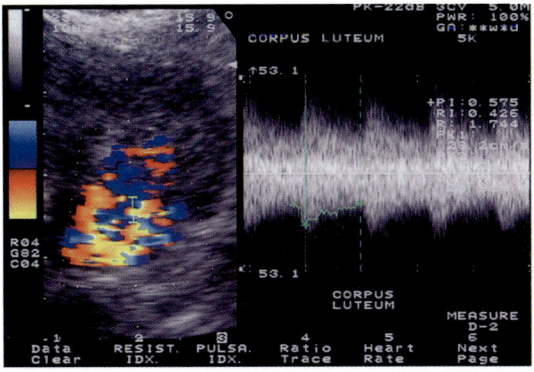

Figure 8 A high blood velocity and a decreased resistance index represent typical signs of ovulation and early corpus luteum blood flow

The qualitative postovulatory changes in intraovarian flow velocity waveforms are exciting: increased turbulent flow accompanying morphological changes in the intraovarian vascular network[25] and the appearance of numerous arteriovenous shunts during the luteal phase[26]. After ovulation, the RI shows a significant difference from the preovulatory values. Each woman with documented ovulation showed an RI of 0.43 ± 0.04 shortly after ovulation[11] (Figure 8). The RI remained at the low level for 4 to 5 days and then gradually climbed to a value of 0.50, still lower than that seen in the early follicular phase. Luteal conversion can be detected in all normal ovulatory cycles[20], independently of the corpus luteum identification. Converted blood flow signals are maintained throughout the luteal phase and are not observed on the non-dominant side, or in patients with anovulatory cycles or luteinized unruptured follicles[27].

Changes in the intraovarian flow velocity therefore occur before ovulation, implying a complexity of these changes that may involve both angiogenesis and hormonal factors, while postovulatory vascular accommodation is potentially important in the luteal phase. Using transvaginal color Doppler, corpus luteum blood flow, characterized by low impedance and high flow requirements, can easily be detected in normal early pregnancy, ectopic pregnancy and non-pregnant women[28]. It is not clear currently whether inadequate vascularization plays a role in luteal phase deficiency and whether luteal flow can be used as an accurate predictor for the evaluation of normal and pathological pregnancy.

ANGIOGENESIS AND NEOVASCULARIZATION

It was long believed that simple dilatation of existing host blood vessels accounted for increased tumor vascularity[29]. Vasodilatation was generally thought to be a 'side-effect' of tumor metabolites or of necrotic tumor products escaping from the tumor. However, some authors suggested that the tumor hyperemia could be related to new blood vessel growth. A report published in 1945 revealed that new vessels in the neighborhood of a tumor implant arose from host vessels and not from the tumor itself[30]. After that report, the debate continued in the literature for two more decades about whether tumors were supplied by existing vessels or by neovascularization[31–35].

Angiogenesis and neovascularization are terms that are entering the vocabulary of every ultrasonographer. Angiogenesis occurs during embryonic development and during several physiological and pathological conditions in adult life[36–38]. As mentioned before, angiogenesis is important in the process of ovulation and the development of the corpus luteum. It accompanies numerous non-malignant diseases such as acute or chronic inflammation (Figure 9) and ectopic pregnancy (Figure 10). However, tumor angiogenesis differs at least in a temporal manner from other types of angiogenesis described. In physiological conditions, angiogenesis is turned off once the process is completed. In non-malignant processes, angiogenesis is prolonged, but still self-limiting (Figure 11). In contrast, tumor angiogenesis is not self-limiting[39]. The malignant tumor microvasculature does not conform to the vasculature of normal tissues. It contains giant capillaries and arteriovenous shunts without intervening capillaries. Newly formed vessels contain no smooth muscle in their walls, but instead contain only a small amount of fibrous connective tissue[39].

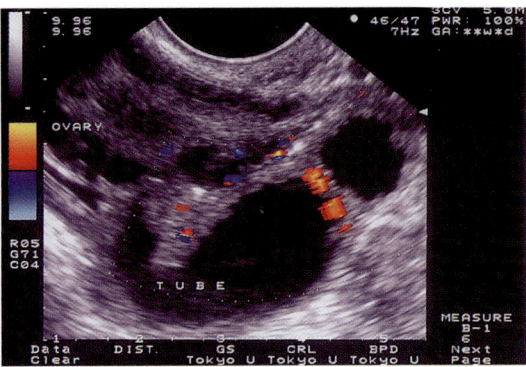

Figure 9 A complex adnexal mass occupying the pouch of Douglas in a patient with acute pelvic inflammation. Note the increased tubal diameter, the thickened tubal mucosa and the fluid within the tubal lumen. The increased vascularity is a response to various bacterial antigens and inflammatory products, and is easily detectable using the color Doppler modality

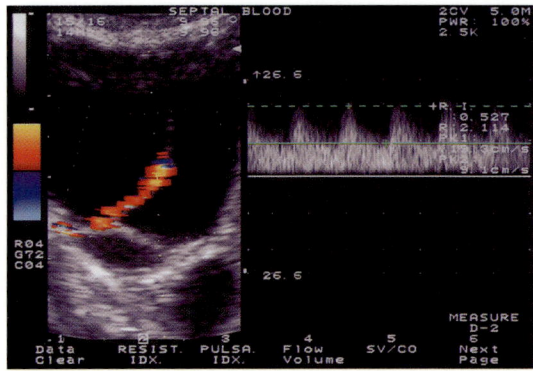

Figure 11 A transvaginal sonogram of a multilocular ovarian cyst. Color Doppler imaging demonstrates septal blood flow with a moderate resistance index (0.53)

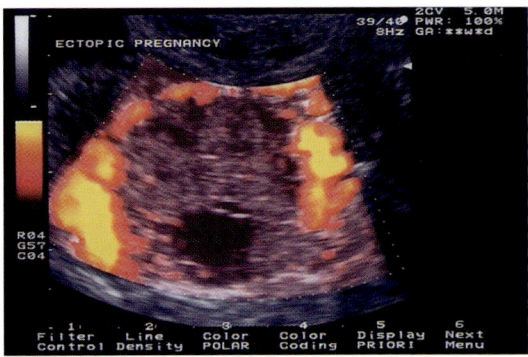

Figure 10 A transvaginal ultrasound scan of a highly vascularized adnexal mass suspected to be an ectopic pregnancy. Power Doppler helps in the diagnosis of ectopic gestation by exposing small and randomly dispersed tubal arteries indicative of trophoblastic activity and invasiveness

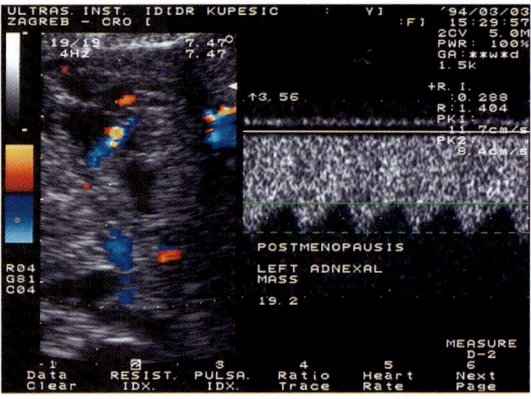

Figure 12 Neovascular signals detected in the central parts of a complex tumor. The pulsed Doppler signal is typical of ovarian malignancy. This flow has high velocity and a low resistance index (0.29), and lacks a diastolic notch

These vascular changes can be detected using color Doppler. Blood flow can be demonstrated throughout diastole, reflecting significantly decreased impedance to flow distal to the point of sampling (Figure 12). Because very similar indices of impedance to blood flow are seen from the preovulatory follicle and corpus luteum, vascular information derived from the premenopausal ovary must always be related to the patient's menstrual cycle. Accordingly, physiological ovarian angiogenic activity could be excluded by carrying out the examination during the early proliferative phase (from the 3rd to the 10th menstrual day). In ovarian lesions which demonstrate low impedance and high diastolic flow, it is important to determine whether the waveform has a diastolic notch. Existence of a notch indicates persistence of an initial resistance from the muscular lining of pre-existing arterioles, and is typical of benign tumors.

Quantitative morphometric studies in induced animal tumors show that vascular volume, length and surface area increase during the early stages of tumor growth, and then decrease after the onset of necrosis[40]. The number of vessels of large diameter increases in the later stages of growth[41]. It is not clear whether the same process happens in cancer metastasis[42]. Tumor cells must gain access to the vasculature in the primary tumor, survive the circulation, stop in the microvasculature of the target organ[43,44], exit from this vasculature[45], grow in the target organ and induce angiogenesis[46]. Small vessels that feed growing ovarian tumors or metastases could not be seen before the transvaginal application of color Doppler. The clinical application of this new modality and characterization of benign and malignant ovarian lesions on the basis of their vascularity have opened exciting avenues in the field of gynecological oncology.

References

1. Reynolds, S. R. M. (1973). Blood and lymph vascular systems of the ovary. In Greep, S. R. (ed.) *Female Reproductive System*, Part 1, pp. 261–316. (Washington: American Physiological Society)
2. Ginther, O. J., Diersche, D. K. J., Walsh, S. W. and Del Campo, C. H. (1974). Anatomy of arteries and veins of uterus and ovaries in rhesus monkeys. *Biol. Reprod.*, **11**, 204–19
3. Gillet, J. Y., Koritke, J. G., Muller, P. and Juliens, C. (1968). On the microvascularization of the rabbit ovary. *Compt. Rend. Soc. Biol.*, **162**, 762–6
4. Merce, L. T. A. (1993). Bases anatomicas de la circulacion utero-ovarica. In Merce, L. T. A. (ed.) *Ecografia Doppler en Obstetricia y Ginecologia*, pp. 1–7. (Madrid: Interamericana McGraw-Hill)
5. Gratton, A. D. T., Hodge, C. and Callamander, R. (1990). Basic physics and instrumentation of transvaginal color imaging. In Kurjak, A. (ed.). *Transvaginal Color Doppler*, 1st edn., pp. 9–15 (Carnforth, UK: Parthenon Publishing)
6. Taylor, K. Y. W., Burns, P. N., Woodlock, J. P. and Wells, P. N. (1985). Blood flow in deep abdominal and pelvic vessels: ultrasonic pulsed Doppler analysis. *Radiology*, **154**, 487–93
7. Eik Nes, S. H., Brubakk, A. O. and Ulstein, M. K. (1980). Measurement of human fetal blood flow. *Br. Med. J.*, **280**, 283–4
8. Kurjak, A., Zalud, I., Jurkovic, D., Alfirevic, Z. and Miljan, M. (1989). Transvaginal color Doppler for the assessment of pelvic circulation. *Acta Obstet. Gynecol. Scand.*, **68**, 131–3
9. Kurjak, A., Zalud, I., Alfirevic, Z. and Jurkovic, D. (1991). The assessment of pelvic blood flow by transvaginal color Doppler. *Ultrasound Med. Biol.*, **16**, 437–50
10. Bourne, T. H. (1991). Transvaginal color Doppler in gynecology. *Ultrasound Obstet. Gynecol.*, **1**, 359–73
11. Kurjak, A., Kupesic-Urek, S., Schulman, H. and Zalud, I. (1992). Transvaginal color Doppler in the assessment of ovarian and uterine blood flow in infertile women. *Fertil. Steril.*, **56**, 870–3
12. Scholtes, M. C. W., Wladimiroff, J., van Rijen, H. J. M. and Hop, W. C. J. (1989). Uterine and ovarian flow velocity waveforms in the normal menstrual cycle; a transvaginal color Doppler study. *Fertil. Steril.*, **52**, 981–5
13. Janson, P. O., Damber, B. E. and Axen, C. (1981). Luteal blood flow and progesterone secretion in pseudopregnant rabbits. *J. Reprod. Fertil.*, **63**, 491–3
14. Ford, S. P. and Chenalult, J. R. (1981). Blood flow to the corpus luteum-bearing ovary and ipsilateral uterine horn of cows during estrous cycle and early pregnancy. *J. Reprod. Fertil.*, **62**, 555–9
15. Taylor, K. J. W. and Burns, P. N. (1985). Duplex Doppler scanning in the pelvis and abdomen. *Ultrasound Med. Biol.*, **11**, 643 7
16. Bruce, N. W. and Hillier, K. (1974). The effect of prostaglandin F on ovarian blood flow and corpus luteum regression in the rabbit. *Nature (London)*, **249**, 176–7
17. Brown, B. W., Emery, M. J. and Mattner, E. (1980). Ovarian arterial blood velocity measured with Doppler ultrasonic transducers in conscious ewes. *J. Reprod. Fertil.*, **58**, 295–300
18. Wary, M. J. and Cook, M. J. (1973). Redistribution of blood flow by prostaglandin F2-alpha in the rabbit ovary. *Am. J. Obstet. Gynecol.*, **117**, 381–5
19. Nell, T. M. and Niswender, G. D. (1981). Luteal blood flow and receptors for LH during PGF2-alpha-induced luteolysis: production of PGF2-alpha during early pregnancy. *Acta Vet. Scand.*, **77** (Suppl.), 117–30
20. Kurjak, A. and Kupesic-Urek, S. (1991). Infertility. In Kurjak, A. (ed.) *Transvaginal Color Doppler*, pp. 33–8. (Carnforth, UK: Parthenon Publishing)

21. Bourne, T. H., Jurkovic, D., Waterstone, J., Campbell, S. and Collins, W. P. (1991). Intra-follicular blood flow during human ovulation. *Ultrasound Obstet. Gynecol.*, **1**, 53–9

22. Collins, W., Jurkovic, D., Bourne, T. H., Kurjak, A. and Campbell, S. (1991). Ovarian morphology, endocrine function and intra-follicular blood flow during the preovulatory period. *Hum. Reprod.*, **6**, 319–24

23. Sladkevicius, P., Valentin, L. and Marsal, K. (1993). Blood flow velocity in the uterine and ovarian arteries during the normal menstrual cycle. *Ultrasound Obstet. Gynecol.*, **3**, 199–201

24. Inger, D. E., Madri, J. A. and Folkman, J. (1986). A possible mechanism for inhibition of angiogenesis by angiostatic steroids: induction of capillary basement membrane dissolution. *Endocrinology*, **119**, 1768–75

25. Reynolds, S. R. M. (1948). Morphological determinations of the flow characteristics between an artery and its branch with special reference to the ovarian spiral artery in the rabbit. *Acta. Anat.*, **5**, 1–6

26. Niswender, G. D., Reiners, T. J., Dickmann, M. A. and Nett, Y. T. M. (1976). Blood flow: a mediator of ovarian function. *Biol. Reprod.*, **14**, 64–81

27. Merce, L. T., Andrino, R., Barco, M. J. and De la Fuente, F. (1990). Cyclic changes of the functional ovarian compartments: echographic assessment. *Acta Obstet. Gynecol. Scand.*, **69**, 327–32

28. Zalud, I. and Kurjak, A. (1990). The assessment of luteal blood flow in pregnant and non-pregnant women by transvaginal color Doppler. *J. Perinat. Med.*, **18**, 215–18

29. Coman, D. R. and Sheldon, W. F. (1946). The significance of hyperemia around tumor implants. *Am. J. Pathol.*, **22**, 821–6

30. Algire, G. H., Chalkey, H. W., Legallais, F. Y. and Park, H. D. (1945). Vascular reactions of mice to wounds and to normal and neoplastic transplants. *J. Natl. Cancer Inst.*, **6**, 73–85

31. Day, E. D. (1964). Vascular relationships of tumor and host. *Prog. Exp. Tumor Res.*, **4**, 57–9

32. Folkman, J., Long, D. and Becker, F. (1963). Growth and metastasis of tumors in organ culture. *Tumor Res.*, **16**, 453–67

33. Folkman, J., Cole, P. and Yimmerman, S. (1966). Tumor behavior in isolated perfused organs: *in vitro* growth and metastasis of biopsy material in rabbit thyroid and canine intestinal segment. *Ann. Surg.*, **164**, 491–502

34. Folkman, J. and Gimbrone, M. (1972). Perfusion of the thyroid. *Acta Endocrinol.*, **4**, 237–48

35. Folkman, J. (1970). The intestine as an organ culture. In Burdette, J. and Thomas, C. C. (eds.) *Carcinoma of the Colon and Antecedent Epithelium*, pp. 113–27. (Springfield, Illinois: Charles C. Thomas)

36. Folkman, J. and Shing, Y. (1992). Minireview. *J. Biol. Chem.*, **267**, 10931–4

37. Klagsbrun, M. and D'Amore, P. A. (1991). Regulators of angiogenesis. *Annu. Rev. Physiol.*, **52**, 217

38. Folkman, J., Melrel, E., Abernethy, C. and Williams, G. (1971). Isolation of tumor factor responsible for angiogenesis. *J. Exp. Med.*, **133**, 275–8

39. Kurjak, A., Shalan, H., Kupesic, S., Predanic, M., Zalud, I., Breyer, B. and Jukic, S. (1993). Transvaginal color Doppler sonography in the assessment of pelvic tumor vascularity. *Ultrasound Obstet. Gynecol.*, **3**, 137–54

40. Gamil, S. L., Shipkey, F. H., Himmelfarb, E. H., Parvey, L. S. and Rabinowity, J. G. (1976). Roentgenology – pathology correlation study of neovascularization. *Am. J. Radiol.*, **126**, 376–85

41. Jain, R. K. and Ward Hartley, K. A. (1987). Dynamics of cancer cell interaction with microvasculature and interstitium. *Biorheology*, **24**, 117–23

42. Folkman, J. (1985). Tumor angiogenesis. *Adv. Cancer Res.*, **43**, 175–80

43. Netland, P. and Letter, B. (1984). Organ-specific adhesion and metastatic tumor cells *in vitro*. *Science*, **224**, 113–15

44. Nicholson, G. L. (1988). Organ specificity of tumor metastasis: role of preferential adhesion, invasion and growth of malignant cells at specific secondary sites. *Cancer Metastasis Rev.*, **7**, 143–88

45. Boxberger, H. J., Pawelety, N., Speiss, E. and Kniehuber, R. (1989). An *in vitro* model study of BS p73 rat tumor cell invasion into endothelial monolayer. *Anticancer Res.*, **9**, 1777–86

46. Weidner, N., Semple, J. P., Welch, W. R. and Folkman, J. (1991). Tumor angiogenesis and metastasis – correlation in invasive breast carcinoma. *N. Engl. J. Med.*, **324**, 1–8

Ultrasound and Doppler studies in polycystic ovarian syndrome

4

C. Battaglia and A. Volpe

INTRODUCTION

In 1721 Antonio Vallisneri, an Italian scientist, described for the first time the clinical and anatomo-pathological features of polycystic ovarian syndrome (PCOS)[1]. Since then, PCOS has been one of the most discussed, controversial and studied areas of endocrinological gynecology. In its classic form it is characterized by infertility, oligo- or amenorrhea, hirsutism, acne or seborrhea, and obesity. In 1935 the syndrome was recognized by Stein and Leventhal in a group of seven hirsute, amenorrheic women on the basis of typical ovarian morphology: fibrotic thickening of the tunica albuginea and outer cortex, and multiple cystic follicles with prominent theca[2].

The incidence of the syndrome is greatly different in various reports. In 1951 Vara and Niemineva, in a series of 12 160 unselected gynecological laparotomies, found polycystic ovaries in 1.4% of patients[3]. Sommers and Wadman, a few years later, diagnosed in 740 autopsies the typical ovarian expression of PCOS in 3.5% of the cases[4]. Clayton and colleagues recently claimed that the finding of polycystic ovaries is more common, with 22% of the younger female population showing a polycystic pattern on ultrasound scanning of the ovaries[5]. Adams and colleagues, by transabdominal ultrasound, found polycystic ovaries in 26% of patients with amenorrhea, in 87% with oligomenorrhea, and in 92% of women with hirsutism[6]. Furthermore, using an epidemiological approach, Hull calculated a possible incidence of PCOS in 90% of infertile oligomenorrheic, and in 37% of infertile amenorrheic patients[7].

From the above reported studies it is possible to conclude that polycystic ovaries are relatively common in the female population[8], and that there is a correlation between ovarian appearance, cycle history and clinical evidence of androgen excess.

PATHOPHYSIOLOGY

Polycystic ovarian syndrome may result from disturbances of various endocrine systems. It has been diagnosed in patients with adult-onset adrenal 21-hydroxylase deficiency, Cushing's syndrome, adrenal hyperplasia, hypo- and hyperthyroidism, adrenal or ovarian tumors, and hyperprolactinemia[9-15]. However, excluding these conditions, and despite a large number of epidemiological, clinical, laboratory and experimental studies, the etiology and pathophysiology of the syndrome still remain obscure[16].

Increased pre- or peripubertal adrenal function may result in elevated circulating androgens, which, by peripheral conversion (in fat and/or brain tissue), are changed into estrogens. The excessive estrogen levels are responsible for a disturbed (pulse frequency and/or amplitude) pattern of luteinizing hormone (LH) secretion. This, in turn, stimulates the ovarian thecal compartment to secrete androgens[17]. When this vicious circle is established, it is possible to appreciate the typical structural changes in the ovary.

To complicate the pathophysiological picture of the syndrome, it has been observed by Adashi and associates that insulin may potentiate the LH secretion in PCOS patients[18]. It is well known that hyperinsulinemia may lead to increased ovarian androgen production and to an enhanced conversion of testosterone to 5α-dihydrotestosterone. In addition, it has been shown that hyperandrogenism may result from an increased activity of cytochrome P-450c17-α, and that it may inhibit the liver production of sex hormone-binding globulin, resulting in a further increase of circulating androgens[19]. Finally, insulin-like growth factor-1 (IGF-1) increases the expression of LH receptors and stimulates LH-induced androgen production and their ovarian accumulation. Although no significant differences in IGF-1 have been shown in PCOS vs. non-PCOS patients, the biological IGF-1 activity may be increased by a decrease of the specific binding globulin[20].

Recently, Poretsky and Piper postulated that elevated LH and hyperinsulinemia, acting synergistically, induce ovarian stromal and thecal hyperplasia, hyperandrogenism and follicular atresia[21]. The subsequent predominance of androgen-secreting cells is responsible for the vicious circle with consequent PCOS clinical manifestations. It seems that both the elevated LH secretion and the insulin resistance of PCOS are genetically determined (the insulin receptor gene and the β-LH subunit gene have been mapped to chromosome 19)[21–23] (Figure 1).

DIAGNOSIS

A detailed history concerning the chronobiological symptom development is mandatory in establishing the true diagnosis. PCOS patients generally have a history of peripubertal onset of increased hair growth, oligo- or amenorrhea, and obesity. An adequate estrogen activity is, however, confirmed by breast development and secondary signs of sexual maturation.

The various clinical manifestations of PCOS, as analyzed by Goldzieher and Axelrod[24], are listed in Table 1. The incidence of symptoms can vary enormously, complicating the diagnosis. The symptoms which present the highest average incidence are: hirsutism (69%), infertility (74%), and menstrual disorders (79%).

The complexity of the pathophysiological interactions and the heterogeneity of the clinical expression are responsible for the lack of a specific hormonal test useful for the diagnosis. In fact, the endocrinological findings generally correlated with PCOS (elevated LH or LH/follicle-stimulating hormone (FSH) ratio, abnormally high androstenedione and/or testosterone levels), are often inconsistent. The discrepancy may be due to the fact that LH and steroid hormones oscillate in pulses of relatively high frequency and are subject to circadian rhythms[25]. Furthermore, plasma testosterone levels are in part determined by peripheral androstenedione conversion and by the amount bound to both circulating sex hormone-binding globulin and albumin[9]. Elevated estrogen plasma levels are also of limited diagnostic value for classifying PCOS. It should in fact be remembered that about 25% of PCOS patients ovulate and that estrone and estradiol plasma levels may derive from the ovary and/or adrenal and from androstenedione peripheral conversion[9]. However, several authors have shown that the simultaneous use of different markers (LH, FSH and androstenedione) may be useful and cost-effective in the diagnosis of PCOS[26]. Nevertheless, the typical appearance of polycystic ovaries at laparoscopy, whether or not associated with ovarian biopsy, is still widely considered essential for a correct diagnosis[27,28].

The advent of ultrasonographic examination of the ovaries has provided the biggest single contribution to PCOS diagnosis. This non-invasive technique, performed by a skilled operator, has a high concordance rate with laparoscopy and histological examination and may be considered the 'gold standard' for the diagnosis of the syndrome.

Identification of polycystic ovaries on pelvic ultrasound

The histo-anatomical features of PCOS are characterized by a discrete variability, although an increased number of follicles and increased stromal ovarian tissue may be considered

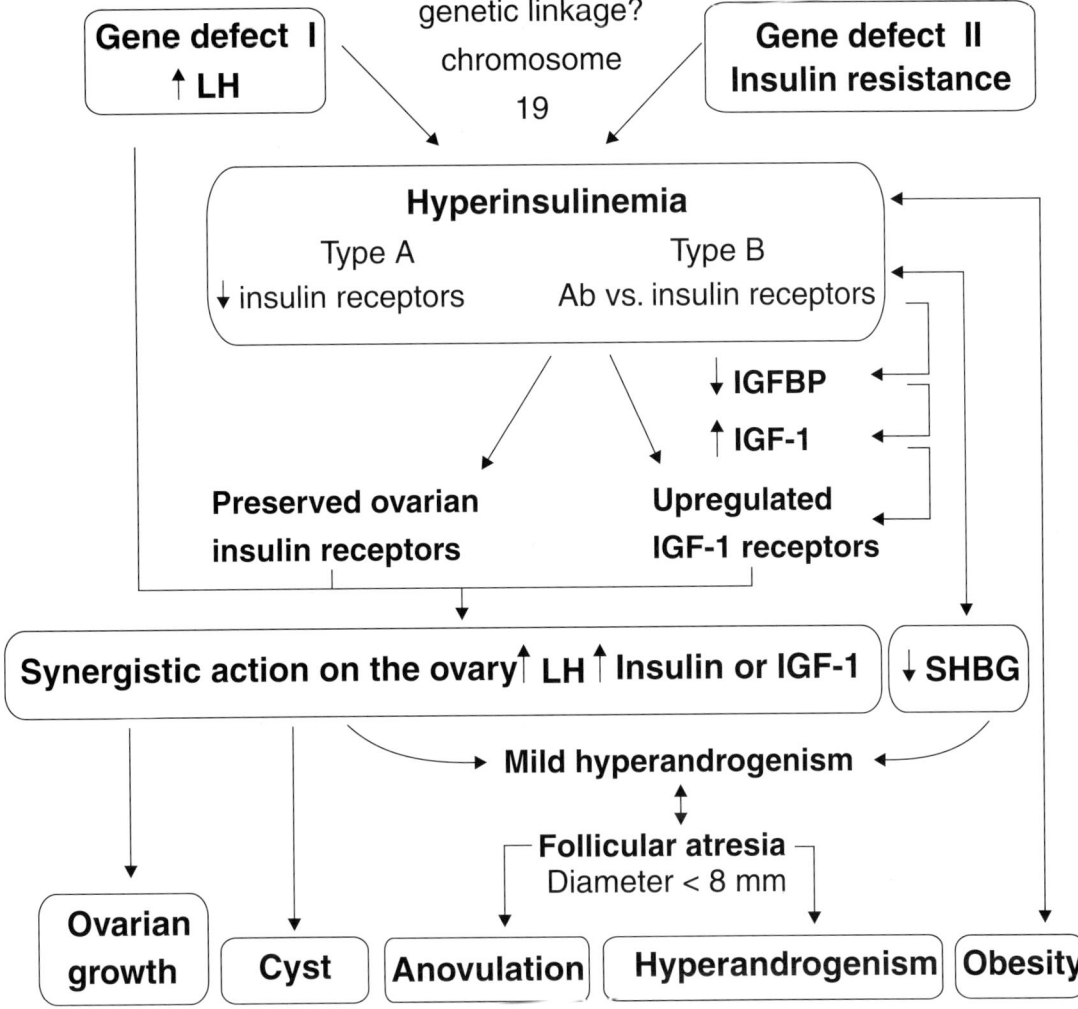

Figure 1 Dual-defect hypothesis of polycystic ovarian syndrome (PCOS). The two hypothesized genetic defects may be responsible for all features of PCOS. Ab, antibody; LH, luteinizing hormone; IGF-1, insulin-like growth factor-1; IGFBP, insulin-like growth factor binding protein; SHBG, sex hormone-binding globulin. Modified from reference 21

constant. These features can be identified with pelvic ultrasound[29].

The possibility of studying the female pelvic structures, namely the uterus and ovaries, using ultrasound was first demonstrated by Kratochwil and colleagues, who also described the ultrasound uterine and ovarian changes in relation to the menstrual cycle[30]. Since then, ultrasound scanning has emerged as an essential method for monitoring utero-ovarian activity in many clinical conditions.

In 1986, Adams and colleagues defined the criteria for ultrasonographic diagnosis of polycystic ovaries: multiple ($n > 10$), small (2–8 mm) peripheral cysts around a dense core of stroma in enlarged ($\geqslant 8$ ml) ovaries[31]. However, ovaries which are normal in volume can be polycystic, as demonstrated by histological and biochemical studies. Transabdominal echography has revealed enlarged ovaries (8–14 ml) in up to 70% of symptomatic patients, and has shown that the follicles

Table 1 Frequency of clinical manifestations of polycystic ovarian syndrome (PCOS)

Clinical manifestation	Frequency (%)	
	Mean	Range
Obesity	41	16–49
Hirsutism	69	17–83
Virilization	21	0–28
Amenorrhea	51	15–77
Infertility	74	35–94
Functional bleeding	29	6–65
Biphasic basal temperature	15	14–40
Corpus luteum at operation	22	0–71

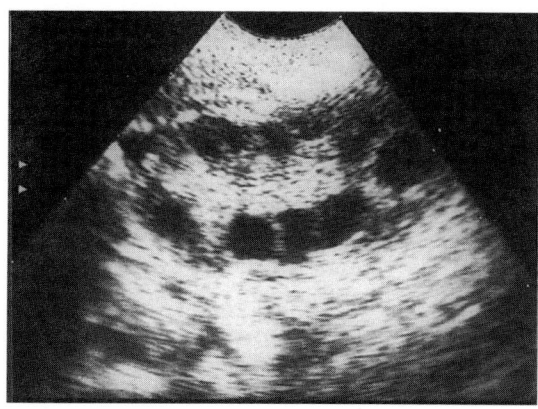

Figure 2 Typical ultrasonographic evidence of polycystic ovarian syndrome of the peripheral cystic pattern: a high number of small subcapsular follicles (10 follicles with maximum diameter < 8 mm), increased ovarian volume (12.3 ml) and increased echodensity of the ovarian stroma

(usually peripherally dislocated) may also be scattered throughout the hyperechogenic stroma[32,33]. These findings are based on transabdominal sonography, which although showing a good specificity, as confirmed in patients undergoing ovarian wedge resection[34], shows variable results in terms of follicular number, ovarian size and stromal ovarian echodensity[35]. It has recently been stated that the anatomic structure of the ovaries can not adequately be assessed with the transabdominal approach in about 42% of cases[36]. Underlying causes are obesity, limited resolution of low-frequency transducers, a full bladder distorting pelvic anatomy, and bowel loops covering the adjacent ovary[37,38].

More recently, the transvaginal approach for ultrasound scanning of pelvic organs has been used. The high frequency of the transvaginal probe avoids the need for a full bladder and bypasses the problems of attenuation and artifacts associated with obesity. Furthermore, transvaginal ultrasonography has the advantage of improved resolution, better visualization of pelvic organs, and greater acceptance among patients[37–42]. The transvaginal approach gives more precise sonographic criteria for diagnosis of polycystic ovaries, bringing transvaginal data into closer agreement with histologic parameters[43,44] (Figure 2).

The number of follicles necessary to establish the diagnosis of polycystic ovaries by ultrasonography has been reported to vary between five and 15[31,45,46]. However, in many reports the highest number of atretic follicles

obtained in normal control patients was five per ovary, so it may conventionally be established that in polycystic ovaries the number of atretic follicles per ovary would be at least six. Matsunaga and colleagues identified two types of polycystic ovary on the basis of ultrasonographic follicular distribution: the peripheral cystic pattern (PCP) and the general cystic pattern (GCP)[32]. In the PCP, small cysts are distributed in the subcapsular region of the ovary (Figure 2), whereas in the GCP they are scattered through the entire ovarian parenchyma (Figure 3). Recently, Takahashi and colleagues showed that these two different ovarian morphologies reflect histopathological differences, and that the PCP and GCP appearances reflect specific endocrine PCOS patterns[43].

Another parameter considered in the diagnosis of polycystic ovaries is the ovarian volume. However, the wide volume overlap between normal and PCOS patients suggests that the discriminative capacity of ovarian volume alone is not sufficient for ultrasound diagnosis of PCOS. The role of a hyperechogenic ovarian stroma has been emphasized, but appraisal of the ovarian stroma echodensity[47], although comparable with computerized quantification[48], is absolutely subjective and may be differently interpreted by the operator.

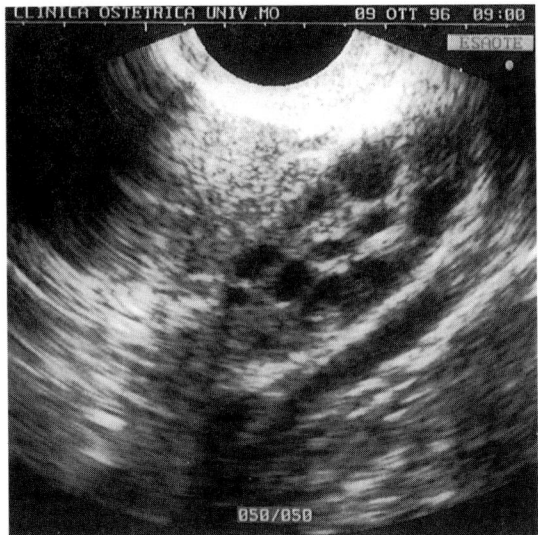

CLINICA OSTETRICA UNIV.MO   09 OTT 96   09:00

050/050

Figure 3 The general cystic pattern in polycystic ovarian syndrome: the numerous ($n = 13$) small cysts are scattered through the entire ovarian parenchyma, the stroma is echodense, and the volume is increased (14.0 ml)

From the above considerations it is evident that great biological variability expresses an equally wide range of echographic patterns and that it is not possible to obtain a cut-off level for any of the analyzed parameters, even in the presence of good sensitivity and specificity. A specific diagnosis can probably be obtained by the combined analysis of all the studied parameters.

Doppler analysis and color flow mapping

The introduction of transvaginal Doppler sonography has contributed markedly to the refinement of ultrasound diagnosis. In addition, it has provided much new morphological and pathophysiological information on blood flow dynamics within the female pelvis[49–53].

In general, blood flow studies have been confined to arteries. The vessels most often analyzed in reproductive endocrinology are the uterine and ovarian arteries. Color flow images of ascending branches of uterine arteries may be obtained, both transvaginally and transabdominally, lateral to the cervix in a longitudinal plane. The ovarian arteries may be evaluated at the level of the ovarian hilum[49,54–60]. Recently, attention has been extended to small vessels supplying the ovarian stroma[61,62] (Figure 4).

It has been shown that in patients with polycystic ovarian syndrome important changes in ovarian vascularization occur at the level of the intraovarian arteries. Although intraovarian arteries are usually not seen before day 8 to 10 of the 28-day cycle[61], we detected distinct arteries with characteristic low vascular impedance as early as cycle day 3 to 5[63]. In the studied population the results were associated with typical PCOS hormonal parameters and were inversely correlated with the LH/FSH ratio. Tonic hypersecretion of LH during the follicular phase of the menstrual cycle occurs in PCOS and is associated with theca cells and stromal hyperplasia with consequent androgen overproduction. Elevated LH levels may be responsible for increased stromal vascularization by different mechanisms that may act individually or in a cumulative way: neoangiogenesis, catecholaminergic stimulation, and leukocyte and cytokine activation[64–66]. In the same study the PCOS patients showed higher uterine pulsatility index (PI) values than nonhirsute normally menstruating women. This finding was correlated with androstenedione levels, confirming a possible direct androgen vasoconstrictive effect due to activation of specific receptors present in the arterial vessel walls and collagen and elastin deposition in smooth muscle cells[67,68]. The increased resistance at the level of the uterine arteries, by reducing the uterine perfusion, has been supposed to be the cause that prevents blastocyst implantation, increasing the incidence of miscarriages in PCOS patients. Similar results were obtained by Zaidi and colleagues[69] and Aleem and Predanic[70], confirming that the Doppler analysis of stromal arteries in PCOS may be useful to improve the diagnosis, and to provide further information about the pathophysiology and evolution of the syndrome. These hypotheses have been recently confirmed[71].

In contrast to the results of Takahashi and colleagues[43], who reported that the GCP appearance is associated with ovarian steroid disorders whereas the PCP is associated with

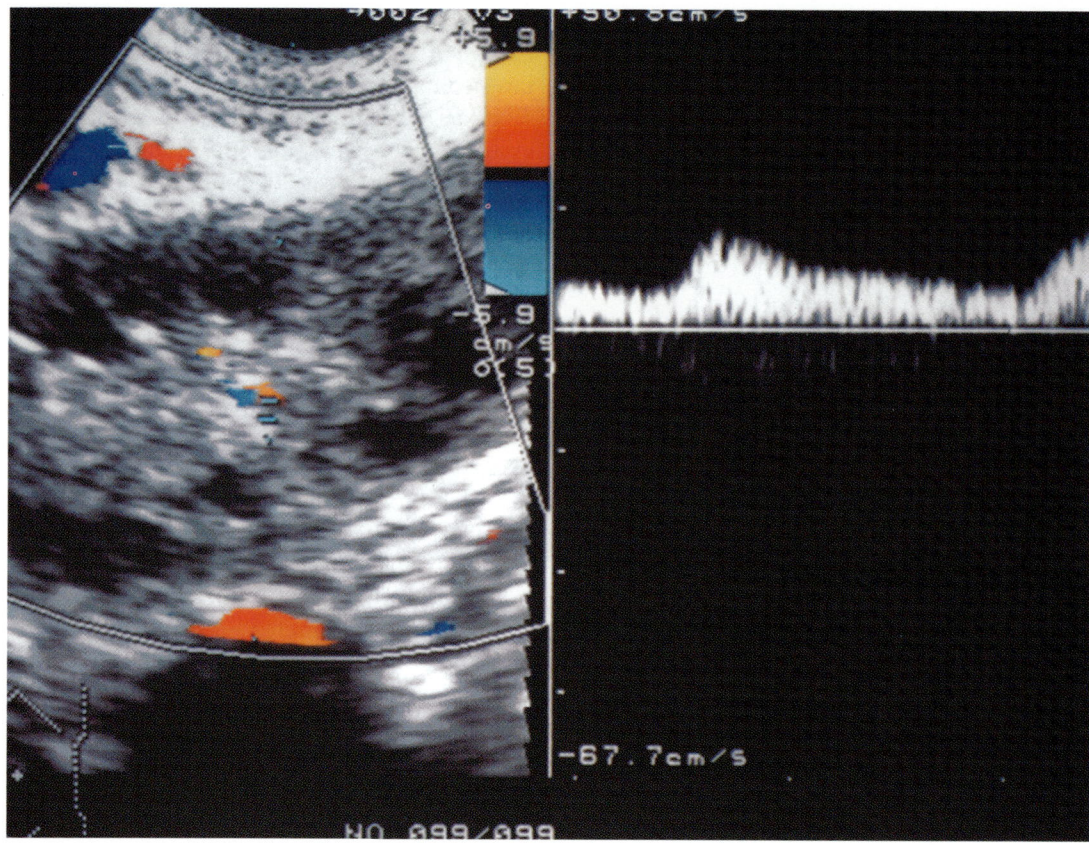

Figure 4 Intraovarian stromal vascularization in polycystic ovarian syndrome: small stromal vessels with low downstream impedance (resistance index 0.52)

abnormal gonadotropin secretion, we suggest that the different ovarian morphologies do not reflect different endocrine patterns but may be considered an evolution of the same endocrinological alteration. In fact, Doppler evaluation showed that PCP patients, in comparison with GCP patients, present significantly lower resistance index (RI) values at the level of the ovarian stromal arteries and that in 22% of GCP patients the intraovarian vessels are not recognized[72] (Table 2). In addition, the GCP appearance of the ovary is more common in the early phase of the disease[32,43] during the peripubertal period. Thus, the ovarian morphology may evolve from a normal multicystic to a polycystic PCP pattern, passing through an ovarian GCP aspect, and untreated PCOS may be regarded as a progressive syndrome. Furthermore, by comparing

Table 2 Doppler findings in the general cystic pattern (GCP) and peripheral cystic pattern (PCP) of polycystic ovarian syndrome (PCOS)

Ovarian stromal artery	GCP (n = 18)	PCP (n = 16)
Resistance index	0.66 ± 0.13	0.54 ± 0.05**
Visualization (%)	78	100*

*$p < 0.05$; **$p < 0.01$

oligo- vs. amenorrheic PCOS patients, it has recently been shown that amenorrheic patients are older and present higher PI values in uterine arteries and lower RI values in intraovarian vessels than oligomenorrheic patients[73]. This finding is associated with higher plasma LH and androstenedione levels and with a more elevated LH/FSH ratio. Furthermore, significantly higher ovarian volumes and subcapsular small-sized follicles are

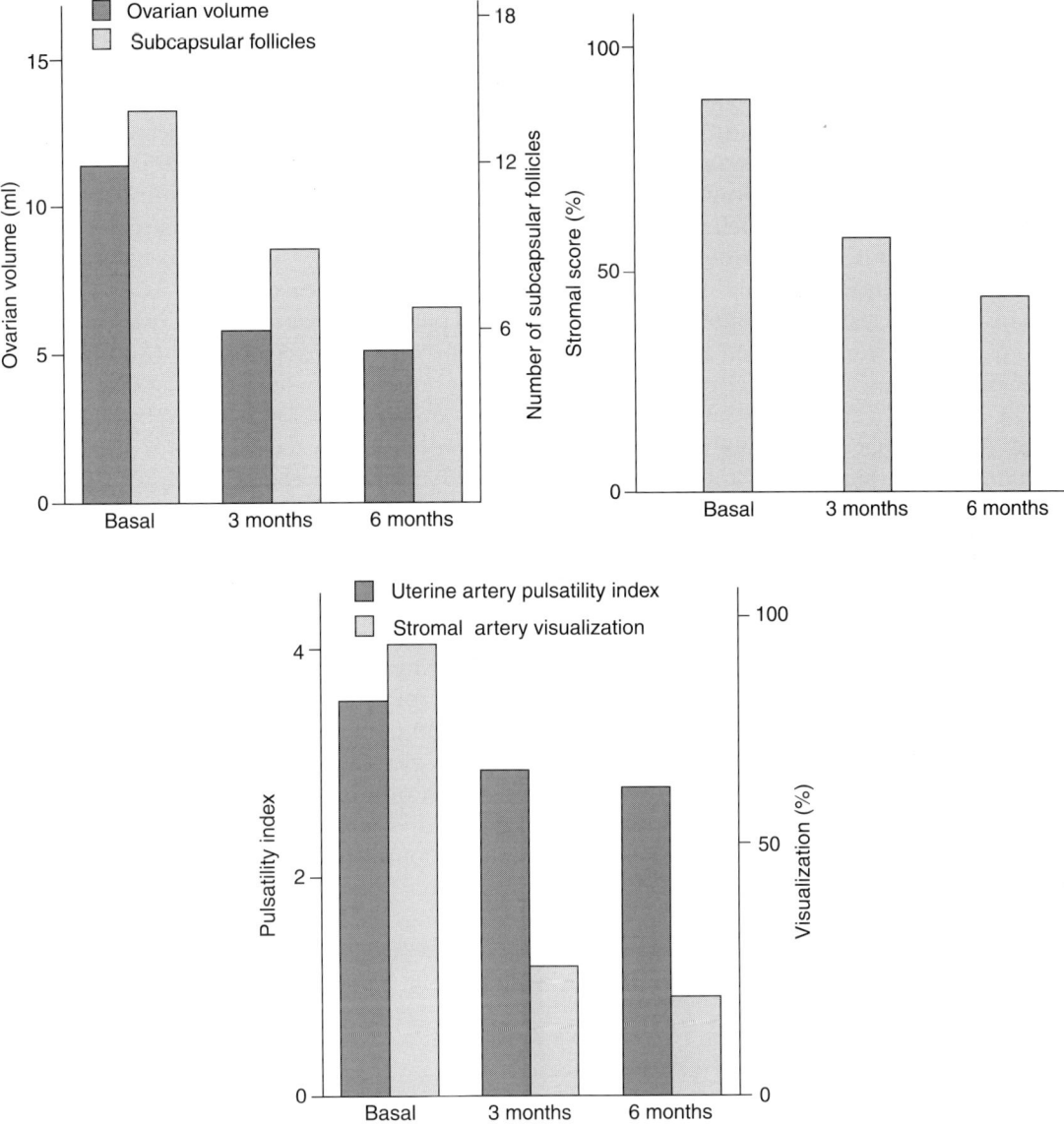

Figure 5 Ultrasonographic and Doppler analysis of uterine and ovarian intraparenchymal arteries, and modifications due to a 6-month treatment with a gonadotropin-releasing hormone (GnRH) analog plus an oral contraceptive in 20 patients with polycystic ovarian syndrome (PCOS)

observed in amenorrheic PCOS patients. These data show that as the number of ovarian microcysts increases, ovarian volume enlarges and Doppler indices worsen, the clinical and endocrine abnormalities become more remarkable, and the menstrual disturbances become more severe. An early therapeutic intervention would probably not only temporarily alleviate symptoms, but may delay the progression of the syndrome.

It is well known that assessment of ovarian morphological and functional changes during the treatment of PCOS has been generally lacking, or contradictory results have been reported. With the use of color Doppler, we recently showed that the association of gonadotropin-releasing hormone (GnRH) analog with an oral contraceptive is effective in improving PCOS symptoms[74]. Both clinical (Ferriman–Gallwey score) and hormonal (androgens, LH/FSH ratio) parameters improved during the therapy and follow-up period. The changes of hormonal findings were associated with complementary ultrasound (decreased ovarian volume and stromal density, and reduced number of small-sized subcapsular follicles) and Doppler (disappearance of stromal vascularization and improvement of PI values at the level of the uterine arteries) modifications (Figure 5). These results showed that it is possible, probably by expanding the duration of the therapy, to reach the main 'goal' of therapy in PCOS: to reduce the elevated androgen plasma levels and regularize the associated sequelae.

Recently, it has been demonstrated that obese PCOS women show higher PI values within the uterine arteries than do lean patients[75]. This is associated with higher hematocrit values, hyperinsulinemia, higher triglyceride levels and lower high-density lipid (HDL) concentrations. Furthermore, in the obese patients, an inverse correlation is observed between HDL concentrations and uterine artery resistance. Insulin resistance is considered to be a risk factor for coronary heart disease, as it is often associated with diabetes mellitus, hypertension and an adverse lipid profile. In addition, Wild and colleagues have shown that in women undergoing coronary angiography, hirsute patients are more likely to have significant atheroma than the non-hirsute[76]. In overweight patients, hyperinsulinemia may be proposed as the uniting factor between increased vascular resistance, obesity, lipid abnormalities and cardiovascular disease. Thus, assuming that PCOS patients are at increased risk for cardiovascular disease, it is possible to affirm that obesity may further increase the risk. In this case transvaginal color Doppler, by evaluating vascular blood flow modifications, may be considered another surrogate marker for possible cardiovascular disease.

CONCLUSION

The assessment of ovarian morphology by transvaginal ultrasound and Doppler flow analysis of both intraovarian and uterine arteries in patients with PCOS may provide an insight into the pathological state and the degree of progression of the disease. However, further and extensive studies are necessary before Doppler studies can be added to the traditional clinical, endocrinological and ultrasonographic parameters used for the diagnosis of polycystic ovarian syndrome.

References

1. Vallisneri, A. (1721). Storia della generazione dell'uomo e dell'animale. Cited in Cooke, I. D. and Lunenfeld, B. (1989). *Res Clin Forums*, **11**, 109–13
2. Stein, I. F. and Leventhal, M. L. (1935). Amenorrhea associated with bilateral polycystic ovaries. *Am. J. Obstet. Gynecol.*, **29**, 181–91
3. Vara, P. and Niemineva, K. (1951). Small cystic degeneration of ovaries as incidental finding in gynecological laparotomies. *Acta Obstet. Gynecol. Scand.*, **31**, 94–9
4. Sommers, S. C. and Wadman, P. J. (1956). Pathogenesis of polycystic ovaries. *Am. J. Obstet. Gynecol.*, **29**, 181–7
5. Clayton, R. N., Ogden, V., Hodgkinson, J., Worswich, L., Rodin, D. A., Dyer, S. and Meade, T. W. (1992). How common are polycystic ovaries in normal women and what is their significance for the fertility of the population. *Clin. Endocrinol.*, **37**, 127–34
6. Adams, J., Polson, D. W. and Franks, S. (1986). Prevalence of polycystic ovaries in women with anovulation and idiopathic hirsutism. *Br. Med. J.*, **293**, 335–59
7. Hull, M. G. R. (1987). Epidemiology of infertility and polycystic ovarian disease: endocrinological and demographic studies. *Gynecol. Endocrinol.*, **1**, 235–45

8. Polson, D. W., Wadszworth, J., Adams, J. and Franks, S. (1988). Polycystic ovaries: a common finding in normal women. *Lancet*, **1**, 870–2

9. Yen, S. S. C. (1991). Chronic anovulation caused by peripheral endocrine disorders. In Yen, S. S. C. and Jaffe, R. (eds.) *Reproductive Endocrinology*, pp. 593–625. (W. B. Saunders Company)

10. Axelrod, L. R., Goldzieher, J. W. and Ross, S. D. (1965). Concurrent 3-beta-hydroxysteroid dehydrogenase deficiency in adrenal and sclerocystic ovary. *Acta Endocrinol.*, **48**, 392–412

11. Futterweit, W. and Krieger, D. T. (1979). Pituitary tumor associated with hyperprolactinemia and polycystic ovarian disease. *Fertil. Steril.*, **31**, 608–13

12. Alger, M., Vazquez-Matute, L., Mason, M., Canales, E. and Zarate, A. (1980). Polycystic ovarian disease associated with hyperprolactinemia and defective metoclopramide response. *Fertil. Steril.*, **34**, 70–1

13. Lisse, K., Schurenkamper, P., Friedrich, W. and Rutkowsky, J. (1980). Diurnal change of serum androstenedione and testosterone and response to hCG and dexamethasone in women with polycystic ovaries, adrenal hyperandrogenism and unexplained hirsutism. *Acta Endocrinol.*, **93**, 216–22

14. Lobo, R. A. and Goebelsmann, U. (1980). Adult manifestation of congenital adrenal hyperplasia due to incomplete 21-hydroxylase deficiency mimicking polycystic ovarian disease. *Am. J. Obstet. Gynecol.*, **138**, 720–6

15. Stevens, V. C. and Goldzieher, J. V. (1986). Urinary excretion of gonadotropins in congenital hyperplasia. *Pediatrics*, **41**, 421–7

16. Insler, V., Shoham, Z., Barash, A., Koistinen, R., Seppala, M., Hen, M., Lunenfeld, B. and Zadik, Z. (1993). Polycystic ovaries in non-obese and obese patients: possible pathophysiological mechanism based on new interpretation of facts and findings. *Hum. Reprod.*, **8**, 379–84

17. Insler, V. and Lunenfeld, B. (1991). Pathophysiology of polycystic ovarian disease: new insights. *Hum. Reprod.*, **6**, 1025–9

18. Adashi, E., Hsueh, A. and Yen, S. S. C. (1981). Insulin enhancement of luteinizing hormone and follicle-stimulating hormone release by cultured pituitary cells. *Endocrinology*, **108**, 1441–9

19. Dahlgren, E. and Janson, P. O. (1994). Polycystic ovary syndrome – long-term metabolic consequences. *Int. J. Gynecol. Obstet.*, **44**, 3–8

20. Homburg, R. (1996). Polycystic ovary syndrome – from gynecological curiosity to multisystem endocrinopathy. *Hum. Reprod.*, **11**, 29–39

21. Poretsky, L. and Piper, B. (1994). Insulin resistance, hypersecretion of LH, and a dual-defect hypothesis for the pathogenesis of polycystic ovary syndrome. *Obstet. Gynecol.*, **84**, 613–21

22. Seino, S., Seino, M. and Bell, G. I. (1990). Human insulin-receptor gene. *Diabetes*, **39**, 129–33

23. Julier, C., Weil, D., Couillin, P., Cote, J. C., Nguyen, V. C., Foubert, C., Boue, A., Thirion, J. P., Kaplan, J. C. and Junien, C. (1984). The beta chorionic gonadotropin-beta luteinizing gene cluster maps to human chromosome 19. *Hum. Genet.*, **67**, 174–7

24. Goldzieher, J. W. and Axelrod, L. R. (1963). Clinical and biochemical features of polycystic ovarian disease. *Fertil. Steril.*, **14**, 631–53

25. Kazer, R., Kessel, B. and Yen, S. (1987). Circulating luteinizing hormone pulse frequency in women with polycystic ovary syndrome. *J. Clin. Endocrinol. Metab.*, **65**, 233–6

26. Koskinen, P., Penttila, T. A., Anttila, L., Erkkola, R. and Irjala, K. (1996). Optimal use of hormone determinations in the biochemical diagnosis of the polycystic ovary syndrome. *Fertil. Steril.*, **65**, 517–22

27. Eden, J. A. (1988). Which is the best way to detect the polycystic ovary? *Aust. N. Z. J. Obstet. Gynaecol.*, **28**, 221–4

28. Saxton, D. W., Farquhar, C. M., Rae, T., Beard, R. W., Anderson, M. C. and Wadsworth, J. (1990). Accuracy of ultrasound measurements of female pelvic organs. *Br. J. Obstet. Gynaecol.*, **97**, 695–9

29. Cheung, A. P. and Chang, R. J. (1990). Polycystic ovary syndrome. *Clin. Obstet. Gynecol.*, **33**, 655–67

30. Kratochwil, A., Urban, G. U. and Friedrich, F. (1972). Ultrasonic tomography of the ovaries. *Ann. Chir. Gynecol.*, **61**, 211–14

31. Adams, J., Franks, S., Polson, D. W., Mason, H. D., Abdulwahid, N., Tucker, M., Morris, D. V., Price, J. and Jacobs, H. S. (1985). Multifollicular ovaries: clinical and endocrine features and response to pulsatile gonadotropin-releasing hormone. *Lancet*, **2**, 1375–8

32. Matsunaga, I., Hata, T. and Kitao, M. (1985). Ultrasonographic identification of polycystic ovary. *Asia-Oceania J. Obstet. Gynecol.*, **11**, 227–32

33. Parisi, L., Tramonti, M., Derchi, L. E., Castiano, S., Zurli, A. and Rocchi, P. (1984). Polycystic ovarian disease: ultrasonic evaluation and correlations with clinical and hormonal data. *J. Clin. Ultrasound.*, **12**, 21–6

34. Yee, B., Barnes, R. B., Vargyas, J. M. and Marrs, R. P. (1987). Correlation of transabdominal and transvaginal ultrasound measurements of follicle size and number with laparoscopic findings for *in vitro* fertilization. *Fertil. Steril.*, **47**, 828–32

35. Fauser, B. C. J. M. (1991). Classification of chronic hyperandrogenic anovulation. In Coeling-Bennink, H. J. T., Vemer, H. M. and van Keep, P. A. (eds.) *Chronic Hyperandrogenic*

Anovulation, pp. 11–15. (New York: Parthenon Publishing)

36. Hull, M. G. R. (1989). Polycystic ovarian disease: clinical aspects and prevalence. *Res. Clin. Forums*, **11**, 21–34

37. Timor-Tritsch, I. E., Bar-Yam, Y., Elgali, S. and Rottem, S. (1988). The technique of transvaginal sonography with the use of a 6.5-MHz probe. *Am. J. Obstet. Gynecol.*, **158**, 1019–24

38. Pache, T. D., Wladimiroff, J. W., Hop, W. C. J. and Fauser, B. C. J. (1992). How to discriminate between normal and polycystic ovaries: transvaginal ultrasound study. *Radiology*, **183**, 421–3

39. Goldstein, S. R. (1990). Incorporating endovaginal ultrasonography into the overall gynecologic examination. *Am. J. Obstet. Gynecol.*, **162**, 625–32

40. Mendelson, E. B., Bohm-Velez, M., Neiman, H. L. and Russo, J. (1988). Transvaginal sonography in gynecologic imaging. *Semin. Ultrasound. Comput. Tomogr. Magn. Reson.*, **9**, 102–21

41. Feichtinger, W. and Kemeter, P. (1986). Transvaginal sector scan sonography for needle-guided transvaginal follicle aspiration and other applications in gynecologic routine and research. *Fertil. Steril.*, **45**, 722–5

42. Battaglia, C., Artini, P. G., D'Ambrogio, G., Galli, P. A. and Genazzani, A. R. (1994). Uterine and ovarian blood flow measurement. Does the full bladder modify the flow resistance? *Acta Obstet. Gynecol. Scand.*, **73**, 716–18

43. Takahashi, K., Ozaki, T., Okada, M., Uchida, A. and Kitao, M. (1994). Relationship between ultrasonography and histopathological changes in polycystic ovarian syndrome. *Hum. Reprod.*, **9**, 2255–8

44. Takahashi, K., Eda, Y., Okada, S., Abu-Musa, A., Yoshino, K. and Kitao, M. (1993). Morphological assessment of polycystic ovary using transvaginal ultrasound. *Hum. Reprod.*, **8**, 844–9

45. Yeh, H. C., Futterweit, W. and Thornton, J. C. (1987). Polycystic ovarian disease: ultrasound features in 104 patients. *Radiology*, **163**, 111–16

46. Fox, R., Corrigan, E., Thomas, P. A. and Hull, M. G. R. (1991). The diagnosis of polycystic ovaries in women with oligo-amenorrhea: predictive power of endocrine tests. *Clin. Endocrinol.*, **34**, 127–31

47. Ardaens, Y., Robet, Y., Lemaitre L., Fossati, P. and Dewailly, D. (1991). Polycystic ovarian disease: contribution of vaginal endosonography and reassessment of ultrasonic diagnosis. *Fertil. Steril.*, **55**, 1062–8

48. Robert, Y., Dubrulle, F., Gaillandre, L., Ardaens Y., Thomas-Desrousseaux, P., Lemaitre, L. and Dewailly, D. (1995). Ultrasound assessment of ovarian stroma hypertrophy in hyperandrogenism and ovulation disorders: visual analysis versus computerized quantification. *Fertil. Steril.*, **64**, 307–12

49. Goswamy, R. K. and Steptoe, P. (1988). Doppler ultrasound studies of the uterine artery in spontaneous ovarian cycles. *Hum. Reprod.*, **3**, 721–6

50. Collins, W., Jurkovic, D., Bourne, T., Kurjak, A. and Campbell, S. (1991). Ovarian morphology, endocrine function and intra-follicular blood flow during the periovulatory period. *Hum. Reprod.*, **3**, 319–24

51. Bourne, T. H., Campbell, S., Steer, C. V., Whitehead, M. I. and Collins, W. P. (1989). Transvaginal colour flow imaging: a possible new screening technique for ovarian cancer. *Br. Med. J.*, **299**, 1367–70

52. Kurjak, A., Zalud, I., Jurkovic, D., Alfirovic, Z. and Miljan, M. (1989). Transvaginal color flow Doppler for the assessment of pelvic circulation. *Acta Obstet. Gynecol.*, **68**, 131–5

53. Kurjak, A., Jurkovic, D., Alfirovic, Z. and Zalud, I. (1990). Transvaginal color Doppler. *J. Clin. Ultrasound*, **18**, 227–34

54. Kurjak, A., Kupesic-Urek, S., Schulman, H. and Zalad, I. (1991). Transvaginal color flow Doppler in the assessment of ovarian and uterine blood flow in infertile women. *Fertil. Steril.*, **56**, 870–3

55. Kurjak, A., Jurkovic, D., Alfirevic, Z. and Zalud, I. (1990). Transvaginal color Doppler flow imaging. *J. Clin. Ultrasound*, **18**, 227–31

56. Kurjak, A., Zalud, I. and Crvenkovic, G. (1990). The assessment of pelvic circulation by transvaginal colour Doppler. *Jpn. J. Med. Ultrasound*, **17**, 116–20

57. Fleischer, A. C. (1991). Assessment of utero-ovarian blood flow with transvaginal color Doppler sonography. *Fertil. Steril.*, **53**, 684–9

58. Steer, C. V., Campbell, S., Pampiglione, J., Kingsland, C. R., Mason, B. A. and Collins, W. P. (1990). Transvaginal color flow imaging of the uterine arteries during the ovarian and menstrual cycles. *Hum. Reprod.*, **5**, 391–5

59. Battaglia, C., Larocca, E., Lanzani, A., Valentini, M. and Genazzani, A. R. (1990). Doppler ultrasound studies of the uterine arteries in spontaneous and IVF stimulated ovarian cycles. *Gynecol. Endocrinol.*, **4**, 245–50

60. Goswamy, R. K., Williams, G. and Steptoe, P. C. (1988). Decreased uterine perfusion – a cause of infertility. *Hum. Reprod.*, **3**, 955–9

61. Mercè L. T., Garcès, D., Barco, M. J. and De la Fuente, F. (1992). Intraovarian Doppler velocimetry in ovulatory, dysovulatory and anovulatory cycles. *Ultrasound Obstet. Gynecol.*, **2**, 197–202

62. Sladkevicius, P., Valentin, L. and Marsàl, K. (1993). Blood flow velocity in the uterine and ovarian arteries during the normal menstrual cycle. *Ultrasound Obstet. Gynecol.*, **3**, 199–208

63. Battaglia, C., Artini, P. G., D'Ambrogio, G., Genazzani, A. D. and Genazzani, A. R. (1995). The role of color Doppler imaging in the diagnosis of polycystic ovary syndrome. *Am. J. Obstet. Gynecol.*, **172**, 108–13

64. Findlay, J. K. (1986). Angiogenesis in reproductive tissues. *J. Endocrinol.*, **111**, 357–66

65. Kawakami, M., Kubo, K., Uemura, T., Nagase, M. and Hayashi, R. (1981). Involvement in ovarian innervation in steroid secretion. *Endocrinology*, **109**, 136–45

66. Brannstrom, M. and Norman, R. J. (1993). Involvement of leukocytes and cytokines in the ovulatory process and corpus luteum function. *Hum. Reprod.*, **8**, 1762–75

67. Horwitz, K. B. and Horwitz, L. D. (1982). Canine vascular tissues are targets for androgens, estrogens, progestins and glucocorticoids. *J. Clin. Invest.*, **69**, 740–8

68. Fisher, G. M. and Swain, M. L. (1977). Effect of sex hormones on blood pressure and vascular connective tissue in castrated and non-castrated rats. *Am. J. Physiol.*, **232**, 617–21

69. Zaidi, J., Campbell, S., Pittrof, R., Kyei-Mensah, A., Shaker, A., Jacobs, H. S. and Lin Tan, S. (1995). Ovarian stromal blood flow in women with polycystic ovaries – a possible new marker for diagnosis? *Hum. Reprod.*, **10**, 1992–5

70. Aleem, F. A. and Predanic, M. (1996). Transvaginal color Doppler determination of the ovarian and uterine blood flow characteristics in polycystic ovary disease. *Fertil. Steril.*, **65**, 510–16

71. Battaglia, C., Genazzani, A. D., Salvatori, M., Giulini, S., Artini, P. G., Genazzani, A. R. and Volpe, A. (1999). Doppler, ultrasonographic and endocrinological environment with regard to the number of small subcapsular follicles in polycystic ovary syndrome. *Gynecol. Endocrinol.*, **13**, 123–9

72. Battaglia, C., Artini, P. G., Salvatori, M., Giulini, S., Petraglia, F., Maxia, N. and Volpe, A. (1998). Ultrasonographic patterns of polycystic ovaries. Color Doppler and hormonal correlations. *Ultrasound Obstet. Gynecol.*, **11**, 332–6

73. Battaglia, C., Artini, P. G., Genazzani, A. D., Florio, P., Salvatori, M., Sgherzi, M. R., Giulini, S., Lombardo, M. and Volpe, A. (1997). Color Doppler analysis in oligo- and amenorrheic women with polycystic ovary syndrome. *Gynecol. Endocrinol.*, **11**, 105–10

74. Battaglia, C., Genazzani, A. D., Artini, P. G., Salvatori, M., Giulini, S. and Volpe, A. (1998). Ultrasonography and color Doppler analysis in the treatment of polycystic ovary syndrome. *Ultrasound Obstet. Gynecol.*, **12**, 180–7

75. Battaglia, C., Artini, P. G., Genazzani, A. D., Sgherzi, M. R., Salvatori, M., Giulini, S., and Volpe, A. (1996). Color Doppler analysis in lean and obese women with polycystic ovary syndrome. *Ultrasound Obstet. Gynecol.*, **7**, 342–6

76. Wild, R. A., Van Nort, J. J., Grubb, B., Bachman, W., Hartz, A. and Bartholomew, M. (1990). Clinical signs of androgen excess as risk factors for coronary artery disease. *Fertil. Steril.*, **54**, 255–9

Normal and abnormal corpus luteum function

5

S. Kupesic, L. T. Merce, T. Zodan and A. Kurjak

INTRODUCTION

The clinical importance of the corpus luteum for a successful establishment of pregnancy is strongly supported by many lines of investigation[1]. A luteal phase defect has been defined as a deficit of more than 2 days in histological development of the endometrium with reference to the day of the cycle. Although a luteal phase defect is often a direct result of hormone production by the corpus luteum, the underlying causes of this dysfunction can be multiple. Decreased levels of follicle-stimulating hormone (FSH) in the follicular phase of the cycle, abnormal patterns of luteinizing hormone (LH) secretion, decreased levels of LH and FSH at the time of the ovulatory surge, or a decreased response of the endometrium to progesterone have all been implicated.

MORPHOLOGICAL AND BIOCHEMICAL CHARACTERISTICS OF THE CORPUS LUTEUM

The formation of a corpus luteum is an important event in the reproductive cycle and one of the crucial factors in early pregnancy support. After ovulation, blood vessels of the theca layer invade the cavity of the ruptured follicle, starting the formation of the corpus luteum (Figure 1). Once formed, the corpus luteum consists of several cell types: K-cells, large luteal cells and small luteal cells. Large luteal cells originate from granulosa cells, whereas small luteal cells originate from theca cells. Large luteal cells produce more progesterone than small luteal cells, but the latter seem to be more responsive to stimulation by LH or human chorionic gonadotropin (hCG). In

addition, small luteal cells are thought to produce the so-called 'corpus luteum angiogenic factor' responsible for the neovascularization of the luteal tissue. Possibly, this function of small luteal cells is totally independent from their steroidogenic function. It has been shown that human luteal cells in culture produce prostaglandin I2, prostaglandin E2 and prostaglandin F2α. Prostaglandins, the production of which is under the control of lypoxygenase products of arachidonic acid such as 5-hydroxyeicosatetraenoic acid (5-HETE), and not under the control of hCG, have a direct impact on progesterone production. Prostaglandins I2 and E2 promote progesterone formation, in contrast to prostaglandin F2α which has a distinct luteolytic effect. Although basically regulated by the hypothalamus (gonadotropin-releasing hormone) and the hypophysis (FSH, LH), the corpus luteum definitely has its own fine-tuning paracrine regulation, which has yet to be elucidated. The luteal phase of the cycle begins with ovulation and formation of the corpus luteum, and ends with the beginning of menstruation. The first event is a significant FSH and LH surge. After that the formation of the corpus luteum takes place. Small luteal cells produce more and more LH receptors and thus amplify the production of progesterone. This chain reaction continues until the so-called mid-luteal phase, which is characterized by peak values of blood LH and progesterone, and the lowest resistance index (RI) in the corpus luteum blood vessels, as proven by transvaginal color and pulsed Doppler ultrasonography by Kupesic and colleagues[1] (Figure 2). Consequently, progesterone suppresses the secretion of gonadotropins, LH and progesterone levels

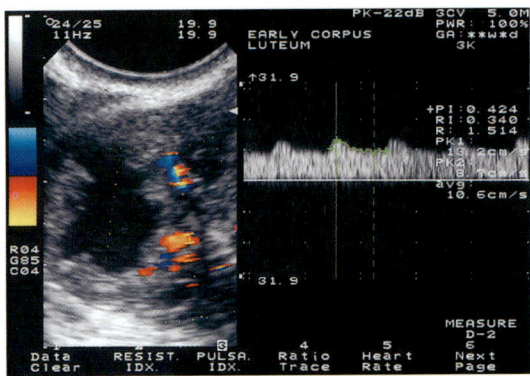

Figure 1 A transvaginal sonogram of the ruptured follicle. An increased blood flow velocity and a decreased resistance index (0.34) represent typical signs of ovulation and
early corpus luteum formation

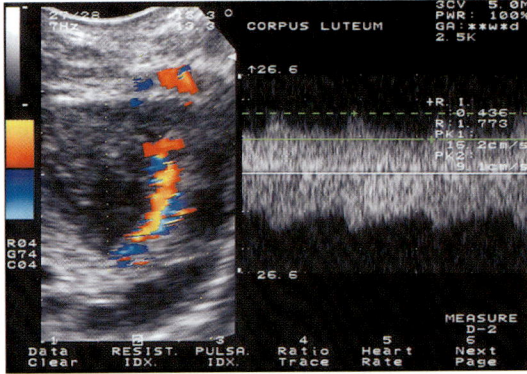

Figure 2 Demonstration of increased vascularity in the
mature corpus luteum. Pulsed Doppler waveform analysis
shows a high velocity and a low resistance index (0.44)

decrease, and the RI in the vessels of the corpus luteum increases. Whether because of
'intrinsic error of mechanism', or because of
the interference of external factors (e.g. strenuous exercise, ovulation-stimulating drugs),
a condition called luteal phase deficiency
(LPD) occurs.

LUTEAL PHASE DEFICIENCY:
CONVENTIONAL METHODS
OF DIAGNOSIS AND TREATMENT

Various names have been assigned to this disorder: short luteal phase, luteal insufficiency,
inadequate luteal phase, luteal defect and
luteal phase deficiency (LPD). All these names
describe the same condition: lack of progesterone, a luteal phase of the cycle shorter
than 11 days, and, when, related to the endometrium, an endometrium out of phase by
> 2 days.

Zeleznik and Little-Ihrig[2] used rhesus
monkeys with sectioned pituitary stalks to
establish the role of LH in supporting corpus
luteum function. Pulsatile administration of
gonadotropin-releasing hormone (GnRH) was
able to re-establish gonadotropin secretion. By
adjusting the height of the GnRH pulses,
plasma LH concentrations could be changed
according to the experimental design. It was
shown that plasma LH levels (determined by
bioassay), reduced to 50% of the standard
values, still sustained progesterone production
during the early luteal phase. These results are
consistent with the hypothesis that luteal
regression during the nonfertile cycles of primates is due primarily to an alteration in
luteal cell responsiveness to LH rather than to
the magnitude of the gonadotropin secretion.

Jones[3] states that an imbalance between
FSH and LH levels is to blame for poor folliculogenesis and inadequate transformation of
the granulosa and theca cells into granulosa-
lutein and theca-lutein cells of the corpus
luteum. Therefore, corpus luteum insufficiency could arise. Corpus luteum deficiency
with normal luteal phase length is concluded
to be a result of either inadequate granulosa
cell function or of an inadequate LH surge,
but a fairly normal LH pulse and theca cell
response; a short luteal phase is related to a
poor LH surge and absent or poor LH pulsatility. It seems that a critical level of LH secretion preceding ovulation is essential for the
morphological and functional transformation
of the granulosa and theca cells with induction
of enzymes for steroidogenesis, regulatory
peptides, and various peptide receptors.

Beitinis and colleagues[4] examined 28
volunteer university students with a history of
normal, regular menstrual cycles who entered
a program of strenuous physical exercise for
2 months. All participants collected serial

overnight urine samples over a period of 3 months: one control cycle and two subsequent training cycles. The urine samples were examined for FSH, LH, estriol and free progesterone. All hormonal values were calculated in relation to creatinine excretion. In 18 of the participants, 20 cycles with luteal phase disturbances were observed. Four women developed inadequate luteal phase (i.e. decreased free progesterone values as well as a luteal phase duration of less than 9 days) in the first exercise month. Two inadequate and four short luteal phases were observed during the second month of exercise. Since abnormalities were also observed in subjects with short luteal phase and LH and estriol secretion, it could be presumed that strenuous exercise, combined in 12 cases with a significant weight loss, actually leads to anovulation. Of special interest is the finding that in only two women did the luteal phase (or ovulation) disturbances appear in two consecutive cycles. This indicates that in normal women strenuous exercise, change of living conditions, stress, or other extraneous impacts may result in menstrual disturbances affecting either the entire cycle course or the luteal phase only. However, in the majority of cases these effects are transient. Clinical practice proves that many women observed over a period of several months have sporadic, apparently abnormal cycles, but only in very few women is the disturbance persistent.

There is still disagreement over whether ovarian stimulation causes LPD. Hecht and colleagues[5] concluded that LPD is infrequent in clomiphene-stimulated cycles, whereas Reshef and associates[6] found that in 30 women treated with human menopausal gonadotropin (hMG) and hCG, the incidence of endometrial inadequacy was 27%.

One of the biggest problems for scientists in this field of research, and also for clinicians, is how to evaluate LPD. One of the possible methods is histologic dating of endometrial biopsies. This method is thought to be accurate because it should reflect the amount of progesterone secreted by the corpus luteum and morphological transformation of the endometrium by progesterone in preparation for implantation and early pregnancy. Timing of the endometrial biopsy depends on the onset of the next menstrual bleeding, assuming a cycle length of 28 days and a luteal phase length of 14 days. However, the length of the luteal phase can vary between 12 and 14 days. The preferred time for endometrial biopsy is also disputed. Early and mid-luteal phase biopsies may give wider variation in histologic dating than late luteal phase biopsies. Endometrial biopsy closer to the next menses will better reflect cumulative progesterone action. According to some studies, biopsies taken on days 25 through to 28 of the cycle give an out-of-phase endometrium in 38.6%, increasing to 53.6% if the biopsies are taken before day 25. This does not mean that a biopsy taken in the peri-implantation period, yielding a higher prevalence of LPD, is a better one. There might be a catch-up in the biological effect of progesterone which is not accounted for. A further disadvantage is an interobserver and intraobserver variance.

Gibson and colleagues[7] recently ran an interesting study. Twenty-five women had endometrial biopsies within the framework of routine infertility investigation. Each subject underwent two endometrial biopsies on the same occasion, yielding 50 slides of paired biopsies from 25 women. Five evaluators observed each slide on two occasions at least 2 weeks apart. The results were puzzling. readings of the same slide by the same evaluator were in exact agreement only in 43.1% of instances and a discordance of $\geqslant 3$ days was found in 5% of cases. The inter-evaluator differences were much larger. Evaluators assigned the same date to 25% of examinations only, and readings discordant by more than 2 days were encountered in 22% of observations. The exact site in the endometrium where a biopsy should be performed has not yet been established.

Measurement of single or selected multiple serum progesterone levels is also used in the assessment of LPD. A minimum progesterone level of 2.5–5.0 ng/ml during the mid-luteal phase has been reported as indicative of ovulation, although a minimum mid-luteal phase level of 10–15 ng/ml has been considered to reflect normal corpus luteum function[8]. Due to diurnal variation and pulsatile secretion with an amplitude of 30% over mean values, a single mid-luteal phase progesterone measurement is not reflective of the functional capacity of the corpus luteum nor of the true amount of progesterone that the endometrium may be subjected to.

Recently, a placental protein 14 has been discovered in the endometrium. It is secreted by endometrial glands and it is rarely detected in blood during the anovulatory cycle[9]. Its reliability when used as a test has not yet been established. Dawood[10] suggests that only by combining all the methods and regarding the results with healthy scepticism can relevant conclusions be drawn.

Current treatment for corpus luteum insufficiency includes optimal recruitment of follicles with clomiphene and hCG or hMG. Response to hCG is dependent on the luteal age of the corpus luteum. Optimum and significant increases in progesterone secretion were obtained when 5000 IU hCG was given 8 and 12 days after the LH surge, but only a modest increase occurred when hCG was given 4 days after the LH surge, and no increase was observed if hCG was given on the day of the LH surge[11]. Based on recent findings, augmentation of corpus luteum function with hCG should be started at the mid-luteal phase, about 7–8 days after the LH surge, or 6–7 days after the basal body temperature shift (i.e. day 21 of the menstrual cycle when the cycle is 28 days)[10]. Statistically, an insignificant benefit of treatment with progesterone suppositories or oral dehydrogesterone compared with no treatment was found in a randomized, controlled trial, and no significant benefit was found in three comparative studies[5,6,10].

Insler[12] explains that LPD represents only one of a whole series of disturbances including unbalanced extra- and intraovarian hormonal and peptide interaction, ill-timed follicular development, and flawed ovum maturation. Among women subjected to various studies, only a small number of those treated with 'pure' FSH during the early follicular phase corrected the endometrial defect observed in previous cycles.

The luteinized unruptured follicle (LUF) syndrome should be mentioned. This is a dysfunctional response of the ovary characterized by a cyclical hormone pattern that is similar to that found in normal ovulatory cycles or LPD. In LUF syndrome the preovulatory follicle does not rupture, although it luteinizes. Follicular luteinization can produce normal or impaired progesterone secretion, and thus the postovulatory parameters do not always show important abnormalities. Furthermore, a 'false' ovulatory cycle can occur, making it difficult to make a diagnosis of this syndrome. Several possible causes of this syndrome have been proposed: an abnormality of the LH peak, the absence of a preovulatory discharge of progesterone, primary abnormality of the oocyte, alterations in prostaglandin synthesis, or alterations in the synthesis of other mediators that lead to the rupture of the follicle. This condition was first diagnosed laparoscopically, and later on low concentrations of ovarian steroids in peritoneal fluid were said to be of diagnostic value. Some new data on this rare condition will hopefully be obtained by ultrasonography measurements.

THE ROLE OF ULTRASOUND AND DOPPLER STUDIES IN DETECTION OF LUTEAL PHASE DEFICIENCY

It is clear that none of the techniques used so far to assess LPD have been absolutely reliable, and that a new method must be introduced in order to keep the research going. The new method is ultrasonography. For a better visualization of the corpus luteum, the transvaginal approach is used. As an addition to B-mode and real-time imaging, sophisticated ultrasound equipment includes color and pulsed Doppler sonography (Figure 3). Research into the corpus luteum, LPD, early pregnancy and early pregnancy failures has already taken a new direction.

Until recently, research in this field was carried out mainly using B-mode and real-time

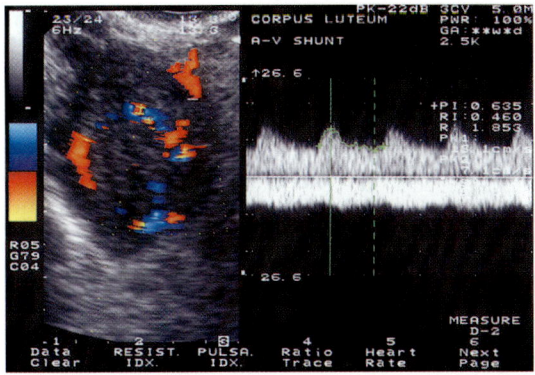

Figure 3 A transvaginal scan of the ovary containing a corpus luteum. Using B-mode sonography it was impossible to gain any information about the functional state of the ovary. However, increased vascularity of the corpus luteum was easily depicted by conventional color Doppler, as shown here. A low resistance index (0.46) and demonstration of the arterio-venous shunts were the typical features of the corpus luteum

imaging. Glock and colleagues[13] tried to determine whether the size, or change in size, of the corpus luteum of early pregnancy correlated with serum progesterone, estradiol or 17-hydroxyprogesterone, or were even predictive of pregnancy outcome. Their hypotheses were that corpus luteum volumes of early human pregnancy would correlate with the serum concentrations of steroids produced in the corpus luteum, that the appearance of the corpus luteum, based on the amount of cystic component, would correlate with serum hormone concentrations or pregnancy outcome, and that a decrease in corpus luteum volume would be associated with pregnancy loss. Disappointingly, the acquired data showed a lack of correlation between corpus luteum size and steroid products, and no correlation between changes in volume and changes in steroid products in early human pregnancy. However, a decreasing corpus luteum volume before 8 weeks of gestation was associated with a higher probability of pregnancy loss. Color flow pulsed Doppler was only used to determine the dominant ovary with the corpus luteum. The dominant ovary showed a low-impedance waveform with a resistance index (RI) of 0.39–0.49, characteristic of blood flow

in early pregnancy. The contralateral ovary in each patient demonstrated a high-impedance flow with an RI of 0.69–1.00, characteristic of a non-dominant ovary. One patient had an RI value of 0.74 in the ovary identified as having the corpus luteum, and an RI of 0.79 in the opposite ovary; this high RI in both ovaries was associated with a nonviable outcome.

Kupesic and Kurjak[14] tried to evaluate the intraovarian resistance index in 47 healthy fertile volunteers with ovulatory cycles, and compare them to 28 patients with luteal phase deficiency and four patients with luteinized unruptured follicle syndrome. Serial sonography allowed daily measurement of the mean follicular diameter, visualization of the follicular collapse, demarcation of the hypoechoic structure representing the corpus luteum, observation of the thickened endometrium, and observation of the presence of free fluid in the cul-de-sac. All these findings were suggestive of ovulation (Figure 4). Doubtful cases (non-visualization of the corpus luteum and/or lack of serial measurements) were excluded from the study. LPD was diagnosed by measuring progesterone levels and performing endometrial biopsy during the mid-luteal phase of the menstrual cycle (Figure 4). Sonographic and Doppler findings were correlated to hormonal and histopathological data. LUF syndrome was documented by daily ultrasound observations and endocrinological measurements. There was evidence of normal follicular development and normal diameter of the preovulatory follicle in all four cases of LUF syndrome (Figure 4). During the period of expected ovulation the follicle remained the same size and maintained its tense appearance. Luteinization of the unruptured follicle was seen as a progressive accumulation of strong echoes located on its periphery. In the group with regular ovulatory cycles, different ovarian RI values were observed. During the stage of follicular growth and development, moderate to high RI values (mean 0.56 ± 0.06) were obtained at the rim of the follicle. A significant decline of the RI ($p < 0.001$) occurred on the day of the LH peak (RI 0.44 ± 0.04). The lowest RI values were obtained during the

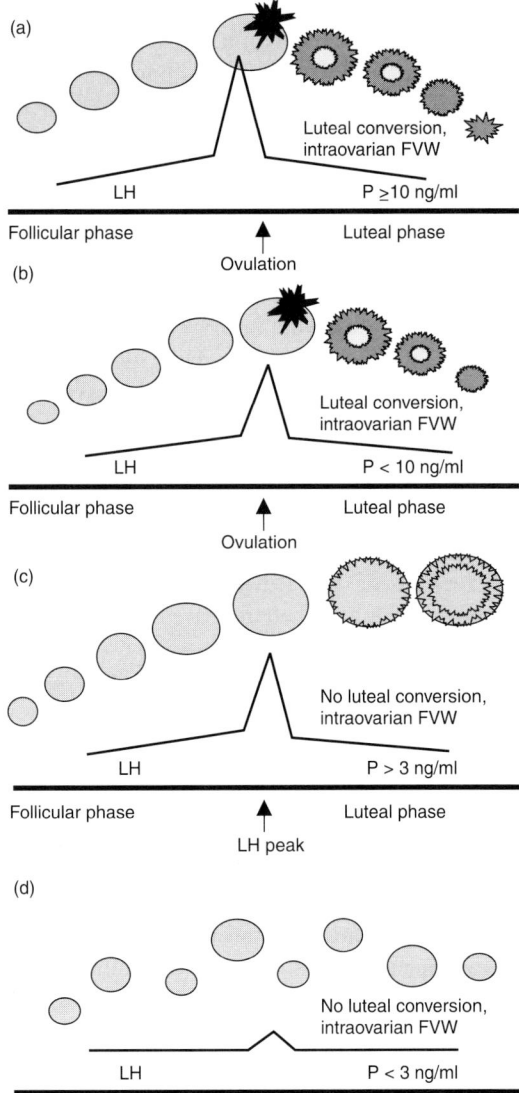

(a)

Luteal conversion, intraovarian FVW

LH   P ≥10 ng/ml

Follicular phase   Luteal phase

↑ Ovulation

(b)

Luteal conversion, intraovarian FVW

LH   P < 10 ng/ml

Follicular phase   Luteal phase

↑ Ovulation

(c)

No luteal conversion, intraovarian FVW

LH   P > 3 ng/ml

Follicular phase   Luteal phase

↑ LH peak

(d)

No luteal conversion, intraovarian FVW

LH   P < 3 ng/ml

Figure 4 Functional and dysfunctional patterns of the ovarian cycle based on sonographic, Doppler and hormonal studies. (a) Normal ovulatory cycle, (b) luteal phase deficiency, (c) luteinized unruptured follicle syndrome, and (d) anovulatory ovarian cycle. LH, luteinizing hormone; P, progesterone; FVW, flow velocity waveform

mid-luteal phase (RI 0.42 ± 0.06), with a return to higher vascular resistance (0.50 ± 0.04) during the late luteal phase. In 15 patients, endometrial biopsy was performed, and normal endometrial dating was detected. In the LPD group, no difference ($p > 0.05$) was obtained in terms of intraovarian RI

during the follicular phase. However, the mean RI throughout the luteal phase (0.56 ± 0.04) was significantly higher ($p < 0.001$) compared to that in the normal women. Furthermore, it did not show any difference between the early, middle and late luteal phase in the LPD group ($p < 0.05$). In the control group, both the follicular and the luteal RI was significantly lower ($p < 0.001$) on the dominant side. However, in the LPD group no difference ($p > 0.05$) occurred in terms of intraovarian RI between the sides. Mean progesterone levels were significantly lower ($p < 0.001$) in the LPD group (6.9 ± 2.3 ng/ml) than in the controls (24.1 ± 11.4 ng/ml), while histopathology revealed a delayed endometrial pattern in all the patients with LPD. A correlation was observed between progesterone levels and RI during the mid-luteal phase ($r = -0.09$, $p < 0.83$). In the patients with LUF syndrome, no difference in terms of intraovarian RI was obtained after the LH peak. Similar RI values were obtained during the follicular and luteal phases (0.55 ± 0.04 vs. 0.54 ± 0.06). There was no difference between the sides in terms of intraovarian vascular resistance. The mean progesterone level in this group was 14.1 ± 6.2 ng/ml.

Merce and colleagues[15] elaborate on all aspects of transvaginal color and pulsed Doppler ultrasonography: its advantages, disadvantages, current possibilities and future directions. In their study of luteal ovarian blood flow they introduce the term 'luteal conversion' to describe Doppler findings during the luteal phase: easily obtained Doppler signals, an increase in the intensity of the frequency spectrum, an increase in turbulence of the blood flow with extensive dispersion of the maximum frequencies and superposition of multiple waveforms presenting variable maximum systolic velocities, and, finally, an increase in the surface area and intensity of the color signal in the ovary. The same authors, in their study of LPD, observed that the resistance index of the dominant ovary drops during the luteal phase with respect to the follicular phase, as also occurs in normal cycles, and no differences were noted in this respect when comparing with any phase of the normal cycle[15]. No significant correlation was demonstrated between the resistance index values and serum progesterone levels.

Merce and colleagues[15] also deal with LUF syndrome. They did not observe any drop in perifollicular intraovarian resistance after the LH peak. During the 4-day period following the LH surge, and while the follicle increased in size and its luteinization was set up, the RI rose to values in the upper limit of the normal curve. Later on, and in spite of the fact that the resistance dropped, the RI values were close to those of the follicular phase. The development of the RI in the LUF syndrome was therefore similar to that of anovulatory cycles, showing a loss in the cyclical rhythm and post-peak LH values similar to those of the follicular growth phase. The other interesting observation is that 'luteal conversion' did not take place, indicating that the changes described in the intraovarian and perifollicular microvascularization were either not produced or were altered in LUF syndrome, probably because the follicle failed to rupture. Merce and colleagues also point out the importance of endometrial and ovarian blood flow regarding implantation. They strongly advocate the use of Doppler techniques in future studies of peri-implantatory flow phenomena and their relations to pregnancy outcome[15].

Glock and Brumsted[16] correlated ovarian blood flow with values of progesterone throughout the cycle. Mean progesterone levels were significantly lower for LPD patients than for normal women throughout the luteal phase ($p < 0.001$). The mean resistance index in LPD patients was significantly higher compared with normal women throughout the follicular and luteal phases ($p = 0.02$). Although systolic and diastolic velocities were observed to be lower in LPD patients compared with normal women, these differences were not statistically different ($p = 0.54$ and $p = 0.11$, respectively). A high correlation was observed between the progesterone level and the resistance index within each of the luteal time-points, achieving the highest value during the mid-luteal phase (early luteal, $r = -0.73$,

$p = 0.03$; mid-luteal, $r = -0.80$, $p < 0.01$; late luteal, $r = -0.63$, $p = 0.07$). The mean resistance index in the dominant ovary was significantly lower than in the non-dominant ovary throughout the cycle in normal women (0.50 vs. 0.65, $p = 0.001$), but not in those with LPD (0.60 vs. 0.66, $p = 0.37$). In the single anovulatory subject, resistance index values remained high (mean 0.76, range 0.70–0.82) in both ovaries. The whole study showed a correlation between the resistance index of corpus luteum blood flow and plasma progesterone in the natural cycle. The strongest correlation was seen in the mid-luteal phase, the period that corresponds to peak neovascularization of the corpus luteum. Consistent with this finding, the authors showed an increase in blood flow impedance in the late luteal phase, the period associated with the onset of corpus luteum regression. These findings suggest the possibility of using the resistance index of corpus luteum blood flow as an adjunct to plasma progesterone assay, as an index of luteal function.

Tinkanen[17], on the other hand, found no difference between the blood flow in the corpus luteum in controls with a normal luteal phase and infertility patients with an abnormal luteal phase. A short luteal phase, claims the author, is not due to premature vascular regression of the corpus luteum as evaluated by measurement of the vascular resistance. Strigini and colleagues[18] observed the change of impedance during the luteal phase of FSH-treated cycles. The uterine pulsatility index during stimulated cycles, both before and after ovulation, was significantly reduced compared with spontaneous cycles. This was explained by the increase of plasma estradiol. Furthermore, the authors advocate administration of exogenous progesterone as a supplementation to FSH-treated cycles, stating that the uterine pulsatility index after administration of progesterone drops even more than in spontaneous or FSH-treated cycles.

Kupesic and colleagues[1] correlated Doppler velocimetry, histological and hormonal markers. They presumed that when combined together, ultrasound results, measurement of hormone values and endometrial biopsy could

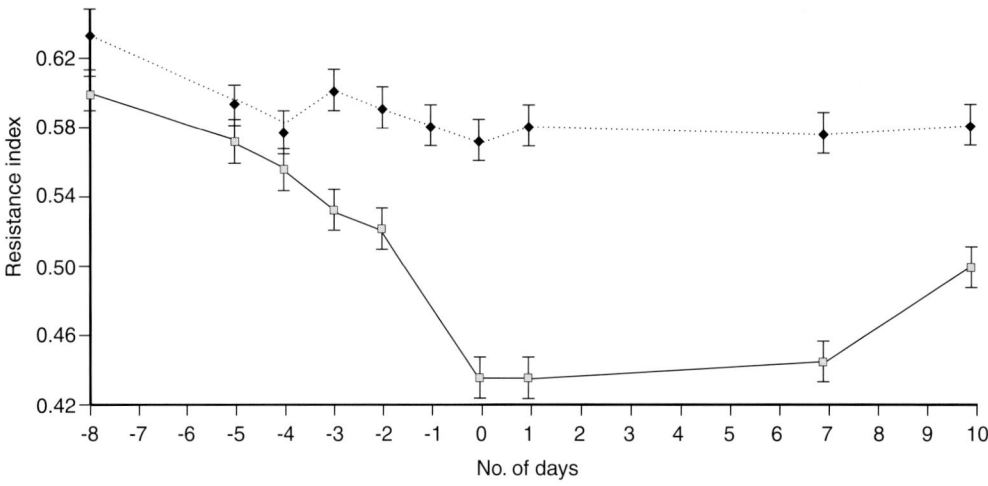

Figure 5 Intraovarian blood flow changes in patients with luteal phase deficiency (♦) and controls (□)

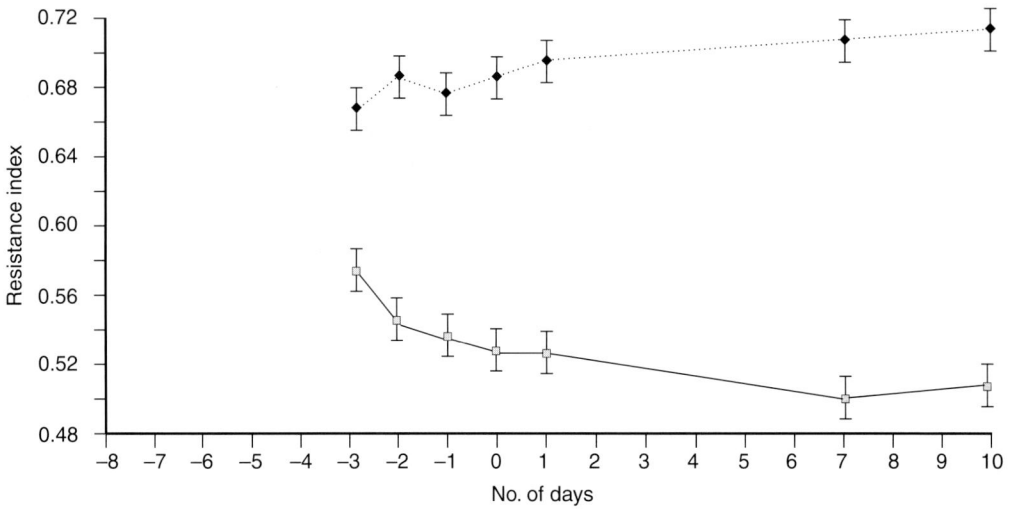

Figure 6 Spiral artery blood flow changes in patients with luteal phase deficiency (♦) and controls (□)

explain more about LPD. They found out that mean progesterone levels were significantly lower in a group with luteal phase deficiency (10.2 ± 4.3 ng/ml) than in controls (21 ± 4.2 ng/ml) ($p < 0.01$). The FSH/LH ratio was significantly lower ($p < 0.001$) in the group with a delayed endometrial pattern compared to normal subjects during follicular and periovulatory phases (0.70 vs. 1.24 and 0.58 vs. 0.75, respectively). There was a close correlation between estradiol levels and the mean diameter of the dominant follicle from days −5 to −1 relative to the day of sonographically observed ovulation. An increase in follicular diameter and endometrial thickness was noted for both normal and LPD groups. Intraovarian blood flow resistance showed no difference ($p > 0.05$) between the groups during the proliferative phase. A significant decline of the RI ($p < 0.05$) occurred in the control group for the day of the LH peak (RI 0.45 ± 0.04), with a return to the follicular phase level of 0.49 ± 0.02 during the second phase of the menstrual cycle. The mean intraovarian RI for the luteal phase defect group (0.58 ± 0.04) was significantly higher ($p < 0.001$) than in the control group throughout the luteal phase (Figure 5). Patients in the control group had a significantly lower RI in the dominant than in the non-dominant ovary, whereas LPD patients had almost the same RI in both ovaries. The authors measured blood flow in spiral arteries as well. Spiral arteries in the control group demonstrated an RI of 0.53 ± 0.04 during the periovulatory phase, and RI values of 0.50 ± 0.02 and 0.51 ± 0.04 were obtained during the mid-luteal and late luteal phases, respectively (Figure 6). Higher impedance values during the periovulatory phase (RI 0.70 ± 0.06, $p < 0.001$), mid-luteal phase (RI 0.72 ± 0.06, $p < 0.001$) and late luteal phase (RI 0.72 ± 0.04, $p < 0.001$) were obtained from the spiral arteries in the LPD group. A close correlation has been found between plasma levels of estradiol and the mean diameter of the follicle. The study demonstrates that patients with normal endometrial development show a similar trend of regression for uterine, radial and spiral artery impedance from the follicular to the luteal phase. In contrast, patients with a delayed endometrial pattern are characterized by increased uterine vascular resistance during the luteal phase. Since the most significant difference in terms of RI is obtained for spiral arteries, it might be expected that endometrial blood flow changes could be used to predict the development of the endometrium and the likelihood of pregnancy.

CORPUS LUTEUM BLOOD FLOW IN EARLY PREGNANCY

Salim and colleagues[19] compared luteal blood flow in normal pregnancies with the flow in abnormal pregnancies. Their study proved the hypothesis that an absence of luteal flow can not coexist with normal pregnancy. Impedance to intraovarian blood flow was significantly higher in patients with abnormal early pregnancy (missed, incomplete and threatened abortion) than in women with normal pregnancy ($p < 0.01$). However, this was not confirmed in patients with blighted ovum and molar and ectopic pregnancies. The impedance to luteal blood flow was almost the same as in normal pregnancy. This difference among subgroups of abnormal early pregnancy may relate to a different natural history of the disease. Missed and incomplete abortions are manifested as failed early pregnancy with no prospects for further development. Threatened abortion is a potentially similar condition. Whether decreased corpus luteum blood flow is a potential cause or a consequence of the disease remains unclear. Anembryonic pregnancies, and molar or ectopic pregnancies are somewhat different. These pathologic conditions are usually progressive and not self-limited. This can explain why impedance to luteal blood flow in these women is similar to that in women with normally progressing pregnancies.

Alcazar and colleagues[20] agree only partially with the results of Salim and associates[19]. Alcazar and colleagues found that the mean RI in missed abortion is higher than in controls. This increased vascular resistance could be explained by the fact that missed abortion consists of a failure of early pregnancy to develop, in which the production of hCG is impaired, which in turn could have a negative effect on luteal function. On the other hand, they found no statistically significant difference in the RI of patients with threatened abortion.

CONCLUSION

The true possibilities of transvaginal color and pulsed Doppler sonography in research into corpus luteum and ovarian blood flow are yet to be realized. Scientific ideas, supported by new equipment, will lead to a better understanding of human reproductive physiology, and also to a better treatment of pathological conditions which are still uncurable.

References

1. Kupesic, S., Kurjak, A., Vujisic, S. and Petrovic, Z. (1997). Luteal phase defect: comparison between Doppler velocimetry, histological and hormonal markers. *Ultrasound Obstet. Gynecol.*, **9**, 1–8

2. Zeleznik, A. J. and Little-Ihrig, L. L. (1990). Effect of reduced luteinizing hormone concentrations on corpus luteum function during the menstrual cycle of rhesus monkeys. *Endocrinology*, **126**, 2237–44

3. Jones, G. S. (1991). Luteal phase defect: a review of pathophysiology. *Curr. Opin. Obstet. Gynecol.*, **3**, 641–8

4. Beitinis, I. Z., McArthur, J. W., Turnbull, B. A., Skrinar, G. S. and Bullen, B. A. (1991). Exercise induces two types of human luteal dysfunction: confirmation by urinary free progesterone. *J. Clin. Endocrinol. Metab.*, **72**, 1350–8

5. Hecht, B. R., Bardawil, W .A., Khan-Dawood, F. S. and Dawood, M. Y. (1990). Luteal insufficiency: correlation between endometrial dating and integrated progesterone output in clomiphene citrate-induced cycles. *Am. J. Obstet. Gynecol.*, **163**, 1986–91

6. Reshef, E., Segars, J. H., Hill, G. A., Pridham, D. D., Jussman, M. A. and Colston-Wentz, A. (1990). Endometrial inadequacy after treatment with human menopausal gonadotropin/human chorionic gonadotropin. *Fertil. Steril.*, **54**, 1012–16

7. Gibson, M., Badger, G. J., Byrn, F., Lee, K. R., Korson, R. and Trainer, T. D. (1991). Error in histologic dating of secretory endometrium: variance component analysis. *Fertil. Steril.*, **56**, 242–7

8. McNeely, M. J. and Soules, M. R. (1988). The diagnosis of luteal phase deficiency: a critical review. *Fertil. Steril.*, **50**, 1–15

9. Fay, T. N., Jacobs, I. J., Teisner, B., Westergaard, J. G. and Grudzinskas, J. G. (1990). A biochemical test for direct assessment of endometrial function: measurement of the major secretory endometrial protein PP14 in serum during menstruation in relation to ovulation and luteal function. *Hum. Reprod.*, **5**, 382–6

10. Dawood, M. Y. (1994). Corpus luteal insufficiency. *Curr. Opin. Obstet. Gynecol.*, **6**, 121–7

11. Yeko, T. R., Khan-Dawood, F. S. and Dawood, M. Y. (1989). Human corpus luteum: luteinizing hormone and chorionic gonadotropin receptors during the menstrual cycle. *J. Clin. Endocrinol. Metab.*, **68**, 529–34

12. Insler, V. (1992). Corpus luteum defects. *Curr. Opin. Obstet. Gynecol.*, **4**, 203–11

13. Glock, J. L., Blackman, J. A., Badger, G. J. and Brumsted, J. R. (1995). Prognostic significance of morphologic changes of the corpus luteum by transvaginal ultrasound in early pregnancy monitoring. *Obstet. Gynecol.*, **85**, 37–41

14. Kupesic, S. and Kurjak, A. (1997). The assessment of normal and abnormal luteal function by transvaginal color Doppler sonography. *Eur. J. Obstet. Gynecol. Reprod. Biol.*, **72**, 83–7

15. Merce, L. T., Garces, D. and De la Fuente, F. (1989). Conversion lutea de la onda de velocidad de fluio ovarica: nuevo parametro ecografico de ovulacion y function lutea. *Acta Obstet. Gynecol. Scand.*, **2**, 113–14

16. Glock, J. L. and Brumsted, J. R. (1995). Color flow pulsed Doppler ultrasound in diagnosing luteal phase defect. *Fertil. Steril.*, **64**, 500–4

17. Tinkanen, H. (1994). The role of vascularization of the corpus luteum in the short luteal phase studied by Doppler ultrasound. *Acta. Obstet. Gynecol. Scand.*, **73**, 321–3

18. Strigini, F. A. L., Scida, P. A. M., Parri, C., Visconti, A., Susini, S. and Genazzani, A. R. (1995). Modifications in uterine and intraovarian artery impedance in cycles of treatment with exogenous gonadotropins: effects of luteal phase support. *Fertil. Steril.*, **64**, 76–80

19. Salim, A., Zalud, I., Farmakides, G., Schulmal, H., Kurjak, A. and Latin, V. (1994). Corpus luteum blood flow in normal and abnormal early pregnancy: evaluation with transvaginal color and pulsed Doppler sonography. *J. Ultrasound Med.*, **13**, 971–5

20. Alcazar, J. L., Laparte, C. and Lopez-Garcia, G. (1996). Corpus luteum blood flow in abnormal early pregnancy. *J. Ultrasound Med.*, **15**, 645–9

Ovarian stromal blood flow and assisted reproduction

6

J. Zaidi

INTRODUCTION

Since the mid-1980s there have been major technological advances in ultrasound imaging which have enhanced the rapid development of assisted reproductive technologies. The use of high-frequency endovaginal probes in combination with real-time ultrasound has improved the image quality of the pelvic organs without the need for a full bladder. Transvaginal ultrasonography has thus become an integral part in the diagnosis and management of female infertility and, in particular, during assisted conception cycles. During the initial assessment of the infertile female a detailed transvaginal ultrasound scan can be performed (the baseline ultrasound scan), ovarian and uterine morphology assessed and the uterine cavity evaluated. With the recent availability of echo-enhancing agents such as Echovist®, tubal patency may also be accurately checked – a technique known as contrast hysterosalpingo-sonography. It is thus possible that during the initial work-up, ultrasound can direct the reproductive gynecologist towards further investigations and treatment of either mechanical infertility or functional infertility or both.

With the introduction of transvaginal color Doppler ultrasonography, the use of ultrasound in infertility has expanded, with the hope that the measurement of vascular changes in the pelvic circulation may improve diagnosis and treatment, and ultimately lead to increased pregnancy rates. Early studies concentrated on investigating blood flow changes in the uterine artery in *in vitro* fertilization programs[1-3], and suggested that lower uterine artery impedance may be associated with higher pregnancy rates. Certainly during the luteal phase of the menstrual cycle uterine artery resistance falls[4-6], and this would coincide with the timing of the implanting blastocyst. Recent uterine artery studies have, however, given conflicting results[7-9], and in the absence of any prospective randomized studies the widespread clinical use of this technique in assisted reproduction has yet to occur. More recently, Doppler studies have focused on intra-ovarian blood flow and, in particular, the vascularity of the ovarian stroma. It is hoped that the assessment of ovarian stromal blood flow may give us a better understanding of ovarian function and therefore the physiological and pathological processes governing fertility treatment.

ANATOMICAL CONSIDERATION OF THE OVARIAN VESSELS

The anatomy of the female pelvic vessels is relatively constant throughout life. However, the anatomical course and blood flow within vessels may alter with increasing parity and/or after pelvic surgery. The external and internal iliac arteries and veins are easily seen on standard gray-scale ultrasound examination, since they have a relatively large diameter and constant position. The external iliac artery and vein are seen on the lateral pelvic wall as they descend towards the inguinal ligament. The internal iliac artery is identified on an oblique ultrasound scan posterior and infero-laterally to the ovaries. The internal iliac artery and vein are thus useful anatomical landmarks facilitating the ultrasound recognition of the ovaries.

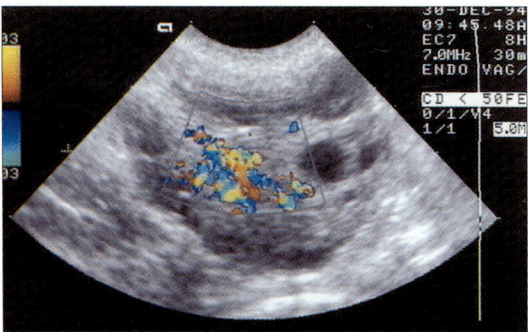

Figure 1   Vessels can be seen coursing through the central medullary part of the stroma towards the ovarian cortex

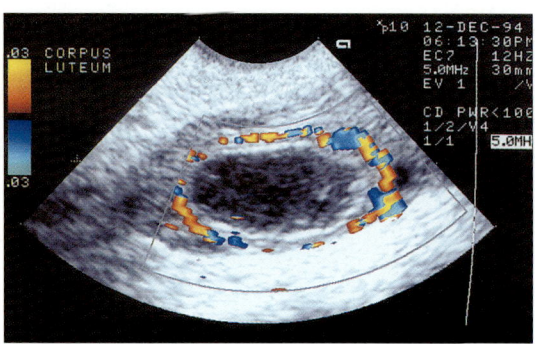

Figure 3   Color Doppler image of the blood supply to the corpus luteum

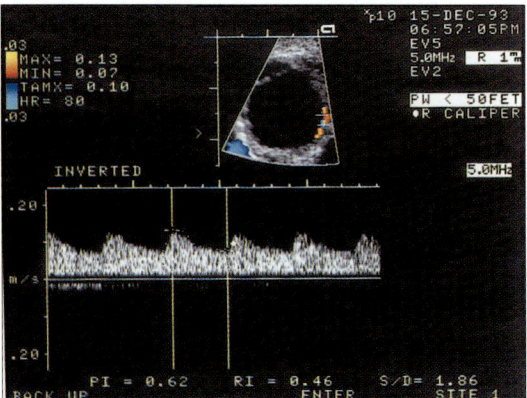

Figure 2   Vessels can be seen developing in the wall of the dominant ovarian follicle during the proliferative phase of the menstrual cycle, with their corresponding flow velocity waveforms

The ovarian artery originates from the abdominal aorta just below the renal artery. The vessel runs down the psoas muscle behind the peritoneum, crossing the brim of the pelvis to enter the infundibulopelvic fold at the lateral extremity of the broad ligament. It gives off a branch to the Fallopian tube which runs medially between the layers of the broad ligament and anastamoses with the tubal branch of the uterine artery. The ovarian artery then enters the ovary at its hilum. It can be noted that the ovary is surrounded by many vessels. The uterine artery lies inferiorly and medially to the ovary, the tubal and ovarian branches of the uterine artery lie above the ovary, while the ovarian and iliac arteries lie laterally to the ovary. Since there are so many vessels surrounding the ovary it is often difficult to accurately identify a particular vessel by color Doppler.

The ovarian artery enters the ovary at the hilum. It divides forming an anastamosing arcade of vessels in the hilar region. The vessels course through the central medullary part of the stroma towards the periphery or ovarian cortex (Figure 1). In the ovarian cortex the vessels form vascular arcades in the stroma surrounding the follicles. During the development of an ovarian follicle during the menstrual cycle a rich, irregular capillary plexus progressively develops in the connective tissue layer or theca surrounding the avascular granulosa cell layer of the ovarian follicle. These vessels can be seen by color Doppler ultrasound during the proliferative phase of the menstrual cycle (Figure 2). Several hours before ovulation, vessels penetrate the granulosa cell layer. Following ovulation there is proliferation of the vessels of the theca to further vascularize the granulosa cell layer as it and the theca merge to form the corpus luteum. Within 3 or 4 days after follicular rupture the corpus luteum is supplied with a dense, multilayered network of sinusoidal capillaries which are drained by numerous superficial venules. Using color Doppler the blood supply to the corpus luteum can be clearly seen as a bright colored ring surrounding the corpus luteum (Figure 3).

In view of the complexity of the ovarian blood supply and the difficulty in identifying the ovarian artery, we therefore preferred to concentrate our studies on the ovarian stromal vessels and follicular vessels. For the purpose of this chapter the blood supply within the ovarian stromal vessels will be described and their significance in assisted reproduction discussed.

ULTRASOUND EQUIPMENT

All ultrasound examinations described in this chapter were performed using an Acuson 128 XP/10 ultrasound system (Acuson Corp., Mountain View, CA, USA). This system was equipped with both EV-519 and EC-7 endovaginal probes. The EV-519 probe emitted an ultrasound frequency of 5 MHz for B-mode imaging while the frequency of the EC-7 probe could be varied between 5 and 7.5 MHz. In both the color and pulsed Doppler modes, the Doppler ultrasound had a frequency of 5 MHz using the EV-519 transducer model while the EC-7 probe frequency was either 5 or 7.5 MHz for color Doppler and 5 MHz for pulsed Doppler ultrasound. The focal range of the transducer could be varied accordingly. The Doppler system was equipped with a high-pass filter to remove signals from vessel wall movements in the path of the Doppler ultrasound pulse. The high-pass filter was set as low as possible so that low blood velocities were still detected. We used a high-pass filter set at 125 Hz.

COLOR DOPPLER ASSESSMENT OF THE OVARIAN STROMAL VESSELS

Using Doppler ultrasound it is possible to estimate absolute velocity (cm/s) but it is essential to know the beam/flow angle of the vessel insonated, keeping the magnitude of the insonation angle to a minimum and thus minimizing error. The velocity measurements that can be made include peak systolic blood flow velocity, time-averaged maximum velocity and time-averaged mean velocity. For larger vessels flow velocity estimations are possible but if vessels are small and tortuous such as the

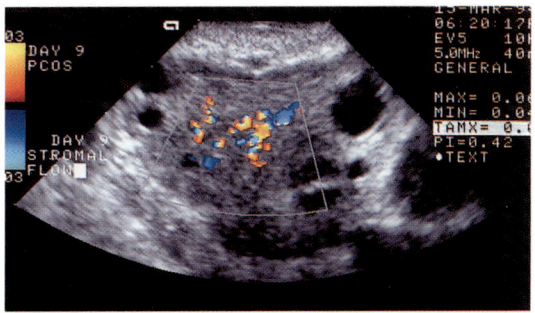

Figure 4 The color Doppler box can be placed over the ovarian stroma, and blood vessels can be clearly visualized

ovarian stroma or follicular vessels, measurement of the beam/flow angle is difficult and true blood flow velocity estimation may be inaccurate. This is especially so with angiogenesis where there are many small, tortuous vessels. However, in practice it may be assumed that at least one vessel in the vascular bed will be located at a low angle, so maximum peak systolic velocities can be measured with minimum error[5,8,10,11].

Intra-ovarian blood flow of each ovary can be assessed by color Doppler ultrasound. The color Doppler box can be placed over the ovarian stroma, and blood vessels can be clearly visualized (Figure 4). An ovarian stromal artery may be defined as any small artery in the ovarian stroma not close to the surface of the ovary or near the wall of a follicle. Areas of maximum color intensity, representing the greatest Doppler frequency shifts, can be selected for pulsed Doppler examination. The resultant flow velocity waveforms produced can be selected for analysis. The optimal flow velocity waveforms (i.e. those with the largest Doppler shift) can be analyzed (Figure 5) and indices of resistance and velocity recorded.

OVARIAN STROMAL BLOOD FLOW AND ASSISTED REPRODUCTION

The ultrasound assessment of ovarian morphology is an essential part of the initial evaluation of the infertile patient. A major reason for this scan is to determine if the patient has polycystic ovaries[12] (Figure 6). Polycystic ovaries may be present in up to 50% of women

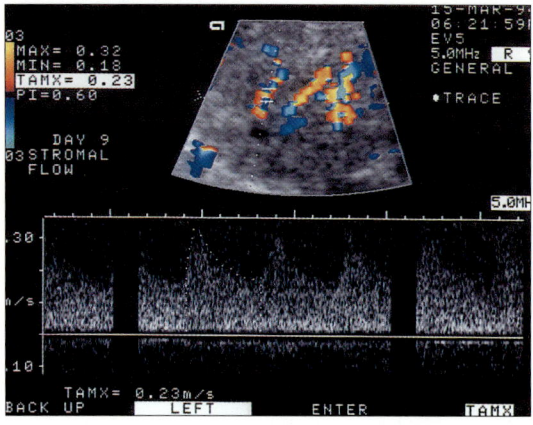

Figure 5 Optimal flow velocity waveforms in the stromal arteries (i.e. those with the largest Doppler shift) can be analyzed, and indices of resistance and velocity can be recorded

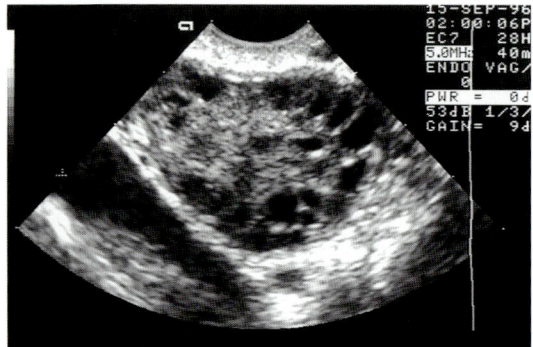

Figure 6 A transvaginal ultrasound image of a polycystic ovary

presenting at infertility clinics[13]. In assisted reproduction, the ultrasound diagnosis of polycystic ovaries is vital and of significant prognostic interest. In a recent case-controlled study of women with polycystic and normal ovaries undergoing superovulation for *in vitro* fertilization, women with polycystic ovaries developed more follicles and more oocytes despite receiving lower quantities of gonadotropins, but had a lower fertilization rate and a higher rate of ovarian hyperstimulation syndrome[14]. In fact, in this study 10.5% of the patients with polycystic ovaries developed moderate or severe ovarian hyperstimulation syndrome, compared with none of the controls[14].

The exact mechanism for this increased sensitivity of the polycystic ovary to exogenous gonadotropins is not clearly understood.

In a recent study, women who were about to undergo *in vitro* fertilization (IVF) treatment underwent transvaginal color Doppler ultrasonography on day 2 or 3 of their menstrual cycle prior to starting treatment with a gonadotropin releasing hormone agonist (GnRH-a) for pituitary desensitization[11]. Based on the clinical history and ultrasound findings, the women were divided into three groups. Group 1 consisted of 63 women who had regular, spontaneous menstrual cycles ranging from 26–32 days with mid-luteal progesterone levels > 30 nmol/l. Transvaginal ultrasonography on day 2 or 3 of the cycle (i.e. the baseline ultrasound scan) showed normal ovaries. Group 2 consisted of 13 women who were similar to Group 1 except that at the baseline ultrasound scan they had polycystic ovaries. Group 3 consisted of 12 women with a history of previous anovulatory menstrual cycles and/or oligomenorrhea and/or elevated serum luteinizing hormone (LH) concentrations (> 10 IU/l) in the early follicular phase and polycystic ovaries on transvaginal ultrasound scan.

Doppler studies of the ovarian stroma of each patient were performed. Typical flow velocity waveforms from arteries within the ovarian stroma in each group of women are shown in Figures 7–9. A subjective assessment by the operator using color Doppler ultrasound showed that the intensity and quantity of colored areas was greater in the ovarian stroma of Groups 2 and 3 than Group 1. Mean ovarian stromal peak systolic blood flow velocity was significantly greater in Groups 2 and 3 when compared with Group 1 but the ovarian stromal pulsatility index (PI) was not significantly different between the three groups of patients.

This study reports significantly greater indices of blood flow velocity in the ovarian stroma of polycystic ovaries compared with normal ovaries at the baseline ultrasound scan. The increased stromal blood flow velocity within the polycystic ovaries is present irrespective of

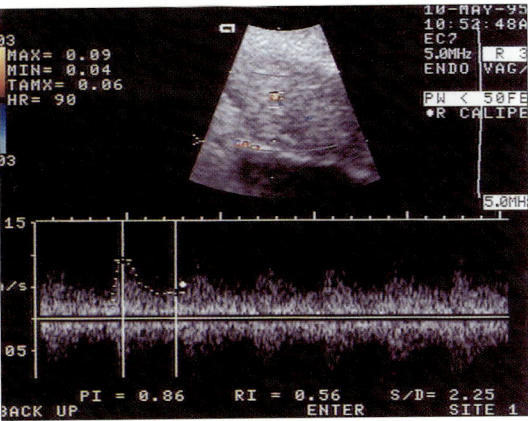

Figure 7 Flow velocity waveforms from the ovarian stroma of a patient in Group 1 (see text)

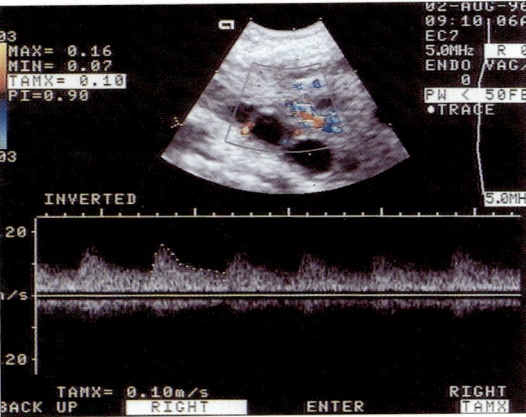

Figure 8 Flow velocity waveforms from the ovarian stroma of a patient in Group 2 (see text)

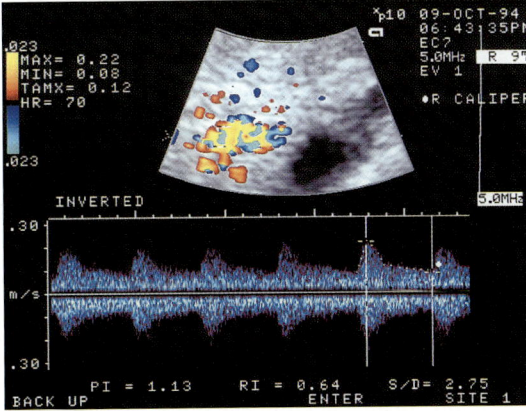

Figure 9 Flow velocity waveforms from the ovarian stroma of a patient in Group 3 (see text)

whether the women had regular or irregular menstrual cycles and/or endocrine disturbances. The subjective assessment of more colored areas in the polycystic ovary was also striking. All women were scanned on the 2nd or 3rd day of their menstrual cycle before recruitment of any follicles, thus ensuring that any contribution of blood flow from developing ovarian follicles was excluded. This increased stromal vascularity observed by Doppler ultrasound is consistent with the histological assessment of the Stein-Leventhal ovary[15]. Furthermore, the Doppler changes suggest that there may be other undetermined factors determining the morphology and vascularity of the ovary. Previous studies have described an increase in intra-ovarian blood flow velocity with minimal change in impedance to blood flow during the peri-ovulatory and luteal phases[5,6,10,16] and have suggested that these observations are likely to be due to angiogenic and/or vasoactive factors within the ovary. The observed increased ovarian stromal velocity in polycystic ovaries may also be due to increased activity of similar factors.

It is therefore suggested that the increased ovarian stromal blood flow velocity in polycystic ovaries, in combination with a relatively unchanged impedance to blood flow, may reflect increased intra-ovarian perfusion and thus a greater delivery of gonadotropins to the granulosa–thecal cell complex with a resultant greater number of follicles being produced. This mechanism may help to explain why patients with polycystic ovaries tend to respond excessively to the administration of gonadotropins[11], and may possibly explain their increased risk of ovarian hyperstimulation syndrome. However, prospective randomized studies evaluating this observation in assisted reproduction are yet to be carried out. Battaglia and associates[17] also studied uterine and ovarian stromal vascularity in women with polycystic ovary syndrome (PCOS) and found significant differences when compared to normal controls. They also discuss interesting insights into the possible pathogenesis of PCOS.

These studies therefore suggest that documentation of ovarian stromal vascularity at the initial baseline scan may be important and may provide useful information for assisted reproductive techniques.

Recently there have been studies to determine if measurement of ovarian stromal blood flow in the early follicular phase is related to subsequent ovarian responsiveness in IVF treatment[18]. This is particularly useful since the ability to predict ovarian response to stimulation by exogenous gonadotropins is still central to success in any IVF program. Most units determine the dose of gonadotropins used for the first attempt based on the chronological age of the patient, with adjustments being made in subsequent attempts depending on their initial response. Unfortunately the ovarian age (capacity of the ovary to produce fertilizable oocytes) and chronological age are not always synchronous, leading to a degree of unpredictability of the number of developing follicles and collected oocytes. Certainly, if an inadequate dose of gonadotropins is used then there may be a relatively poor response which reduces the number of oocytes retrieved, whereas if an excessive dose is used, there may be an increased risk of ovarian hyperstimulation syndrome.

In order to improve prediction of ovarian response to gonadotropins in IVF treatment, a number of strategies may be adopted. Measurement of the plasma follicle-stimulating hormone (FSH) level in the early follicular phase of the menstrual cycle is recognized as a good indicator of altered ovarian function[19], with high basal FSH concentrations, generally greater than 15 IU/l, predicting poor responsiveness to ovarian stimulation[20,21]. Unfortunately, the majority of patients have basal FSH levels less than 15 IU/l and many patients exhibiting a poor response to ovarian stimulation have normal FSH levels. Another technique is to perform an ultrasound scan in the early follicular phase to assess ovarian morphology. Certainly patients with polycystic ovaries are more sensitive to ovarian stimulation and are at higher risk of developing the ovarian hyperstimulation syndrome[22]. Nevertheless, the majority of patients have normal basal FSH levels and normal ovaries on

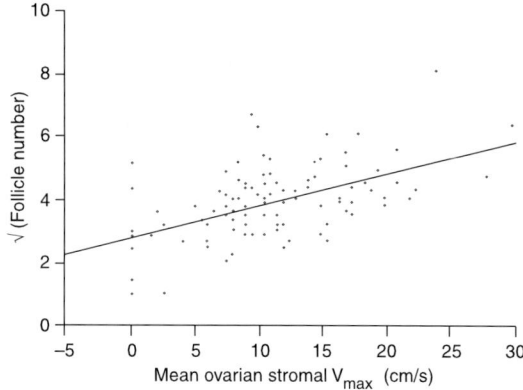

Figure 10 Unadjusted regression analysis of mean ovarian stromal peak systolic blood flow velocity (V_{max}) and the square root of the number of follicles present. Reprinted with permission from the American College of Obstetricians and Gynecologists (*Obstetrics and Gynecology*, 1996; 88: 779–84)

baseline ultrasound scan and, to date, there is no method to predict ovarian response in these patients.

A recent study correlated ovarian stromal blood flow velocity at the initial baseline ultrasound scan with subsequent ovarian response[18] (Figure 10). The results showed that there was a significant positive independent relationship between the maximum ovarian stromal blood flow velocity at the baseline scan and the subsequent ovarian response. There was no relationship between resistance to blood flow and folliculogenesis, implying that the results reflect varying degrees of intra-ovarian perfusion in the stromal arteries at the baseline scan. It is possible that the women with greater ovarian stromal blood flow have increased intra-ovarian perfusion so that, in response to the same dosage of gonadotropins, a relatively greater amount of gonadotropin is delivered to the granulosa–thecal cell complex, which in turn would lead to a greater number of follicles being produced. This observational study goes on to suggest that ovarian stromal blood flow velocity may also be able to predict a poor response to gonadotropins[18]. Prospective randomized studies evaluating these observations have, however, yet to be carried out. Furthermore, it is possible that patients with increased ovarian stromal blood flow velocity at the baseline ultrasound scan may be at an increased risk of the ovarian hyperstimulation syndrome. If this is true, then perhaps the ovarian stromal vascularity *per se* is the real determinant of follicular responsiveness and it may be that the description of ovarian stromal vascularity is more important than describing ovarian morphology. Only further prospective research in this exciting field will tell us the exact place of Doppler assessment of ovarian stromal blood flow in assisted reproduction.

References

1. Sterzik, K., Grab, D., Sasse, S., Hutter, W., Rosenbusch, B. and Terinde, R. (1989). Doppler sonographic findings and their correlation with implantation in an *in vitro* fertilization program. *Fertil. Steril.*, **52**, 825–8
2. Strohmer, J., Herczeg, H., Plockinger, B., Kemeter, P. and Feichtinger, W. (1991). Prognostic appraisal of success and failure in an *in vitro* fertilization program by transvaginal Doppler ultrasound at the time of ovulation induction. *Ultrasound Obstet. Gynecol.*, **1**, 272–4
3. Steer, C. V., Campbell, S., Tan, S. L., Crayford, T., Mills, C., Mason, B. A. *et al.* (1992). The use of transvaginal color flow imaging after *in vitro* fertilization to identify optimum uterine conditions before embryo transfer. *Fertil. Steril.*, **57**, 372–6
4. Steer, C. V., Campbell, S., Pampiglione, J., Mason, B. A. and Collins, W. P. (1990). Transvaginal colour flow imaging of the uterine arteries during the ovarian and menstrual cycles. *Hum. Reprod.*, **5**, 391–5
5. Sladkevicius, P., Valentin, L. and Marsal, K. (1993). Blood flow in the uterine and ovarian arteries during the normal menstrual cycle. *Ultrasound Obstet. Gynecol.*, **3**, 199–208
6. Tan, S. L., Zaidi, J., Campbell, S., Doyle, P. and Collins, W. P. (1996). Blood flow changes in the ovarian and uterine arteries during the normal menstrual cycle. *Am. J. Obstet. Gynecol.*, **175**, 625–31
7. Favre, R., Bettahar, K., Grange, G., Ohl, J., Arbogast, E., Moreau, L. *et al.* (1993). Predictive value of transvaginal uterine Doppler assessment in an *in vitro* fertilization program. *Ultrasound Obstet. Gynecol.*, **3**, 350–3
8. Tekay, A., Martikainen, H. and Jouppila, P. (1995). Blood flow changes in the uterine and ovarian vasculature, and predictive value of transvaginal pulsed colour Doppler ultrasonography in an *in vitro* fertilization programme. *Hum. Reprod.*, **10**, 688–93
9. Zaidi, J., Pittrof, R., Shaker, A., Kyei-Mensah, A., Campbell, S. and Tan, S. L. (1996). Assessment of uterine artery blood flow on the day of human chorionic gonadotropin administration by transvaginal color Doppler ultrasound in an *in vitro* fertilization program. *Fertil. Steril.*, **65**, 377–81
10. Campbell, S., Bourne, T. H., Waterstone, J., Reynolds, K., Crayford, T. J., Jurkovic, D., Okokon, E. and Collins, W. P. (1993). Transvaginal color flow imaging of the periovulatory follicle. *Fertil. Steril.*, **60**, 433–8
11. Zaidi, J., Pittrof, R., Campbell, S., Kyei-Mensah, A., Shaker, A., Jacobs, H. and Tan, S. L. (1995). Ovarian stromal blood flow changes in women with polycystic ovaries. A possible new marker for ultrasound diagnosis? *Hum. Reprod.*, **10**, 1992–6
12. Adams, J., Polson, D. and Franks, S. (1986). Prevalence of polycystic ovaries in women with anovulation and idiopathic hirsutism. *Br. Med. J.*, **293**, 355–9
13. Jacobs, H. S. (1987). Polycystic ovaries and polycystic ovarian syndrome. *Gynecol. Endocrinol.*, **1**, 113–31
14. MacDougall, M. J., Tan, S. L., Balen, A. and Jacobs, H. S. (1993). A controlled study comparing patients with and without polycystic ovaries undergoing *in vitro* fertilization. *Hum. Reprod.*, **8**, 233–7
15. Hughesdon, P. E. (1992). Morphology and morphogenesis of the Stein-Leventhal ovary and of so-called 'hyperthecosis'. *Obstet. Gynecol. Surv.*, **37**, 59–77
16. Collins, W. P., Jurkovic, D., Bourne, T., Kurjak, A. and Campbell, S. (1991). Ovarian morphology, endocrine function and intrafollicular blood flow during the peri-ovulatory period. *Hum. Reprod.*, **6**, 319–24
17. Battaglia, C., Artini, P. G., D'Ambrogio, G., Genazzani, A. and Genazzani, A. (1995). The role of color Doppler imaging in the diagnosis of polycystic ovary syndrome. *Am. J. Obstet. Gynecol.*, **172**, 108–13
18. Zaidi, J., Barber, J., Kyei-Mensah, A., Pittrof, R., Campbell, S. and Tan, S. L. (1996).

Relationship of ovarian stromal blood flow at the baseline ultrasound scan to subsequent follicular response in an *in vitro* fertilization program. *Obstet. Gynecol.*, **88**, 779–84

19. Sherman, B. M. and Korenman, S. G. (1975). Hormonal characteristics of the human menstrual cycle throughout reproductive life. *J. Clin. Invest.*, **55**, 699–706

20. Muasher, S. J., Oehninger, S., Simonetti, S., Matta, J., Ellis, L. M., Liu, H.-C. *et al.* (1988). The value of basal and/or stimulated serum gonadotropin levels in prediction of stimulation response and *in vitro* fertilization outcome. *Fertil. Steril.*, **50**, 298–307

21. Scott, R. T., Toner, J. P., Muasher, S. J., Oehninger, S., Robinson, S. and Rosenwaks, Z. (1989). Follicle-stimulating hormone levels on cycle day 3 are predictive of *in vitro* fertilization outcome. *Fertil. Steril.*, **51**, 651–4

22. MacDougall, M. J., Tan, S. L. and Jacobs, H. S. (1992). *In vitro* fertilization and the ovarian hyperstimulation syndrome. *Hum. Reprod.*, **7**, 597–600

Ultrasonic assessment of ovarian endometriosis

7

A. Kurjak and S. Kupesic

INTRODUCTION

The term endometriosis is defined by the presence of tissue outside the uterus that is pathologically similar to endometrium. Endometrial tissue within the myometrium, termed adenomyosis, is a separate pathological entity with a different patient population, etiology and clinical course[1]. Endometriosis is a unique disease process characterized by its invasive but non-neoplastic growth pattern, the presence of endometrium at ectopic sites, and evidence of hormonal responsiveness with menstrual cyclicity[2]. It is probably a consequence of transplantation of viable endometrial cells regurgitated through the Fallopian tubes at the time of menses. However, the dissemination of viable endometrial cells can occur by other routes, and some cases can only be explained by the metaplasia theory[3]. Although endometriosis is a common benign gynecological condition, there is still much to learn about its etiology and pathogenesis.

ENDOMETRIOSIS IN INFERTILE PATIENTS

Endometriosis is an extremely common disease, and unsuspected endometriosis accounts for approximately 15% of infertility[4]. Many asymptomatic women are found to have endometriosis, and some of them are reported to have severe disease discovered after the incidental detection of an ovarian mass or during laparoscopy for infertility. The classic symptom of endometriosis is pelvic pain associated with menstruation (or the immediate premenstrual phase)[5]. Suspicion is heightened when the infertile patient complains of

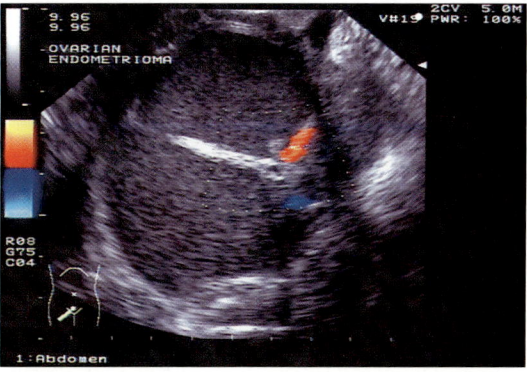

Figure 1 An ovarian endometrioma. Homogeneous high-level internal echoes and prominent vascularization at the level of the ovarian hilus are easily visualized

dysmenorrhea and dyspareunia. Pelvic adhesions, ovarian dysfunction, altered prostaglandin secretion, and peritoneal fluid macrophages are implicated as possible pathophysiological mechanisms[6]. Sonography is accurate in determining the type (cystic, mixed or solid), shape and location of endometriosis[7]. Cystic lesions, which constitute about 30–62%, are seen as irregular cysts with some evidence of septation (Figure 1). The sonographic appearance in the mixed type is compatible with pelvic inflammatory disease of an infectious cause, while a solid pattern may even suggest ovarian malignancy. Sometimes it is difficult to differentiate a 'chocolate cyst' from a hemorrhagic ovarian cyst or corpus luteum cyst (Figure 2). Fibrinolysis of the hemolytic content of a hemorrhagic ovarian cyst may change its pattern[8].

Endometriomas usually remain constant as non-echogenic cysts with a semi-solid content of a 'parenchymatous' texture representing

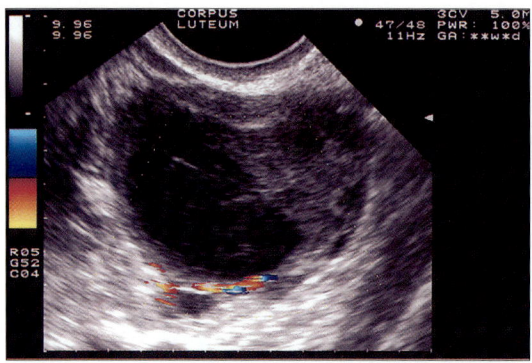

Figure 2 A transvaginal scan of a corpus luteum cyst emphasizing the internal appearance created by a retracting clot

'chocolate' paste-like fluid within a cyst[4]. The most common site of their deposition is the ovaries. Endometriomas may mimic developing follicles or functional cysts. Sometimes endometriomas increase in size during ovulation induction and mimic developing follicles. The experienced ultrasonographer may distinguish them accurately on the basis of low-level echoes, irregular shape, persistence during several cycles and observation of their behavior. Transvaginal sonography can be used for monitoring the regression of these collections under hormonal therapy.

Many years ago Scott and Te Linde[9] presented the sites of endometriosis detected in a series of 516 cases. They showed the ovaries to be the most common site followed by the pelvic peritoneum. In an infertile population of 182 women, Jenkins and colleagues[10] similarly noted the ovary to be a major site (54.9%) followed by the posterior broad ligament (35.2%), the anterior or posterior pouch of Douglas (each 34%), and the uterosacral ligaments (28%).

Common physical findings associated with endometriosis also include fixation of pelvic structures secondary to adhesions. The uterus may be retroverted[11]. Nodularity and tenderness of the uterosacral ligaments are noted in one-third of patients with endometriosis[12]. The condition has aroused much interest and controversy in recent years with regard to its accurate diagnosis, infertility association, and proper treatment. Even with the recent

ongoing achievements in operative endoscopy, clinicians are still faced with a problem of correct diagnosis, both in the sense of missing this pathology and of treating a luteinic cyst as an endometrioma[13,14]. Therefore, any diagnostic technique that could differentiate accurately and reliably between hemorrhagic luteinic cyst, cystadenoma, dermoid cyst, ovarian malignancy and endometrioma would be a useful additional tool for better management of this enigmatic disease.

ULTRASOUND DIAGNOSIS

The outside characteristics of the ovarian endometrioma are well known but they do not always suffice for reliable diagnosis. There have been several reports on the diagnosis of endometriosis by transabdominal sonography[7,15–18]. Typically, ovarian endometriomas have been described as cystic masses that are entirely or predominantly anechoic[16,17]. In other reports[15,18] they have been characterized more commonly as complex masses. In the recent transvaginal study by Kupfer and colleagues[14], 82% of 32 surgically proven endometriomas showed the presence of a homogeneous hyperechoic 'carpet' of low-level echoes.

The recent introduction of transvaginal color Doppler ultrasound increased the potential for *in vivo* characterization of adnexal masses, particularly in the differentiation between benign and malignant conditions[19]. The addition of color Doppler capabilities to transvaginal transducers enables detection of vascularity within endometriomas[20]. Endometriotic cysts are supported by already existing vessels within the ovarian hilus, showing moderate vascular impedance (Figure 3). If present, inflammatory changes may show alterations in perfusion that are characterized by a marked reduction in blood flow resistance. This finding may be wrongly interpreted as ovarian malignancy[21,22] (Figure 4).

Kurjak and Kupesic[23] were the first to report on the combined use of transvaginal color Doppler and the CA-125 level in patients with ovarian endometriomas. A new non-invasive scoring system (Table 1), using clinical signs

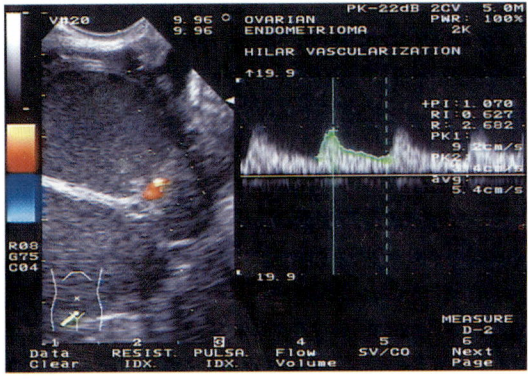

Figure 3 A case of septate ovarian endometrioma in an infertile patient. Pulsed Doppler signals demonstrate moderate vascular resistance (resistance index 0.63)

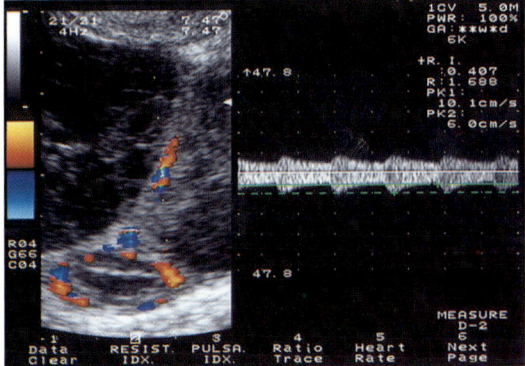

Figure 4 Hilar vascularization of an ovarian endometrioma. Pulsed Doppler signals derived from the early follicular phase of the menstrual cycle show low resistance (resistance index 0.41)

Table 1 Scoring system for endometriosis based on transvaginal color and pulsed Doppler sonography

Characteristic	Score
Reproductive age	2
Chronic pain (premenstrual or menstrual)	1
Infertility	1
B-mode ultrasonography	
Position (medial, retrouterine)	2
Bilaterality	1
Serial sonography positive	2
Thick walls	2
Homogeneous echogenicity	2
Clear demarcation from the ovary	1
Transvaginal color Doppler	
Vascularization	2
Pericystic/hilar location	2
Regularly separated vessels	2
Existence of notching	1
RI < 0.40 (menstrual phase)	2
RI = 0.41 to 0.60 (late follicular/corpus luteum phase)	2
CA-125 > 35 IU/ml	2

RI, resistance index; CA-125, carcino-embryonic antigen 125. From reference 23, with permission

patients. The average age of patients suffering from ovarian endometriosis was 31 years (range 19 to 45 years). At the beginning of the study, a new scoring system was created in an effort to improve sensitivity and specificity in the diagnosis of ovarian endometriosis. The scoring system used age, clinical signs and symptoms (pelvic pain associated with menstruation and presentation of infertility), CA-125 levels, sonographic findings, and transvaginal color and pulsed Doppler parameters. A blood sample for determination of the CA-125 level was obtained on the day before surgery. Patients were examined sonographically at least twice, both when they were admitted to the unit and on the day before the intervention. The peritoneal implants were excluded from the analysis, because no role can be expected from pelvic sonography in the detection of minimal or mild endometriosis. B-mode ultrasonography was used to evaluate the location, appearance and width of the ovarian lesion. The morphological scoring system was based on internal borders, quality of cyst, and fluid echogenicity. It included position and the existence of adnexal mass bilaterality. The sonographic

and symptoms, CA-125 levels, sonographic findings and transvaginal color and pulsed Doppler parameters, was developed and used for the preoperative recognition of ovarian endometriosis. The authors performed a 5-year prospective study in patients undergoing laparotomy and laparoscopy. The study group consisted of 544 women with clinically suspected adnexal masses who were undergoing laparotomy and 112 patients who were undergoing laparoscopy. In the second group, management of the ovarian mass and lysis of adhesions in infertile patients were the indications for diagnostic and/or operative laparoscopy. The mean patient age was 46 years. Ovarian endometriosis was proved histologically in 103

Table 2 The accuracy of the morphological scoring system

	Morphological score	Histopathology
True positive (n = 73)	73 endometriomas	73 endometriomas
False negative (n = 14)	7 hemorrhagic cysts	7 endometriomas
	5 dermoid cysts	5 endometriomas
	2 cystadenomas	2 endometriomas
False positive (n = 15)	7 endometriomas	7 hemorrhagic cysts
	6 endometriomas	6 dermoid cysts
	2 endometriomas	2 cystadenomas
True negative (n = 553)		

From reference 23, with permission

Table 3 Assessment of the combined scoring system for endometriosis

	Combined scoring system	Histopathology
True positive (n = 102)	102 endometriomas	102 endometriomas
False negative (n = 1)	1 hemorrhagic cyst	1 endometrioma
False positive (n = 2)	1 endometrioma	1 hemorrhagic cyst
	1 endometrioma	1 dermoid cyst
True negative (n = 551)		

From reference 23, with permission

criteria for the diagnosis of endometriosis were thick walls, regular margins, and homogeneous low echogenicity of the fluid. The presence of the cyst was confirmed at least twice in different cycles before surgery (the interval between the first and second ultrasound examinations ranged from 42 to 84 days). In 427 patients, serial ultrasound examinations were performed. The part of the scoring system dedicated to color Doppler evaluation was derived from vascular location, type of vascularization, and vascular quality. The vascular location typical for endometriomas is pericystic, at the level of the ovarian hilus. The type of vascularization represents the vascular arrangement within the ovarian endometrioma, and can comprise regularly separated vessels or no vessels seen. The vascular quality is the Doppler waveform signal assessed in terms of the resistance index (RI). The threshold value for discrimination between ovarian endometriosis and other ovarian lesions was a value of 20 in the combined scoring system. The histopathological diagnosis was considered definitive in all cases.

Transvaginal sonography demonstrated 656 adnexal masses: of these, 580 were benign, six were borderline, and 70 were malignant histologically proven ovarian lesions. For each lesion, combined scores for endometriosis were calculated the day before surgery or laparoscopy (Tables 2 and 3). Ovarian endometriomas appeared as thick-walled cystic structures containing marked internal echoes in 86 patients and multilocular cysts in seven patients, whereas a solid-cystic appearance was present in 10 patients. The median diameter of the endometriomas was 55.3 mm. Although at times the internal pattern represented a predominantly solid appearance, some acoustic enhancement was always demonstrated. In such cases, ballotement through the abdominal wall caused movements of the echoes, confirming the liquid mass. Most of the ovarian endometriomas were positioned medially or retrouterine. A well-demarcated separation between the endometrioma and the normal adjacent ovarian stroma was detected ultrasonically and proved surgically in 43.7% of cases. An endometrioma was confused morphologically with an acute hemorrhagic cyst in seven patients, which is not surprising because of the similar blood content. In seven patients with hemorrhagic cysts, sonography indicated endometriomas. An acute onset of symptoms

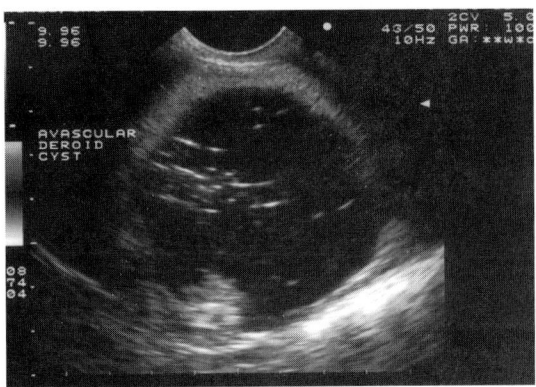

Figure 5 A transvaginal scan of a complex adnexal tumor with prominent echogenicity of the solid tumor parts. Color Doppler does not reveal any vascularity. A dermoid cyst was proved by histopathology

in these patients was suggestive of a hemorrhage, whereas a history of chronic pain was associated with endometriosis. In follow-up, endometriomas remained constant both in size and internal echo pattern, whereas all the hemorrhagic cysts resolved or decreased in size during the one or two ensuing cycles. Seven more false-negative cases were observed: sonographic reports indicated five cystic teratomas and two ovarian cystadenomas (Figure 5). The five false-negative cases by morphological scoring alone were caused by cystic teratomas in patients with a partly solid appearance of endometriosis. In three, the surrounding scarification process was obvious. These structures were confused for high amplitude reflectors with acoustic shadowing typical for dermoid cysts. Two patients with ovoid, huge multilocular endometriomas were interpreted incorrectly as having mucinous cystadenomas. Sonographic evaluation, whether alone or in combination with tumor markers, did not determine the nature of the lesion before Doppler assessment. In one patient with ovarian cystadenocarcinoma, the septations, papillary projections and solid areas were absent. Pelvic sonography demonstrated a small unilocular cyst of 28 mm with a smooth cystic wall, containing homogeneous fluid of low echogenicity. Eight more false-positive cases were observed: the morphological scoring system indicated endometriomas in six patients with homogeneous dermoid cysts and two cystadenomas. The sensitivity of vaginal sonographic characterization of endometriomas was 83.9%. The specificity and positive predictive value of this scoring system were 97.1% and 82.0%, respectively. The negative predictive value of transvaginal sonography was 97.5%. These results of attempts to distinguish ovarian endometriomas by the morphological scoring system alone showed that it is not possible to characterize ovarian lesions with acceptable accuracy.

COMBINED STUDIES BY DOPPLER ULTRASOUND AND TUMOR MARKERS

Even though a combination of transvaginal ultrasonography and color Doppler flow imaging may identify ovarian endometriosis with great reliability, measurement of CA-125 levels seems to enhance the sensitivity of the new scoring system. CA-125 is a cell surface antigen expressed on certain cells derived from embryonic coelomic epithelium, the measurement of which aids in the diagnosis and clinical follow-up of patients with ovarian carcinoma[24].

Elevation of CA-125 levels has been noted in patients with other benign conditions of the pelvis, such as endometriosis, myoma, adenomyosis, acute pelvic inflammatory disease and ovarian cysts[25]. The mechanism by which the elevated serum concentration of CA-125 occurs in women with endometriosis has not yet been clarified. McBean and Brumstead[26] showed that the endometrium of women with advanced endometriosis represents a potential source of elevated serum levels of CA-125. Disruptions of normal barriers between tissue and intravascular space could explain the increased amounts of this antigen. A majority of studies measuring CA-125 values in patients with endometriosis have demonstrated elevation of serum CA-125 levels during menses[27]. Elevation specifically during menses may result from retrograde flow and increased peritoneal inflammation, which is more pronounced than in women without disease.

O'Shaughnessy and associates[25] demonstrated that screening tests based on the variation of multiple CA-125 measurements throughout the menstrual cycle are more sensitive for detection of endometriosis than tests based on a single CA-125 level. When these authors performed CA-125 analysis in 14 false-negative cases by morphological score, they found an increased CA-125 value in nine patients. Color and pulsed Doppler showed vascularization typical for endometriomas in 13 patients: regularly separated vessels at the level of the ovarian hilus with an RI between 0.40 and 0.56. The existence of notching was noticed in 10 of 14 false-negative cases. When the authors analyzed serum CA-125 levels in 16 false-positive cases, they found normal results in 14 patients. Color and pulsed Doppler analysis showed typical luteal blood flow in six hemorrhagic cysts. Five dermoides showed no areas of vascularity, whereas two cystadenomas had an RI > 0.50. The morphological score indicated endometrioma in a patient with endometrioid cystadenocarcinoma (stage Ia). Color Doppler demonstrated massive diastolic flow and an RI of 0.38, suggestive of ovarian malignancy. In 13 of 14 patients with a false-negative diagnosis by B-mode ultrasonography, color Doppler was decisive in definitive diagnosis when used in combined assessment for ovarian endometriosis. Endometrioma-supplying vessels were identified in 91 patients. The most prominent vascular area in these cystic structures was at the level of the ovarian hilus. The resistance index values measured from this location were usually greater then 0.45. Blood flow indices varied between low (RI = 0.36–0.40) in 5.83%, intermediate (RI = 0.41–0.50) in 41.75% and high (RI = 0.51–0.60) in 40.77%. A total absence of blood flow was noticed in the remaining 11.65% of patients. In 11 patients with inflammatory changes surrounding the endometrioma, color Doppler showed intermediate RI values (0.41 to 0.50). Moderate elevation of serum CA-125 has been observed in 63.11% of patients suffering from endometriosis[23]. The sensitivity and specificity of preoperative CA-125 levels, using a cut-off of > 35 IU/ml, were 63.10% and 83.28%, respectively, whereas the positive and negative predictive values were 36.93% and 93.57%, respectively. In 104 patients the combined scoring system suspected an endometrioma (Table 3). The false-positive results were caused by a vascularized homogeneous cystic teratoma and a hemorrhagic cyst. Elevated serum CA-125 levels (40 IU/ml for cystic teratoma and 42 IU/ml for hemorrhagic cyst) were obtained. In both of these cases, color Doppler demonstrated an intermediate RI in visualized tumor vessels: in the first case, within the small bulge on the lateral cystic wall (RI = 0.48), and in the second case, at the edge of the inner wall of the ovarian cyst (RI = 0.45). Both ovarian tumors had a total score value of 21. One false-negative result was observed when the combined noninvasive scoring system for endometriosis indicated a corpus luteum cyst. The serum CA-125 level in this case was 28 IU/ml, whereas color Doppler had not revealed any area of angiogenesis. The sensitivity of the combined scoring system was 99.04%. The specificity and positive predictive values were 99.64% and 98.10%, respectively. The negative predictive value of the new scoring system was 99.82%. Of 103 patients, 45 were diagnosed correctly as having bilateral endometriomas. No malignancy was observed in the group of patients in whom ovarian endometriosis was suggested by the combined score.

Alcazar and colleagues[28] performed a similar study, trying to assess the diagnostic accuracy of transvaginal sonography alone and combined with color flow velocity imaging in differentiating ovarian endometriomas from other non-endometriotic masses. Twenty-seven (32.9%) of 82 masses were proven to be ovarian endometriomas. Morphological assessment correctly diagnosed 24 (88.9%) of the 27 endometriomas. A typical flow pattern (pericystic flow at the level of the ovarian hilus) was present in 90.5% of endometriomas. CA-125 levels in patients with endometriomas (45.6 ± 6.3 IU/ml) were significantly higher than in patients with non-endometriotic masses (26.5 ± 5.5 IU/ml). The sensitivity, specificity and positive and negative predictive values of transvaginal ultrasonography alone were 88.9%, 91%, 84.2%, and 94.5%, respectively, and combined with color velocity imaging and pulsed Doppler were 76.2%, 88.9%, 82.4% and 82.4%, respectively. For CA-125 levels, using a cut-off of $\geqslant 35$ IU/ml, these figures were 79.3%, 84.6%, 79.3% and 84.6%, respectively. The authors concluded that the use of color velocity imaging and pulsed Doppler does not improve the diagnostic accuracy of transvaginal ultrasound in the diagnosis of ovarian endometriomas. However, they did not perform serial ultrasound examinations, the vascular resistance was not related to the phase of the menstrual cycle, and CA-125 levels were evaluated separately.

Aleem and colleagues[29] reported a specific appearance of the vascular pattern of endometriomas: a few spots peripherally located. The values of the RI and pulsatility index (PI) for the endometriomas were 0.59 ± 0.02 and 0.95 ± 0.1, respectively. All endometriomas showed an RI of $\geqslant 0.5$ with a range of 0.5–0.74, while the range for the PI was 0.59–1.59. No significant differences between flow indices for endometriomas and other benign cystic lesions were noted. Scattered vascularity, one feature of adnexal endometriomas, may help to differentiate these endometriomas from other lesions of dense vascular distribution, such as corpora lutea or ovarian neoplasms.

Recently, there have been several multicenter studies on the use of transvaginal color and pulsed Doppler in the early detection of ovarian malignancy[19,30,31]. The highest rate of false-positive results has been found in the ovarian endometriomata group. It seems that this new scoring system for reliable detection of endometriomas can potentially reduce the number of false-positive cases in screening programs for ovarian malignancy.

At laparoscopy or laparotomy, most typical endometriotic lesions are surrounded by a substantial number of blood vessels. According to the transplantation theory of Sampson[32], viable endometrial cells that reach the peritoneal cavity by retrograde menstruation could

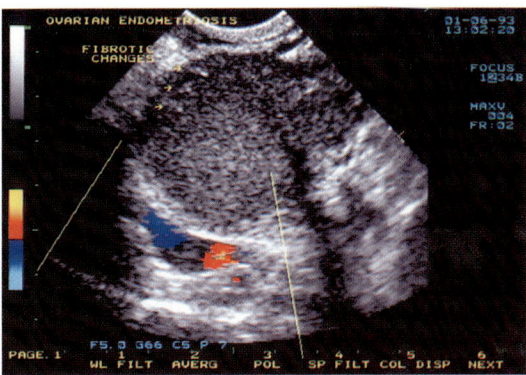

Figure 6 An avascular ovarian endometrioma as detected by transvaginal color Doppler

implant and form endometriotic lesions. Further progression of the lesions depends on different factors: the hormonal, immunologic, and vascular environments. Oosterlynck and colleagues[33] investigated the presence of angiogenetic factors in the peritoneal fluid of women with endometriosis. They found that increased angiogenetic activity could be important for further outgrowth and progression of these ectopic endometrial implants. It seems that the extent of fibrosis and the presence of focal hemorrhage correlate with the hormonal responsiveness of these implants. The collagen layer[34] may alter the vascularity and the diffusion of nutrients and oxygen into the endometrioma. It is possible that toxic factors within the lesion or increased pressure caused by accumulation of chocolate fluid alter the vascularity and result in an impaired response to cyclic endogenous hormones.

Color Doppler ultrasound has good potential in evaluating blood flow patterns in patients with ovarian endometriosis. Low impedance and high diastolic flow (RI = 0.36 to 0.40) are present when there is hemorrhage during the menstrual phase of the cycle[23]. The existence of a notch in such cases indicates the persistence of an initial resistance from the muscular lining of pre-existing arterioles and is suggestive of benign tumors[35]. Therefore, to distinguish this condition from ovarian malignancy, a careful study of ovarian endometrioma vascularity during the late follicular phase or early luteal phase is recommended. Serial color and pulsed Doppler evaluation is useful in doubtful cases.

It has been postulated that the effect of medical treatment is highly dependent on the arrival of metabolically active products via a blood-supplying network. Based on our experience[23], varying vascularity between lesions may determine the efficacy of therapy. Medical treatment of ovarian endometriomas with fibrotic plaques is never successful[36] (Figure 6). Intraperitoneal injection of gonadotropin-releasing hormone analogs could be used successfully in patients with an optimal vascular pattern. The scarification process surrounding the implants modifies the vascularization, which it is possible to detect using transvaginal color Doppler. An avascular lesion must be removed surgically.

CONCLUSION

Transvaginal color Doppler is a promising non-invasive method for highlighting women who might have endometriosis. It is hoped that combined scoring systems that use both transvaginal color flow and the CA-125 level can replace laparoscopy in obvious cases. Furthermore, study of the vascularity seems to be a guideline for the management of patients suffering from endometriosis. Reliable blood flow analysis of the endometriotic implant has overwhelming advantages, after which an effective treatment can be instituted. The success of medical treatment is dependent upon delivering metabolically active products via the endometrioma blood supply. Surrounding inflammation and scarification processes change the delivery of the medication. Therefore, in avascular lesions, surgical therapy should be recommended.

Transvaginal color Doppler has already been proved to be the method of choice for analysis of regional blood flow in patients with adnexal masses[19], and is complementary to laparoscopy. It seems that the introduction of three-dimensional color Doppler will be of additional help in the study of ovarian endometrioma vascularization. These most exciting developments in the field of gynecology in recent years might change the approach and can help the clinician to determine the best treatment options available to infertile patients suffering from endometriosis.

References

1. Flowers, C. E. Jr and Wilborn, W. H. (1978). New observation in the physiology of menstruation. *Obstet. Gynecol.*, **51**, 16–24
2. Ridley, J. H. (1968). The histogenesis of endometriosis: a review of facts and fancies. *Obstet. Gynecol. Surv.*, **23**, 1–25
3. Donnez, J., Nisolle, M., Casanas-Roux, G. and Grandjean, P. (1989). Endometriosis: pathogenesis and pathophysiology. In Shaw, R. W. (ed.) *Endometriosis*, pp. 11–29. (Carnforth, UK: Parthenon Publishing)
4. Hill, M. L. (1992). Infertility and reproductive assistance. In Nyberg, D. A., Hill, L. M., Bohm-Valez, M. and Mendelson, E. B. (eds.) *Transvaginal Ultrasound*, pp. 43–6. (St. Louis: Mosby Year Book)
5. Barlow, D. H. and Kennedy, W. (1989). Endometriosis: clinical presentation and diagnosis. In Shaw, R. W. (ed.) *Endometriosis*, pp. 1–10. (Carnforth, UK: Parthenon Publishing)
6. Doody, M. C., Gibbons, W. E. and Buttram, V. C. Jr. (1988). Linear regression analysis of ultrasound growth series: evidence for an abnormality of follicular growth in endometriosis patients. *Fertil. Steril.*, **49**, 47–51
7. Friedman, H., Vogelzang, R. L., Mendelson, E. B., Neiman, H. L. and Cohen, M. (1985). Endometriosis detection by ultrasound with laparoscopic correlation. *Radiology*, **157**, 217–20
8. Kupesic, S., Kurjak, A. and Stilinovic, K. (1994). The assessment of female infertility. In Kurjak, A. (ed.) *An Atlas of Transvaginal Color Doppler*, pp. 171–97. (London: Parthenon Publishing)
9. Scott, R. B. and Te Linde, R. W. (1950). External endometriosis: the scourge of the private patient. *Ann. Surg.*, **131**, 706–9

10. Jenkins, S., Olive, D. L. and Haney, A. F. (1986) Endometriosis: pathogenic implications of anatomic distribution. *Obstet. Gynecol.*, **67**, 335–8

11. Dodson, M. G. (1995). Infertility. In Dodson, M. G. (ed.) *Transvaginal Ultrasound*, pp. 157–62. (New York: Churchill Livingstone)

12. Speroff, L., Glass, R. H. and Kase, N. G. (1989). Endometriosis and infertility. In *Clinical Gynecology, Endocrinology and Infertility*, 4th edn. (Baltimore: Williams and Wilkins)

13. Brosens, I. A. (1993). Classification of endometriosis revisited. *Lancet*, **341**, 630

14. Kupfer, M. C., Schwimer, R. S. and Lebovic, J. (1992). Transvaginal sonographic appearance of endometriomata: spectrum of findings. *J. Ultrasound Med.*, **11**, 129–32

15. Sandler, M. A. and Karo, J. J. (1978). The spectrum of ultrasonic findings in endometriosis. *Radiology*, **127**, 229–32

16. Coleman, B. G., Arger, P. H. and Mulhern, C. B. (1979). Endometriosis: clinical and ultrasonic correlation. *Am. J. Radiol.*, **132**, 747–50

17. Athey, A. and Diment, D. D. (1989). The spectrum of sonographic findings in endometriosis. *J. Ultrasound Med.*, **8**, 847–9

18. Goldman, S. M. and Minkin, S. I. (1980). Diagnosing endometriosis with ultrasound: accuracy and specificity. *J. Reprod. Med.*, **25**, 4–8

19. Kurjak, A., Shalan, H., Kupesic, S., Predanic, M., Zalud, I., Breyer, B. and Jukic, S. (1993). Transvaginal color Doppler sonography in the assessment of pelvic tumor vascularity. *Ultrasound Obstet. Gynecol.*, **3**, 1–8

20. Kurjak, A., Jurkovic, D., Alfirevic, Z. and Zalud, I. (1991). Transvaginal color Doppler imaging. *J. Clin. Ultrasound*, **18**, 227–34

21. Kurjak, A., Zalud, I. and Alfirevic, Z. (1991). Evaluation of adnexal masses with transvaginal color ultrasound. *J. Ultrasound Med.*, **10**, 295–9

22. Kurjak, A., Schulman, H., Sosic, A., Zalud, I. and Shalan, H. (1992). Transvaginal ultrasound, color flow and Doppler waveform analysis of the postmenopausal adnexal mass. *Obstet. Gynecol.*, **80**, 917–21

23. Kurjak, A. and Kupesic, S. (1994). Scoring system for prediction of ovarian endometriosis based on transvaginal color and pulsed Doppler sonography. *Fertil. Steril.*, **62**, 81–8

24. Bast, R. C. Jr, Klug, T. L. and St. John, E. (1983). A radioimmunoassay using monoclonal antibody to monitor course of epithelial ovarian cancer. *N. Engl. J. Med.*, **309**, 883–7

25. O'Shaughnessy, A., Check, J. H., Nowroozi, K. and Lurie, D. (1993). CA 125 levels measured in different phases of the menstrual cycle in screening for endometriosis. *Obstet. Gynecol.*, **81**, 99–103

26. McBean, J. H. and Brumstead, J. R. (1993). *In vitro* CA 125 secretion by endometrium from women with advanced endometriosis. *Fertil. Steril.*, **59**, 89–92

27. Jager, W., Meier, C., Wildt, L., Sauerbrei, W. and Lang, N. (1988). CA-125 serum concentrations during the menstrual cycle. *Fertil. Steril.*, **50**, 223–7

28. Alcazar, J. L., Laparte, C., Jurado, M. and Lopez-Garcia, G. (1997). The role of transvaginal ultrasonography combined with color velocity imaging and pulsed Doppler in the diagnosis of endometrioma. *Fertil. Steril.*, **67**, 487–91

29. Aleem, F., Pennisi, J., Zeitoum, K. and Predanic, M. (1995). The role of color Doppler in diagnosis of endometriomas. *Ultrasound Obstet. Gynecol.*, **5**, 51–4

30. Campbell, S., Bourne, T. H., Reynolds, K., Hampson, J., Royston, P. and Whitehead, M. I. (1992). Role of color Doppler in an ultrasound-based screening programme. In Sharp, F., Mason, W. P. and Creasman, W. (eds.) *Ovarian Cancer. Biology, Diagnosis and Management*, pp. 237–47. (London: Chapman and Hall Medical)

31. Kurjak, A. and Predanic, M. (1992). New scoring system for prediction of ovarian malignancy based on transvaginal color Doppler sonography. *J. Ultrasound Med.*, **11**, 631–8

32. Sampson, J. A. (1921). Perforating hemorrhagic (chocolate) cysts of the ovary. *Arch. Surg.*, **3**, 245–323

33. Oosterlynck, D. J., Meuleman, C., Sobis, H., Vandeputte, M. and Konincky, P. R. (1993). Angiogenic activity of peritoneal fluid from women with endometriosis. *Fertil. Steril.*, **59**, 779–82

34. Metzger, D. A., Szpk, C. A. and Haney, A. F. (1993). Histologic features associated with hormonal responsiveness of ectopic endometrium. *Fertil. Steril.*, **59**, 83–8

35. Fleischer, A. C. (1998). Color Doppler sonography of benign and malignant pelvic masses: the spectrum of findings. In Kurjak, A. and Fleischer, A. C. (eds.) *Doppler Ultrasound in Gynecology*, pp. 27–37. (London: Parthenon Publishing)

36. Malinak, L. R. and Wheeler, J. M. (1990). Combination medical–surgical therapy for endometriosis. In Shaw, R. E. (ed.) *Endometriosis*, pp. 85–91. (Carnforth, UK: Parthenon Publishing)

Hormonal normalization of baseline ovarian ultrasound scans in infertility

8

D. de Ziegler, P.-A. Brioschi and P.-J. Ditesheim

INTRODUCTION

Cyclical changes in ovarian activity make it difficult to normalize ultrasound assessments in infertility. During the follicular phase the successive processes of follicular recruitment, selection and maturation are responsible for day-to-day changes in the ultrasound appearance of the ovary, and these changes have hampered all attempts at normalizing the echographic characteristics of the ovarian tissue, and even attempts at assessing ovarian volume. Furthermore, the degree of advancement of the follicular maturation at any specific menstrual cycle day varies from patient to patient, depending on whether the follicular phase is short or long. In other words, the menstrual cycle days are counted starting from an event linked to the previous cycle (i.e. the menses), which does not reflect the true functional advancement of the follicular phase. Hence, to be functionally comparable, data need to be normalized according to the subsequent luteinizing hormone (LH) surge. Unfortunately, the normalization of ultrasound findings to the LH surge can only be carried out retrospectively, and multiple hormonal determinations are necessary to identify the actual occurrence of the LH surge. The timing of ultrasound data according to the LH surge is therefore not practically feasible in common clinical evaluations.

Luteal phase assessments of ovarian appearance on ultrasound suffer from the impact of the corpus luteum, which affects follicular growth through paracrine mechanisms[1,2]. The sheer volume of the corpus luteum will also affect the validity of ovarian volume measurements on that side. Furthermore, the corpus luteum may be associated with local phenomena such as intraovarian bleeding and/or cyst formation. Some investigators acknowledging this problem have preferred to use the smallest ovarian volume (the ovary not bearing the active corpus luteum) in their computations[3]. Using this model, Syrop and colleagues[3] have identified a functional correlation between the ovarian volume of the smallest ovary and the response to controlled ovarian hyperstimulation (COH) with human menopausal gonadotropin (hMG) or recombinant follicle-stimulating hormone (FSH). As illustrated in Table 1, an inverse correlation was seen between baseline ovarian volume and COH outcome. Furthermore, as illustrated in Table 2, determination of ovarian volume by ultrasound offers the possibility of anticipating the risk of ovarian hyperstimulation syndrome (OHSS).

Baseline ultrasound assessments of ovarian function in the early follicular phase offer potential for predicting the response to ovarian stimulation, and for adjusting treatments accordingly. Practically speaking, however, this is hampered by two factors:

(1) The clinical sign serving to identify the onset of the menstrual cycle (the menses) is functionally related to the preceding cycle (reflecting the decrease in progesterone levels), and not to the new follicular maturation process. The true functional onset of the cycle is therefore not readily identifiable;

Table 1 Ovarian volumes and outcome measures of controlled ovarian hyperstimulation

Ovarian volume (ml)	n	Mean age (years)	Peak estradiol (pg/ml)	Mean no. of eggs	Mean no. of embryos	Cancellation rate (%)	Clinical pregnancy rate per initiated cycle (%)
Volume of smallest ovary							
< 3	18	34.8	1.524	11.6	8.2	22	28
3–9	144	33.4	1.945	15.8	9.8	14	35
> 9	26	32.7	2.907	21.3	11.6	0	46
Total ovarian volume							
< 8.6	29	33.6	1.497	12.3	7.8	21	31
8.6–22.2	133	33.4	1.994	15.6	10.0	13	34
> 22.2	26	33.3	2.898	23.4	11.4	4	50

Values given are for patients who were not cancelled. Data from reference 3, with permission

Table 2 Comparison of different variables (means ± SD) in patients with and without moderate or severe ovarian hyperstimulation syndrome (OHSS)

	With OHSS	Without OHSS	p
No. of patients	8	86	
Age (years)	29.1 ± 4.2	32.7 ± 4.3	
hMG administered (ml) (%)	2 (7.1)	26 (81.3)	
FSH	6 (9.1)	59 (86.7)	
Days of stimulation	10.5 ± 2.5	10.5 ± 1.8	
Estradiol-17β (pg/ml)	2439 ± 1350	937 ± 686	0.0001
No. of follicles	23.3 ± 4.3	13.8 ± 7.5	0.0025
No. of oocytes	16.4 ± 2.6	5.9 ± 3.0	0.0001
Cycle length (days)	34.1 ± 5.8	28.7 ± 2.2	0.0001
Body weight before stimulation (kg)	55.4 ± 3.8	62.8 ± 11	0.011
Body weight after stimulation (kg)	54.3 ± 4.5	62.9 ± 10.7	0.03
Ovarian baseline volume (ml)	13.2 ± 5.0	8.9 ± 3.7	0.035

hMG, human menopausal gonadotropin; FSH, follicle-stimulating hormone. Data from reference 4, with permission

(2) For most women it is impractical or unpleasant to undergo transvaginal ultrasound examinations during menses.

It is for these two reasons that we designed a hormonal manipulation using physiological hormones to maintain luteal phase levels of estradiol artificially, and to control (postpone) the functional onset of the follicular phase. Our objective was to develop a new approach, offering the potential for true early follicular phase ultrasound assessment of ovarian function.

THE FUNCTIONAL ONSET OF THE FOLLICULAR PHASE

By definition, the follicular phase starts on the first day of menses. The true functional onset of the follicular phase is controlled, however, by the intercycle slight increase in plasma FSH levels, which occurs independently of menses. Unfortunately, the intercycle increase in FSH cannot easily be recognized precisely because of the small magnitude of the FSH elevation. In ideal circumstances, the demise of the corpus luteum of the preceding cycle triggers a concomitant decline of plasma progesterone, estradiol and inhibin A levels. It is, however, solely the decrease in progesterone that is responsible for triggering the clinically identifiable menstrual bleeding through a process called withdrawal bleeding. Indeed, previous studies have shown that the occurrence of withdrawal bleeding in response to declining progesterone levels is independent of estradiol

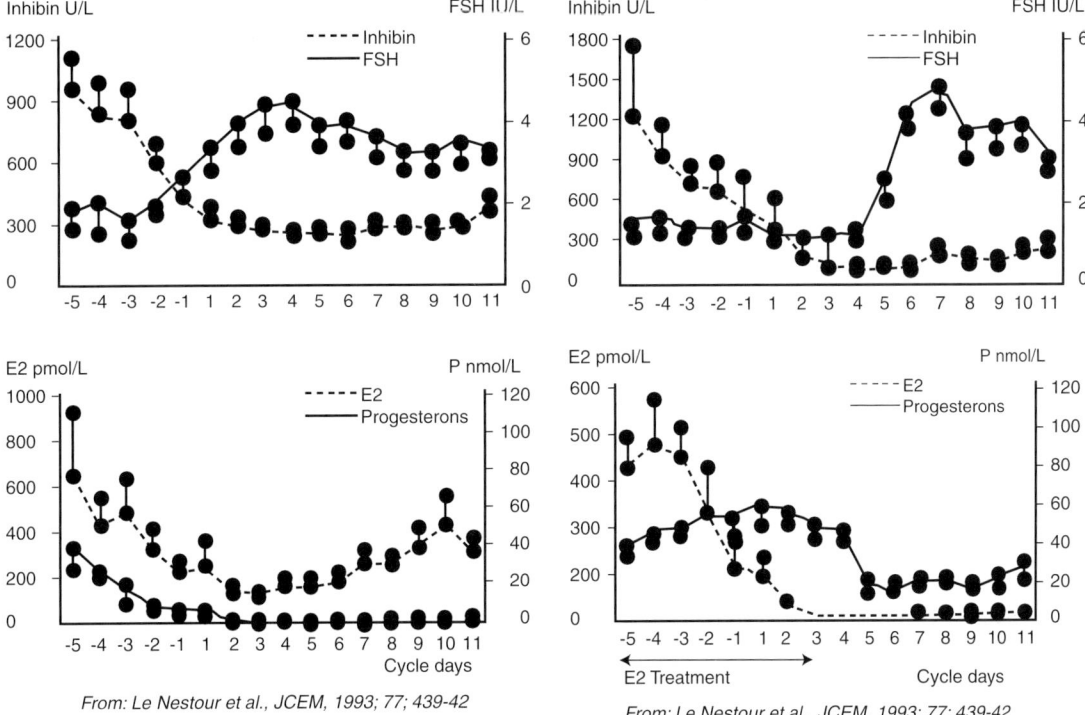

From: Le Nestour et al., JCEM, 1993; 77; 439-42

Figure 1 The luteal–follicular transition under physiological conditions. During the interval the demise of the corpus luteum results in decreasing plasma levels of estradiol, progesterone and inhibin A. This is followed by the intercycle increase in follicle-stimulating hormone, which initiates the ultimate or gonadotropin-dependent phase of follicular maturation

Figure 2 The luteal–follicular transition under the effect of exogenous estradiol. Administration of exogenous estradiol, in quantities maintaining luteal levels of estradiol after the demise of the corpus luteum, postpones the intercycle increase in follicle-stimulating hormone (FSH) until after exogenous estradiol is discontinued. After interrupting estradiol treatment, plasma FSH levels peak 3 days later

levels, which in some instances decrease either before or after the decline in progesterone without impacting on the timing of menstrual bleeding[5,6].

In a prior study we artificially maintained plasma estradiol at luteal phase levels during the demise of the corpus luteum by administering physiological amounts of exogenous estradiol[7]. Results were compared to 'control' cycles, during which the intercycle transition was studied in the same volunteers when they did not receive supplemental hormone. As illustrated in Figures 1 and 2, end luteal phase treatment with estradiol resulted in postponement of the intercycle increase in FSH until the exogenous source of estradiol was interrupted. These results indicate that it is the decrease in estradiol, and not inhibin A as

previously suggested[8], that represents the primary signal for the intercycle increase in FSH. One practical consequence of this phenomenon is the theoretical possibility of using physiological amounts of exogenous estradiol to postpone the intercycle increase in FSH. Potentially, this treatment offers the possibility of controlling the intercycle FSH increase that takes place upon discontinuation of estradiol treatment. For example, by interrupting the estradiol treatment on a set day of the week, it is possible to time true early follicular phase ultrasound scans on another preset day and give advance appointments accordingly. This approach could provide full control of the onset of the increase in FSH and permit normalized early follicular phase ultrasound scans for assessing ovarian function.

EXOGENOUS ESTRADIOL AND PROGESTERONE FOR BLOCKING FOLLICULAR RECRUITMENT

Synthetic estrogens (such as ethinyl estradiol) and progestins (such as norethisterone acetate) have been used as oral contraceptives to block ovulation, with a recent trend towards decreasing the amount of hormone administered without hampering efficacy. In contrast with the abundance of data available on oral contraceptives, little has been learned on the impact of physiological amounts of exogenous estradiol on follicular recruitment and ovulation. We therefore conducted a trial to determine whether exogenous estradiol can prevent follicular recruitment for up to 2 weeks and prime endometrial receptivity[9]. The objective that motivated this early trial was to determine the practicality of this approach for timing the transfers of cryopreserved embryos using exogenous estradiol and progesterone in women whose ovaries remained functional, without down-regulating gonadotropins with a gonadotropin-releasing hormone (GnRH) agonist. We formulated the hypothesis that early follicular phase administration of estradiol would prevent follicular recruitment by interfering with the intercycle slight increase in FSH. In a pilot study[9] we conducted ultrasound scans on cycle days 3, 9 and 14 in women with active ovaries who started to receive exogenous estradiol on cycle day 1. The delivery dose ranged from 0.05 to 0.4 mg/day, following a model duplicating the menstrual cycle pattern of estradiol levels. On cycle day 3, between three and eight small ovarian follicles (< 8 mm in diameter) were counted in each ovary. The total mean number of follicles on that day was 11.1 ± 6.9 per woman (mean ± SD). Repeat ultrasound scans on days 9 and 14 showed no follicular growth, and in particular showed no follicle $\geqslant 12$ mm in diameter. Plasma estradiol and progesterone levels (sampled twice a week) were not different from findings in women suffering from premature ovarian failure and receiving a similar regimen of estradiol and progesterone.

Table 3 Effect of priming of endometrial receptivity with estradiol and progesterone on pregnancy and implantation rates after transfers of cryopreserved embryos

	Natural cycle	GnRH agonist treatment	Estradiol/ progesterone treatment
No. of transfers	53	65	51
No. of embryos	79	103	116
Pregnancy rate per transfer (%)	11	6	17.5
Implantation rate per transfer (%)	8	4	8.6

Data with permission from Lelaidier, C., De Ziegler, D., Gaetano, J., Hazout, A., Fernandez, H. and Frydman, R. (1992). Controlled preparation of the endometrium with oestradiol and progesterone: a novel regimen not using a gonadotrophin-releasing hormone agonist. *Hum. Reprod.*, **7**, 1353–6

Findings were also similar to hormonal values encountered in the menstrual cycle, except for plasma progesterone levels which only reached the lower end of the physiological range for the luteal phase. Plasma LH levels remained low until day 10 and started to increase thereafter. The mid-cycle elevation in mean plasma LH levels resulted from individual increases in plasma LH to pre-ovulatory surge values, with subsequent return to baseline values, displaying individual positive feedback responses to exogenous estradiol. Despite an increase in plasma LH to pre-ovulatory surge levels occurring in all women (in response to exogenous estradiol), plasma progesterone levels remained remarkably low at $\leqslant 0.4$ ng/ml in all subjects prior to exogenous administration of progesterone. Indeed, because of the lack of follicular development, plasma LH surges never resulted in an increase in circulating progesterone, and therefore had no effect on endometrial morphology. From these data we concluded that it is only necessary to inhibit follicular development, and not plasma LH values, to control endometrial receptivity with exogenous hormones in women whose ovaries are functioning. As illustrated in Table 3, pregnancy and implantation rates after transfers of cryopreserved embryos primed with estradiol and progesterone only were similar to those obtained in the natural menstrual cycle or after down-regulation of gonadotropins with a GnRH agonist.

Another practical consequence of our observation that physiological amounts of exogenous estradiol can block follicular recruitment for up to 2 weeks is that estradiol treatment can allow assessment of the ultrasound appearance of ovaries in conditions of 'physiological arrest', and findings can be used to guide the clinical management of COH cycles. This could potentially provide better baseline data for studies correlating ultrasound findings and hormonal parameters with the quality of follicular recruitment and development, and aid in making treatment adjustments.

THE CONCEPT OF THE FUNCTIONAL DAY

As stated earlier, the classical method for counting menstrual days takes the menses as a reference, which is a physiological event triggered by the demise of the corpus luteum of the previous cycle. We reported on the possibility of withholding by simple means the intercycle slight increase in FSH which normally triggers the physiological events (follicular recruitment) initiating the new menstrual cycle. This provides a more meaningful reference for dating the progression of the follicular phase. As stated earlier, we know that the intercycle increase in FSH can be controlled with exogenous estradiol. This approach allows the dating of follicular days from the discontinuation of exogenous estradiol treatment, which represents the trigger for FSH elevation. The last day of exogenous estradiol is called functional day 0 (FD-0) because plasma FSH is still at a resting level. Subsequently, the days that follow the interruption of estradiol treatment are numbered from FD-1 onward. This new approach offers the advantage of anchoring the dating to an event functionally important for the follicular phase, the withdrawal from luteal phase levels of estradiol and the subsequent increase in FSH levels. Hence, this approach is linked to the true phenomenon which initiates the ultimate

phase (or gonadotropin-dependent phase) of follicular recruitment.

SYNCHRONIZATION OF OVARIAN ULTRASOUND SCANS

We used this new approach for timing baseline ultrasound scans and COH in a pilot trial[10]. We prescribed exogenous estradiol (Progynova® 2 mg orally, twice daily, starting on menstrual cycle day 25 or approximately 5 days before the expected onset of menses. Estradiol treatment was arbitrarily interrupted on the first Tuesday following the onset of menses[10]. The last day of estradiol treatment was designated FD-0. In our previous study[7] we observed that plasma FSH peaked 3 days after the interruption of exogenous estradiol treatment. Hence, in this pilot trial[10] looking at the possibility of synchronizing the elevation of endogenous FSH with exogenous estradiol treatments, we started hMG administration 3 days after interrupting estradiol treatment (FD-3). This approach offers an ideal opportunity for 'normalized' echographic assessments of the ovaries at a time when menses are finished.

In this pilot trial, 30 women aged 35.1 ± 6.3 years (mean $\pm$ SD) received estradiol valerate (Progynova). Women underwent a baseline ultrasound scan 3 days later (FD-3). Clinically, performing this scan on FD-3 offers several advantages. First, FD-3 can be compared with cycle day 3 of conventional treatments, the day on which exogenous gonadotropin administration is started. Meaningful comparisons are therefore permitted between results obtained with the new and standard regimens. Second, menses have usually stopped on FD-3 (on average 8 days after the onset of menses in our trial, but this can be set differently when necessary), which makes a vaginal ultrasound scan more acceptable. Also, the corpus luteum has usually regressed fully, and will not alter ultrasound findings. In our trial, estradiol treatment was started 7.1 ± 3.3 days (mean $\pm$ SD) before the onset of menses and continued for 5 ± 2 days after the onset of menses. Plasma FSH, LH and estradiol levels and the FSH/LH ratio on FD-0 and FD-3 are provided in

Table 4 Plasma gonadotropin and estradiol levels (means ± SEM) on functional days 0 and 3 after the last day of estradiol treatment

	Functional day 0	Functional day 3
Estradiol (pg/ml)	171 ± 80	76 ± 42
FSH (mIU/l)	3.8 ± 0.4	6.7 ± 0.7
LH (mIU/l)	5.5 ± 0.8	6.9 ± 0.8
FSH/LH ratio	1.0 ± 0.2	1.2 ± 0.2

FSH, follicle-stimulating hormone; LH, luteinizing hormone. Data from reference 10, with permission

Table 4. It can be seen that plasma estradiol decreased by 55%, falling from 171 ± 80 pg/ml on FD-0 to 76 ± 42 pg/ml on FD-3 (mean ± SEM) after discontinuation of exogenous estradiol treatment. Plasma FSH increased, from 3.8 ± 0.4 mIU/ml to 6.7 ± 0.7 mIU/ml (76% increase from baseline). Plasma LH also increased in response to estradiol withdrawal, but to a lesser extent, from 5.5 ± 0.8 mIU/ml to 6.9 ± 0.8 mIU/ml (26% increase from baseline). The FSH/LH ratio remained remarkably constant, however, at 1.0 ± 0.2 and 1.2 ± 0.2 on FD-0 and FD-3, respectively.

Typical baseline ovarian ultrasound findings on FD-3 are illustrated in Figure 3. In contrast to findings made in the luteal phase, little difference was observed between the left and right ovaries. The control of follicular recruitment provided by timely administration of estradiol valerate also permits prevention of early follicular recruitment and development, which confuses the interpretation of the ovarian ultrasound findings. As illustrated, off-line computer-assisted three-dimensional reconstruction permits an improved evaluation of the cohort of recruitable follicles.

ULTRASOUND ASSESSMENT OF OVARIAN VOLUME

In regularly ovulating women, the mean ovarian volume has been found to be between 5.9 and 9.8 ml by different authors[11-13]. These differences contrast with the high degree of precision of ultrasound measurements of ovarian volume when results are confirmed by actual measurements of organs obtained by surgery[14], or by the follicular fluid content (Table 5)[15]. Furthermore, a high degree of correlation

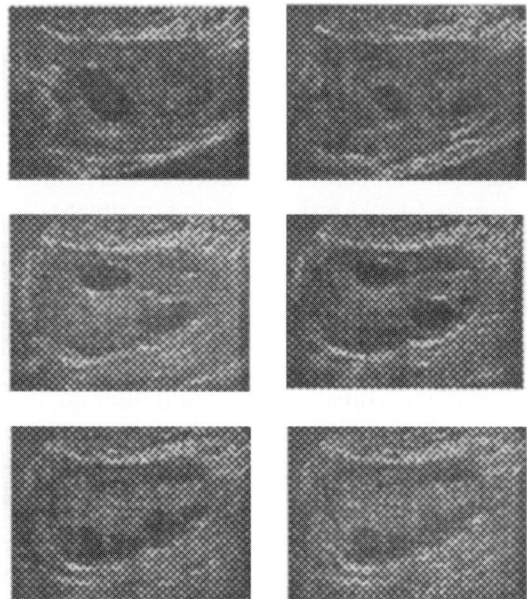

Figure 3 On functional day 3 it is possible to evaluate the size of the pool of recruitable follicles by conducting serial ultrasound sections, possibly with the help of an off-line computer-assisted three-dimensional system. At baseline, three-dimensional reconstruction of ovarian ultrasound scans offers the prospect of predicting the quality of ovarian responses to human menopausal gonadotropin and recombinant follicle-stimulating hormone, and optimizing the dosing regimen in order to limit the risks of hyperstimulation and multiple pregnancy. The ultrasound scans shown are serial sections showing the total number of recruitable follicles

($r = 0.960$) has been found between the ovarian volume measurements made by different examiners[16]. We interpret this apparent paradox by postulating that the differences in baseline ovarian volumes are related to the various characteristics of the population studied and the functional time in the menstrual cycle selected for performing the measurements. Evidently, the latter source of variation can be minimized by conducting baseline measurements of the ovarian volume in normalized conditions such as offered on FD-0. It is important to note that the accuracy of follicular volume measurements can potentially be improved significantly by off-line three-dimensional reconstruction using a computer-based system[4].

(1) Exogenous estradiol allows postponement of the intercycle FSH elevation;

Table 5 Statistical comparison of aspirate volume and follicular volume obtained using two- and three-dimensional ultrasonography

	Two-dimensional ultrasonography	Three-dimensional ultrasonography
Standard deviation of differences between measured volume and aspirate volume (ml)	1.22	0.32
Mean difference from aspirate volume (ml)	0.52 (+0.02 to −1.02)	0.1 (−0.03 to +0.23)
Upper limit of agreement (d + 2s)	2.97 (2.47 to 3.47)	0.74 (0.52 to 0.96)
Lower limit of agreement (d − 2s)	−1.92 (−2.42 to −1.42)	−0.54 (−0.76 to −0.43)

Values in parentheses are 95% confidence intervals. Data from reference 15, with permission

(2) The baseline ultrasound scan is best performed just prior to starting hMG/recombinant FSH treatments (functional day 3);

(3) Exogenous estradiol permits true baseline ultrasound analysis without interferences from the corpus luteum or emerging follicular maturation. Furthermore, it allows one to avoid performing vaginal ultrasound scans during menses;

(4) The baseline ultrasound scan provides information on the recruitable follicles (number of follicles with diameter between 3 and 11 mm). Data provide information on ovarian reserve and permit prospective adjustments of hMG and recombinant FSH doses for COH.

Baseline ovarian assessment with determination of the size of the pool of recruitable follicles has been shown to predict both the quality of ovarian response to COH[3] and the risk of OHSS[4].

It is not surprising that ovarian volume values are markedly different between regularly ovulating women and subjects suffering from polycystic ovarian disease (PCOD)[11]. Furthermore, identification of an increased stromal echogenicity was found to be a valuable surrogate marker for the disease, with high sensitivity and specificity for PCOD at 94% and 90%, respectively. The number of identifiable follicles was increased in PCOD as compared to cycling controls with 9.8 and 5.0 follicles per ovary in the two groups, respectively[11].

Baseline ovarian ultrasound scans can also serve to complement the evaluation of ovarian age and reserve. While early follicular phase FSH levels have long been recognized to carry a predictive value for the remaining reproductive potential of women reaching the transition years, intermittent fluctuation in baseline FSH values have notoriously hampered the predictive value of this parameter. Because ovarian volume progressively decreases when women enter menopause[12], its assessment offers a valuable adjunct to early follicular phase FSH measurements. This latter parameter is indeed far less likely to suffer from intermittent variations, provided that interferences from confounding parameters such as corpus luteum volume and follicular maturation are avoided, as is made possible by hormone normalization. Mehta and colleagues[17] observed that ovarian volume measurement in women suffering from premature ovarian failure permitted the identification of a substantial subset of patients (approximately 40%) who retained ovarian follicles and a potential for fertility, consistent with the diagnosis of resistant ovary syndrome. The preservation of an ovarian volume characteristic of the reproductive years permits the recognition of this subgroup of patients with premature ovarian failure.

In conclusion, a new method for hormonal normalization is proposed, which permits true baseline ovarian ultrasound assessments. This original approach is based on the physiological observation that artificially maintaining the luteal phase levels of estradiol can delay the intercycle increase in plasma FSH. We anticipate that this approach will improve the predictive value and clinical relevance of ovarian volume measurements. Combined with the determination of the size of the pool of recruitable ovarian follicles, this is likely to play a greater role in the future for determining prospectively the reproductive potential of women. These new ultrasound parameters may prove to be particularly useful for distinguishing cases of overt premature menopause (with shrunken ovaries) from other cases of premature ovarian failure that may retain some reproductive potential. Further work will clarify the role played by baseline ultrasound assessment of ovarian volume in the functional assessment of ovarian age.

References

1. Adashi, E. Y. (1991). The ovarian life cycle. In Yen, S. S. C. and Jaffe, R. B. (eds.) *Reproductive Endocrinology: Physiology, Pathophysiology and Clinical Management*, 3rd edn., pp. 181–237. (Philadelphia: W. B. Saunders Company)
2. Gougeon, A. (1996). Regulation of ovarian follicular development in primates: facts and hypotheses. *Endocr. Rev.*, **17**, 121–55
3. Syrop, C. H., Willhoite, A. and Van Voorhis, B. J. (1995). Ovarian volume: a novel outcome predictor for assisted reproduction. *Fertil. Steril.*, **64**, 1167–71
4. Danninger, B., Brunner, M., Obruca, A. and Feichtinger, W. (1996). Prediction of ovarian hyperstimulation syndrome by ultrasound volumetric assessment of baseline ovarian volume prior to stimulation. *Hum. Reprod.*, **11**, 1597–9
5. de Ziegler, D., Cedars, M., Randle, D., Lu, J. H. K., Judd, H. L. and Meldrum, D. R. (1987). Suppression of the ovary using a GnRH agonist prior to stimulation for oocyte retrieval. *Fertil. Steril.*, **48**, 807–10
6. de Ziegler, D., Bergeron, C., Cornel, C., Médalie, A., Massai, M. R., Milgrom, E., Frydman, R. and Bouchard, P. (1992). Effects of luteal estradiol on the secretory transformation of human endometrium and plasma gonadotropins. *J. Clin. Endocrinol. Metab.*, **74**, 322–31
7. Le Nestour, E., Marraoui, J., Lahlou, N., Roger, M., de Ziegler, D. and Bouchard, P. (1993). Role of estradiol in the rise in follicle-stimulating hormone levels during the luteal–follicular transition. *J. Clin. Endocrinol. Metab.*, **77**, 439–42
8. Roseff, S. J., Bangah, M. L., Kettel, L. M., Vale, W., Rivier, J., Burger, H. G. and Yen, S. S. C. (1989). Dynamic changes in circulating inhibin levels during the luteal–follicular transition of the human menstrual cycle. *J. Clin. Endocrinol. Metab.*, **69**, 1033–9
9. de Ziegler, D., Cornel, C., Bergeron, C., Hazout, A., Bouchard, P. and Frydman, R. (1991). Controlled preparation of the endometrium with exogenous estradiol and progesterone in women having functioning ovaries. *Fertil. Steril.*, **56**, 851–5
10. de Ziegler, D., Jääskeläinen, A. S., Brioschi, P. A. and Bulletti, C. (1998). Synchronization of endogenous and exogenous FSH stimuli in controlled ovarian hyperstimulation (COH). *Hum. Reprod.*, **13**, 561–4
11. Pache, T. D., Wladimiroff, J. W., Hop, W. C. and Fauser, B. C. (1992). How to discriminate between normal and polycystic ovaries: transvaginal ultrasound study. *Radiology*, **183**, 421–3
12. Tepper, R., Zalel, Y., Markov, S., Cohen, I. and Beyth, Y. (1995). Ovarian volume in postmenopausal women – suggestions to an ovarian size nomogram for menopausal age. *Acta Obstet. Gynecol. Scand.*, **74**, 208–11
13. Cohen, H. L., Tice, H. M. and Mandel, F. S. (1990). Ovarian volumes measured by ultrasound: bigger than we think. *Radiology*, **177**, 189–92
14. Saxton, D. W., Farquhar, C. M., Rae, T., Beard, R. W., Anderson, M. C. and Wadsworth, J. (1990). Accuracy of ultrasound measurements of female pelvic organs. *Br. J. Obstet. Gynaecol.*, **97**, 695–9
15. Kyei-Mensah, A., Zaidi, J., Pittrof, R., Shaker, A., Campbell, S. and Tan, S. L. (1996). Transvaginal three-dimensional ultrasound: accuracy of follicular volume measurements. *Fertil. Steril.*, **65**, 371–6
16. Higgins, R. V., Van Nagel, J. R., Woods, C. H., Thompson, E. A. and Kryscio, R. J. (1990). Interobserver variation in ovarian measurements using transvaginal sonography. *Gynecol. Oncol.*, **39**, 69–71
17. Mehta, A. E., Matwijiw, I., Lyons, E. A. and Faiman, C. (1992). Noninvasive diagnosis of resistant ovary syndrome by ultrasonography. *Fertil. Steril.*, **57**, 56–61

Uterine causes of infertility

9

S. Kupesic and A. Kurjak

INTRODUCTION

The uterine cavity must provide an environment for successful sperm migration from the cervix to the Fallopian tube. Normality of the mucosal lining, glandular secretion and vascularity are necessary to support implantation and placentation. Uterine anomalies, polyps, myomata, neoplasia, infections and intrauterine scar tissue can lead to poor reproductive performance. Attempts have been made to correlate the sonographic parameters (such as thickness and reflectivity) and endometrial receptivity. This chapter emphasizes the role of transvaginal sonography and color Doppler imaging in evaluation of luteal function and detection of uterine abnormalities.

CONGENITAL ANOMALIES

Diagnosis of anatomic disorders is made in 38–55% of patients with recurrent pregnancy loss[1,2]. Sonographic identification of duplication anomalies of the uterus (such as septate uterus, bicornuate uterus or uterus didelphys) has the highest sensitivity and specificity during the secretory phase of the menstrual cycle. However, the accuracy of ultrasound for diagnosing uterine anomalies depends on the severity of the anomaly[3]. During the secretory phase the endometrium is most prominent: a separated echogenic line representing the endometrium surrounded by hypoechoic myometrium, and contour abnormalities are easily identified (Figure 1). Conversely, a careful search with the transvaginal transducer may demonstrate a single uterine horn and atypical endometrial echoes in a patient with uterus unicollis[4]. Large quantities of intracavitary fluid should raise the suspicion of an underlying obstruction in a case of inperforate hymen or vaginal atresia.

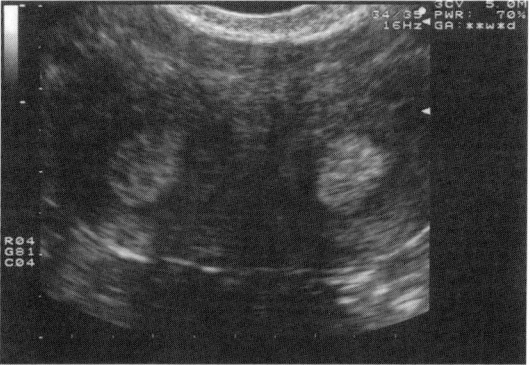

Figure 1 A transvaginal ultrasound scan demonstrating a duplication anomaly of the uterus. Note the two separate endometria during the secretory phase of the menstrual cycle

The use of continuous sonographic visualization for the assessment of the endometrial cavity during and after instillation of a contrast fluid is called sonohysterography[5]. Using this method uterine septa are precisely visualized and the extent of the septum can be delineated. In the hysterosonographic study of Randolph and colleagues[6] the results agreed with those of hysteroscopic examination in 53 out of 54 patients, yielding a sensitivity of 98% and a specificity of 100%.

ENDOMETRIAL POLYPS

Endometrial polyps are anatomic defects that are implicated in the etiology of recurrent pregnancy loss and infertility. Polyps appear as diffuse or focal thickening of the endometrium. Using sonohysterography an intracavitary polyp is seen surrounded by anechoic fluid, and the point of attachment can be visualized[5] (Figure 2). If the examination is performed in the follicular phase, use of the distending medium is not necessary to detect

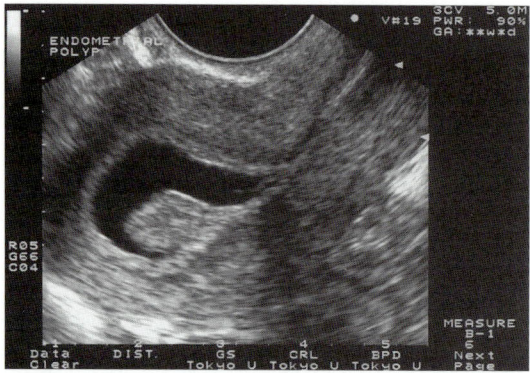

Figure 2 A transvaginal ultrasound scan of the uterus of an infertile patient with irregular menstrual bleeding, after injection of isotonic saline. Note the area of increased endometrial thickening representing a polyp

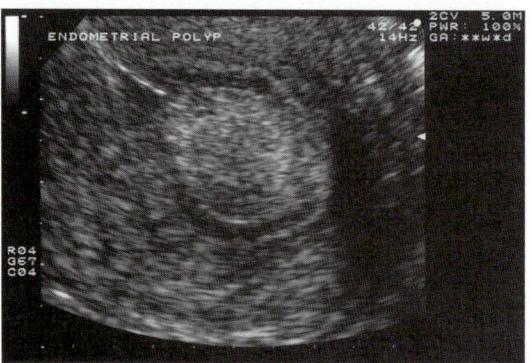

Figure 3 A transvaginal ultrasound scan of the uterus demonstrating a focal area of increased echogenicity. This is a case of an endometrial polyp

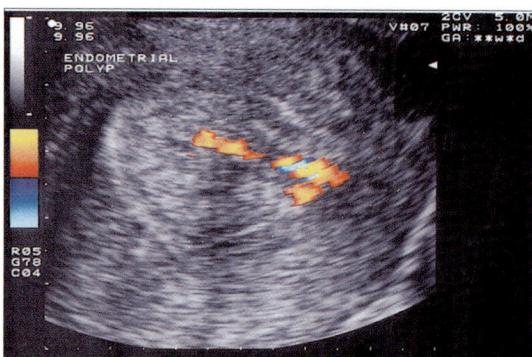

Figure 4 Transvaginal color Doppler demonstrates a focal area of increased echogenicity and a peripheral distribution of regularly separated vessels, typical of an endometrial polyp

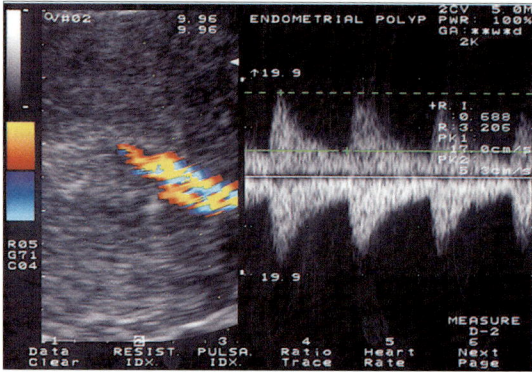

Figure 5 In the same patient as in Figure 4, pulsed Doppler indicates a benign uterine mass represented by the moderate-to-high resistance index (0.69)

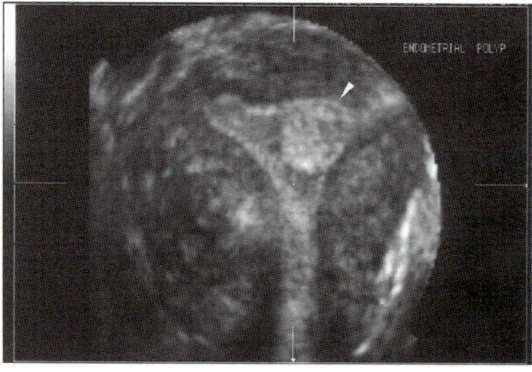

Figure 6 A case of an endometrial polyp as seen by three-dimensional ultrasound. The polyp is demonstrated as localized endometrial thickening which does not affect the whole of the uterine cavity. The volume of the polyp is therefore smaller than the volume of other diffuse endometrial disorders

abnormal endometrial thickening (Figure 3). However, during the periovulatory and secretory phase, polyps are better visualized when outlined by fluid.

By using transvaginal color and pulsed Doppler we can study minor arteries supplying the growth of the endometrial polyp (Figures 4 and 5). Three-dimensional ultrasound allows a detailed analysis of the uterine cavity in frontal reformatted sections which enables clear demarcation of polyps (Figure 6).

SUBMUCOUS FIBROIDS

The diagnosis of a submucous leiomyoma is based on distortion of the uterine contour,

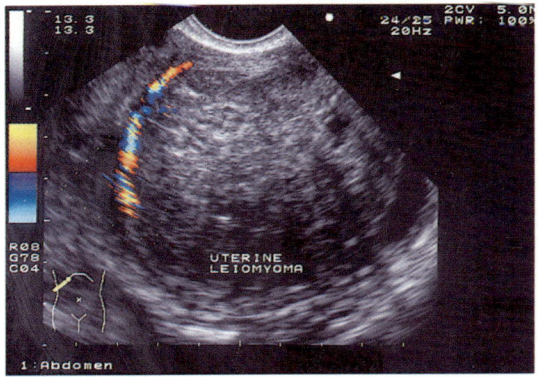

Figure 7 A transvaginal sonogram of a patient with a posterior isoechoic leiomyoma. Color Doppler imaging demonstrates a thick vessel encircling the uterine leiomyoma

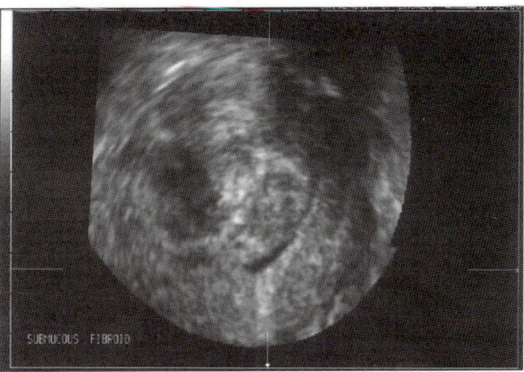

Figure 9 A submucous fibroid occupying the majority of the uterine cavity as seen by three-dimensional ultrasound

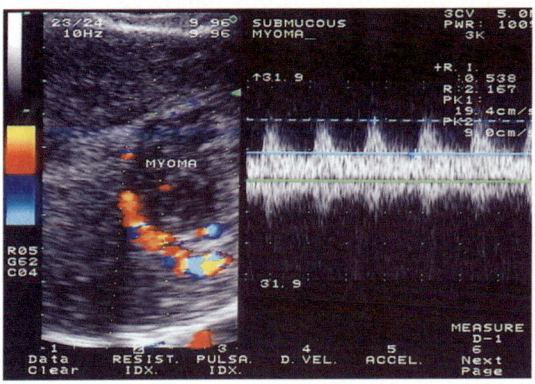

Figure 8 A transvaginal sonogram of a submucous leiomyoma in an infertile patient. Color signals explored by pulsed Doppler waveform analysis show moderate resistance to blood flow (resistance index 0.54)

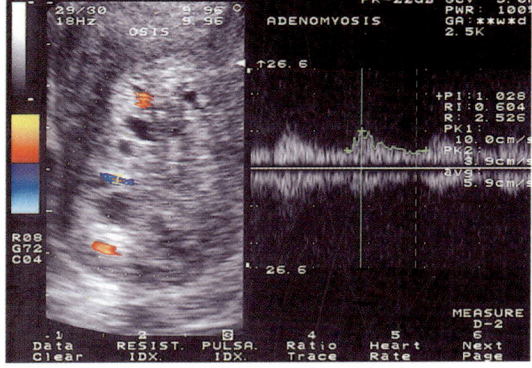

Figure 10 A diffusely enlarged uterus, with a thickened 'Swiss cheese' appearance of the myometrium, shows increased vascularity. Waveform analysis demonstrates low velocity and moderate resistance to blood flow (resistance index 0.60) indicative of adenomyosis

uterine enlargement and textural changes. Since leiomyomas have a varying amount of smooth muscle and connective tissue, these benign tumors also have a variety of sonographic features[6]. Sonographic texture ranges from hypoechoic to echogenic, depending on the amount of smooth muscle and connective tissue. Central ischemia, which is a consequence of tumor enlargement and inadequate blood supply, is usually followed by various stages of degeneration. The most common cause of calcification within the uterus is calcific degeneration within a fibroid. Other types of degeneration include cystic, myxomatous, and hyaline degeneration. Sometimes, because of the variety of appearances, submucous leiomyomas may be mistaken for endometrial polyps, endometrial carcinoma, blood or mucus. Fedele and associates[7] evaluated the accuracy of transvaginal sonography in detection of small submucous myomas in patients who underwent both transvaginal ultrasound examination and hysteroscopy before hysterectomy. The sensitivity and specificity of transvaginal sonography were similar to those of hysteroscopy in that study.

In patients with submucous fibroids the uterine environment is not conducive to implantation of a fertilized ovum and the blood supply might be inadequate[8]. Deligdish and Loewenthal[9] performed a histological study of the endometrium at four sites in uteri containing submucous myomas. They found atrophy of the endometrial glands and stroma in the endometrium overlying or opposite the leiomyoma, while at the border of the leiomyoma, hyperplastic glands were detected. This finding is secondary to increased vascularity and increased estrogen concentrations. Farrer-Brown and colleagues[10] were able to demonstrate vascular obstruction and venous dilatation within the overlying endometrium. Therefore, a submucous leiomyoma may reduce blood flow, cause progressive congestion and reduce the delivery of hormones necessary for normal endometrial development. These changes can result in atrophy of the endometrium and inadequate placentation. Furthermore, submucous leiomyomas may interfere with expansion of the fetus or limit the compliance of the uterus[11].

A leiomyoma grows centripetally as proliferations of smooth muscle cells and fibrous connective tissue, creating a pseudocapsule of compressed muscle fibers. Therefore, color Doppler demonstrates most of the myometrial blood vessels at its periphery (Figure 7). The presence of blood vessels in the central portion of the leiomyoma is usually correlated with necrotic, degenerative and inflammatory changes. These vessels display lower resistance index (RI) values than peripherally located vessels, and can sometimes be misinterpreted as a malignant neovascular pulsed Doppler signal[12]. Vascular impedance to blood flow in myometrial supplying vessels depends not only on size but location within the uterus. A significant difference was shown in blood flow characteristics for leiomyoma-supplying vessels between entirely subserosal versus intramural and submucous leiomyomas. Lower impedance values for subserosal leiomyomas can be explained by the fact that these leiomyomas are supplied with blood vessels through a very small contact area (Figure 8). These blood vessels are surrounded with loose connective tissue and therefore dilated, with very low vascular impedance to blood flow. In contrast, submucous leiomyomas and those located within the myometrium are supplied by blood vessels with higher vascular impedance. A high basal tonus of the myometrial tissue surrounding intramural or submucous leiomyomas could cause a difference in hemodynamic parameters. Three-dimensional ultrasound precisely estimates the relationship between a submucous leiomyoma and the uterine cavity (Figure 9).

Kurjak and colleagues[12] performed transvaginal color flow evaluation in 101 patients with palpable uterine fibroids and 60 healthy volunteers. The mean resistance index from the periphery of the leiomyomas was 0.54, and the mean pulsatility index (PI) was 0.89. The pathohistological finding was a benign uterine tumor in all cases, even when the RI was very low. Lowered resistance indices were present in cases with necrosis and secondary degenerative and inflammatory changes within the fibroid. Increased blood flow velocity and decreased RI (mean 0.74) in both uterine arteries occurred in patients with uterine fibroids.

ADENOMYOSIS

Adenomyosis, characterized by ingrowing of the endometrium into the myometrium, is usually asymptomatic, but may be presented by uterine bleeding, pain and infertility. A difusely enlarged uterus without discrete fibroids and an intact endometrium has been reported as a suggestive appearance of adenomyosis[13]. Disordered echogenicity of the middle layer of the myometrium is present in some severe cases.

Multiple small cysts in the myometrium have been reported as a suggestive finding of adenomyosis[2]. The reported sensitivity and specificity of transvaginal ultrasound in detection of this benign entity are 86% and 50%, respectively[13]. Color Doppler may reveal increased vascularity, mainly characterized by moderate vascular resistance (Figure 10).

ENDOMETRITIS

Chronic endometritis is characterized by increased echogenicity, thickness and vascularity of the endometrium[8]. The most common cause of chronic endometrial infection is *Mycobacterium tuberculosis*. During the activation of infection, pregnancy often terminates ectopically or as an abortion. Transvaginal sonographic findings may include calcified pelvic lymph nodes or smaller irregular calcifications in the adnexa and deformity of the endometrial cavity suggestive of adhesions in the absence of a history of prior curettage or abortion. In the acute stage of endometritis, low- to moderate-impedance blood flow signals are easily obtained on the periphery of the endometrium. Blood flow is usually absent in cases with irreversible tissue damage. Transvaginal sonography allows elucidation of the abnormal endometrial morphology, after which appropriate cultures should be taken and broad-spectrum antibiotic therapy administered. In order to prevent the development of intrauterine adhesions (especially after dilatation and curettage), administration of conjugated estrogens for 1 to 2 months is recommended. This therapy allows regeneration of the healthy endometrium, which is paralleled by a sharp increase in end-diastolic velocities of the spiral arteries at the time of color flow and pulsed Doppler analysis.

ASHERMAN'S SYNDROME

In 1948 Asherman described eight cases of intrauterine stenosis[14]. Destruction of the endometrium may result in scarring and the development of bands of scar tissue, or synechiae, within the uterine cavity. This destruction may occur as a result of vigorous curettage of the uterus following an abortion or, more often, after a curettage of an advanced pregnancy. Tuberculosis may also cause uterine synechiae, but only in rare cases. This may result in formation of adhesive bands of different sizes with a subsequent partial or total obliteration of the endometrial cavity. The menstrual pattern is characterized by amenorrhea or hypomenorrhea.

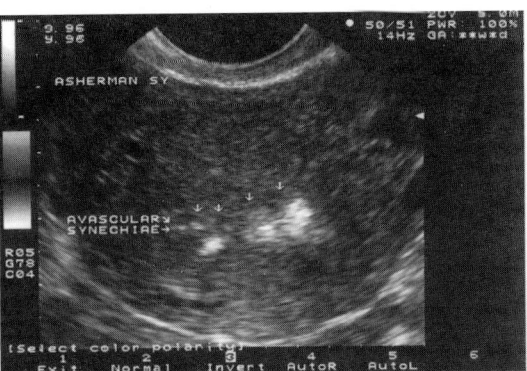

Figure 11 A transvaginal sonogram of an infertile patient with intrauterine synechiae. Note the hyperechoic bridges within the endometrial cavity. Color Doppler does not reveal increased vascularity

Patients with endometrial adhesion such as Asherman's syndrome may have a distorted endometrial pattern with areas where no endometrium can be imaged mixed with areas that appear normal[15]. Adhesions are observed as endometrial irregularities or hyperechoic bridges within the endometrial cavity (Figure 11).

Schlaff and Hurst[16] analyzed seven amenorrheic patients with severe Asherman's syndrome. Transvaginal sonography demonstrated a well-developed endometrial stripe in three of the seven women, while three others had virtually no endometrium seen. All the patients with well-developed endometrium were found to have adhesions excluding the lower uterine segment and had resumption of normal menses and normalization of the cavity after hysteroscopy. The women with minimal endometrium had no cavity identified and derived no benefit from surgery. The conclusion of that study was that endometrial pattern on transvaginal sonography is highly predictive of both surgical and clinical outcome in patients with severe Asherman's syndrome characterized by complete obstruction of the cavity at hysterosalpingography.

Intrauterine synechiae do not present increased vascularity on color Doppler examination (Figure 11). They are better visualized during menstruation when intracavitary fluid outlines them, or following hysterosonography.

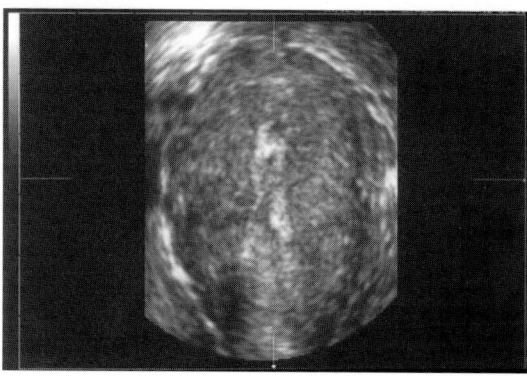

Figure 12 A three-dimensional ultrasound scan demonstrates an irregular uterine cavity with a significantly reduced endometrial volume suggestive of Asherman's syndrome

Three-dimensional ultrasound demonstrates a significant reduction of the endometrial cavity volume in all reformatted sections (Figure 12).

ENDOMETRIAL FACTORS IN INFERTILITY

Ultrasonographic examination is a non-invasive procedure and has the advantage that serial observation of the endometrial texture and thickness may be easily analyzed.

Endometrium, which is the target organ for circulating estradiol and progesterone, displays textural variations during the menstrual cycle. In the postmenstrual period endometrium is visualized as a thin echogenic interface. In the proliferative phase it becomes isoechoic in comparison with the myometrium. As ovulation approaches the endometrium becomes more echogenic secondary to the development of secretions within the endometrial glands[3]. A hypoechoic halo probably arises from the inner layer of the myometrium, while a hypoechoic area within the endometrium results from edema of the compacta. During the secretory phase a progressive increase of acoustic enhancement is observed as a result of progesterone action. This change of the endometrial pattern is due to a progressive increase of the mucous secretions and coiling phenomena of the endometrial glands. These events take place from the endometrial base towards the surface.

Data on the use of sonography to interpret endometrial function are conflicting. Gonen and Casper[17] described three different types of endometrial texture on the day of oocyte retrieval in an *in vitro* fertilization program. They found that triple-line endometrium was more likely to be associated with successful implantation than the two other types (homogeneously hyperechoic or intermediate iso-echogenic pattern). Furthermore, the endometrial thickness was greater in patients who became pregnant (8.7 ± 0.4 mm) than in the group who did not (7.5 ± 0.2 mm). Some publications[18–20] suggest that in cases in which endometrial thickness is less than 6 mm, embryo implantation appears drastically reduced. When it exceeded 9 or 10 mm, optimal implantation rates were obtained. Smith and colleagues[21] felt that both endometrial thickness and pattern were important. Other investigators[22–24] have also analyzed the relationship between the endometrial thickness and texture and the outcome, and have found statistically significant correlations.

Kepic and associates[25] determined that endometrial thickness and pattern, follicle size and estradiol levels correlated to both the likelihood of pregnancy and subsequent outcome. Contrary to these data, studies of Fleischer and co-workers[26,27] found no correlation between endometrial thickness and embryo implantation. Such conflicting results can be explained by the variability of the endometrial appearance according to the timing of the ultrasound scan (day of human chorionic gonadotropin administration, day of oocyte pick-up or day of embryo transfer). It seems that the most promising data are obtained when the study is performed on the day of human chorionic gonadotropin (hCG) administration, since progesterone production does not interfere with endometrial characteristics at this period of the menstrual cycle.

Li and colleagues[28] examined the prevalence of abnormal endometrial development during the luteal phase of an infertile population ($n = 142$) and a fertile population ($n = 68$). The authors used histological dating by traditional criteria. The prevalence of a

Table 1 A comparison of the age, duration of infertility, follicular phase length, luteal phase length, and the prevalence of retarded endometrial development (dated by traditional criteria) among four groups of infertile subjects and a group of normal fertile subjects

	Group I (tubal) (n = 34)	Group II (male) (n = 21)	Group III (endometriosis) (n = 48)	Group IV (unexplained) (n = 48)	Group V (normal) (n = 68)
Age (years)	32.5 ± 4.0	30.8 ± 4.0	34.0 ± 2.9	32.7 ± 4.4	33.4 ± 4.0
Duration of infertility (years)	6.1 ± 3.3	6.8 ± 2.7	6.9 ± 2.9	6.0 ± 3.3	—
Follicular phase length (days)	14.3 ± 3.2	13.7 ± 2.1	13.9 ± 2.1	14.5 ± 2.4	13.6 ± 1.8
Luteal phase length (days)	13.2 ± 1.0	13.1 ± 1.6	11.9 ± 1.5	12.7 ± 1.8	12.9 ± 1.5
Prevalence of retarded endometrium (%)	1/34 (2.9)	3/39 (7.7)	6/21 (29)*	10/48 (21)*	3/68 (4.4)

Data are given as means ± SD or numbers (%). *$p < 0.01$ compared with fertile subjects. From reference 27, with permission

retarded endometrium was significantly higher in infertile than in fertile women (14% vs. 4.4%). The authors subdivided the infertile patients into four subgroups according to the cause of infertility. Patients suffering from endometriosis had a significantly higher prevalence (29%) of abnormal endometrial development, while no difference occurred in patients with tubal or male infertility. Furthermore, 21% of patients with unexplained infertility had out-of-phase endometrium. The summarized results of this study are presented in Table 1.

Further technological development has resulted in a combination of transvaginal color and pulsed Doppler with real-time sonography. This method has been proposed for obtaining valuable information concerning the uterine receptivity by studying the uterine artery perfusion. Furthermore, the uterine artery impedance indices are found to be predictive of pregnancy outcome[29–31]. The blood supply to the endometrium is derived from the branches of the uterine arteries. Radial arteries extend through the myometrium and form two types of terminal branches: straight and coiled. The straight branches, called basal arteries, supply the basalis layer of the endometrium. The coiled branches, called spiral arteries, transverse that endometrium and supply the functionalis layer[32]. The spiral

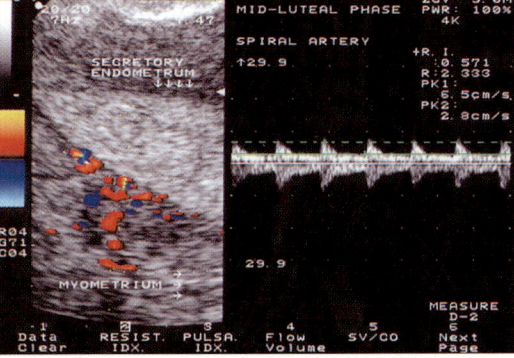

Figure 13 A transvaginal sonogram of the secretory-changed endometrium. The pulsed Doppler waveform analysis obtained from the spiral arteries shows moderate-to-low resistance during the mid-luteal phase of the menstrual cycle

arteries, like the endometrium and unlike the basal arteries, are remarkably responsive to hormonal changes during the menstrual cycle (Figure 13).

Kupesic and Kurjak[33] were the first to report spiral artery perfusion during the periovulatory period in spontaneous and induced ovarian cycles with both sonographically and hormonally confirmed ovulation. Increased blood flow velocity and decreased spiral artery impedance occurred the day before ovulation in the group with spontaneous cycles (PI 1.13) compared with the hormonally stimulated group (PI 2.32). Endometrial thickness was

Table 2 Endometrial thickness (mm) during 27 spontaneous and 51 induced cycles

	Days before and after ovulation				
	−3	−2	−1	0	+1
Spontaneous cycles (n = 27)	8 ± 1.1*	10 ± 1.2	12 ± 1.4	12 ± 1.5	13 ± 1.2
Induced cycles					
CC (n = 15)	7 ± 1.5	9 ± 1.4	11 ± 1.4	12 ± 1.2	13 ± 1.6
CC subsequent cycles (n = 12)	4 ± 1.5	6 ± 2.0	7 ± 2.0	7 ± 1.8	7 ± 2.0
CC/hMG (n = 16)	5 ± 1.5	6 ± 2.0	8 ± 2.0	9 ± 2.5	9 ± 2.0
hMG (n = 8)	6 ± 1.8	8 ± 2.0	11 ± 1.8	12 ± 2.0	12 ± 1.8

Data are given as means ± SD. CC, clomiphene citrate; hMG, human menopausal gonadotropin. From reference 33, with permission

significantly decreased in patients in whom clomiphene citrate was used for follicular stimulation three or more times, compared with spontaneous cycles and those stimulated with clomiphene citrate for the first time (Table 2). Significantly thicker endometrium was observed in human menopausal gonadotropin (hMG) stimulated patients compared with the clomiphene citrate/hMG group throughout the follicular phase of the cycle. Clear flow velocity waveforms were obtained from 80% of the endometria of the patients stimulated for the first time with clomiphene citrate. Spiral artery perfusion was detected and evaluated on a daily basis only in 16.7% of patients with clomiphene citrate stimulation for three or more cycles. Analyzing the spiral artery blood flow according to the type of stimulation, a significant difference ($p < 0.001$) occurred in the clomiphene citrate/hMG-stimulated group compared with the other groups.

Clomiphene citrate is shown to deplete estrogen receptors in estrogen-sensitive tissue, influencing both endometrial growth and pattern[34–37]. Kupesic and Kurjak[33] found a strong correlation between endometrial thickness and flow velocities. However, this does not apply to the group of patients stimulated with clomiphene citrate/hMG and who had normal endometrial growth, where absence of diastolic flow was detected in 55.6% of patients.

Zaidi and colleagues[38] analyzed endometrial thickness, endometrial morphology and presence or absence of subendometrial or intraendometrial color flow in 96 infertile patients undergoing *in vitro* fertilization treatment. The results of the study obtained on the day of hCG administration were related to the pregnancy rates. The overall pregnancy rate was 32.3% and there was no significant difference between pregnant and non-pregnant groups with regard to endometrial thickness. The pregnancy rates were not significantly different for different endometrial morphological patterns ($p > 0.05$). The absence of endometrial blood flow was associated with failure of implantation ($p < 0.05$). However, no difference in pregnancy rates was found related to the zones of vascular penetration (subendometrial, outer hyperechogenic zone or inner hypoechogenic zone). Both studies analyzing endometrial blood flow stated that color and pulsed Doppler can be used to monitor the uterine receptivity and to reveal unexplained infertility problems[33,38].

Another problem of clinical importance is luteal phase deficiency (LPD). Luteal phase deficiency is defined as a lack of more than 2 days in histologic development of the endometrium compared to the day of the cycle[39,40]. Several methods have been developed to evaluate endometrial function, such as quantitative histology, electron microscopy, histochemistry and immunohistochemistry, hysteroscopy and measurement of endometrial protein levels in plasma or endometrial washings. All these methods are invasive and cause some discomfort to the patient and could potentially interrupt implantation in a conception cycle. Therefore, Doherty and colleagues have used transvaginal sonography for the assessment of luteal phase endometrium and non-invasive identification of patients with LPD[41].

A recent Doppler study[42] was undertaken in an attempt to establish a relationship between the color Doppler analysis of the segmental uterine and ovarian circulation and histologic dating on the endometrial biopsy. Spiral arteries in the control group demonstrated an RI of 0.53 ± 0.04 during the periovulatory phase, while RI values of 0.50 ± 0.02 and 0.51 ± 0.04 were obtained during the mid-luteal and late luteal phases, respectively. Higher impedance values during the periovulatory phase (RI 0.70 ± 0.06, $p < 0.001$), mid-luteal phase (RI 0.72 ± 0.06, $p < 0.001$) and late luteal phase (RI 0.72 ± 0.04, $p < 0.001$) were obtained from the spiral arteries in the LPD group. Data on ovarian and intraovarian vascular impedance demonstrated significant differences between the normal and LPD groups. Color and pulsed Doppler analysis of the corpus luteum and minor endometrial vessels may therefore aid in assessing luteal phase adequacy. An interested reader can find more on corpus luteum insufficiency in Chapter 5.

AGE AND ENDOMETRIAL FACTOR

Navot and colleagues[43] and Edwards and associates[44] addressed the relationship between increasing maternal age and a decline in fertility. Both studies found that amenorrheic women or patients over the age of 40 years who received donor oocytes had better implantation and pregnancy rates than those who were cycling but received their own oocytes. Therefore, the main determinant of reproductive outcome in this age group is oocyte quality rather than endometrial receptivity. Decline in fertility potential may be readily restored by oocyte donation in an artificially induced cycle. Recent studies by Batista and colleagues[45] proved normal luteal and endometrial secretory function and normal endometrial maturation in cycling women aged over 40 years. Their results clearly indicate that implantation failure due to a hostile endometrium does not play a significant role in the decline of fertility in this population.

Kurjak and Kupesic[46] performed serial measurements throughout the menstrual cycle in 120 normally cycling women with documented infertility, 85 postmenopausal patients and 45 postmenopausal patients receiving hormone replacement therapy. They found obvious changes in the flow velocity patterns of the ovarian, uterine, radial and spiral arteries with age. The fact that the uterine artery resistance index did not change significantly in the first postmenopausal years strongly supports the thesis that the aging process initially affects the uterus less than the ovary. Furthermore, the uterine environment could be easily manipulated during the menopausal years by proper hormonal stimulation.

ENDOMETRIAL PERISTALSIS

Birnholtz[47] was the first to report endometrial movements as a reflection of myometrial activity. These contractions are most common in the follicular phase and culminate around ovulation. At that time the contractions are towards the fundus and may help sperm transport and maintenance of pregnancy. However, these first observations were made by transabdominal ultrasound, and a quantification of the movement was not attempted.

Oike and associates[48] used transvaginal sonography to observe endometrial movements in the proliferative phase of the menstrual cycle, although they were not able to detect any contractility during the secretory phase of the menstrual cycle. In 1990 Abramowitz and Archer[49] and De Vries and colleagues[50] made a classification of the movements in terms of intensity and frequency using a transvaginal probe. The ideal method to observe this peristaltic motion is by recording the examination on video-tape and later playing back the tape at accelerated speed. De Vries and colleagues[50] performed 46 examinations on 42 consecutive women. Contractions were retrograde in all phases of the menstrual cycles except during menstruation.

The same observations have been made by Lyons and associates[51].

Oike and colleagues[52] correlated endometrial activity with hormonal levels. They found that endometrial peristalsis has a strong correlation with estradiol levels. Rising progesterone levels seem to reduce the frequency of endometrial/myometrial movements. Preliminary data of Abramowitz and Archer[49] suggest that peristaltic contraction disturbance may play a role in some cases of unexplained infertility.

THE CERVICAL FACTOR IN INFERTILITY

Cervical mucus plays an important role in the normal process of fertilization[53]. It enables sperm to survive for up to 48 h despite the harmful acid secretions within the female vagina. The nature of cervical mucus depends on the hormonal state of the woman, so it changes during the menstrual cycle. During infection, it may be densely populated by leukocytes and other phagocytes, which are harmful to sperm survival. Also, in up to 10% of the fertile female population, antisperm antibodies may be found[53]. Although these are not cytotoxic, they interfere with and change the sperm motility.

The female cervix is clearly demonstrated both on transabdominal and transvaginal sonography, but it is also visible on gynecological examination using a speculum. The external and internal cervical canal should be accurately measured by transvaginal sonography; its width is a consequence of hormonal (estrogen) level changes and mucus secretion by the cervical glands. High blood flow velocity waveforms in both uterine arteries measured by transvaginal color Doppler in the periovulatory period parallel the production of watery cervical mucus at mid-cycle.

CONCLUSION

Transvaginal sonography has become an indispensable tool in the detection of uterine causes of infertility. Color Doppler investigation of the uterine perfusion and frontal reformatted sections of the uterus obtained by three-dimensional ultrasound assists the endocrinologist in evaluating the infertile patient. Improved resolution of current ultrasound equipment and recent technological developments reveal unknown causes of infertility and therefore unfold infertility investigation and treatment.

References

1. Kutteh, W. and Carr, B. (1993). Recurrent pregnancy loss. In Carr, B. R. and Blackwell, R. E. (eds.) *Textbook of Reproductive Medicine*, pp. 559–70. (Norwalk: Appleton and Lange)
2. Stray-Pedersen, B. and Stray-Pedersen, S. (1984). Etiological factors and subsequent reproductive performance in 195 couples with a prior history of habitual abortion. *Am. J. Obstet. Gynecol.*, **148**, 140–6
3. Fleischer, A. C. and Keppe, D. M. (1992). Benign conditions of the uterus, cervix and endometrium. In Nyberg, A., Hill, L. M., Bohm-Velez, M. and Mendelson, E. B. (eds.) *Transvaginal Ultrasound*, pp. 21–43. (St Louis: Mosby Year Book)
4. Funk, A. and Fendel, H. (1988). Sonography diagnosis of congenital uterine abnormalities. *Z. Geburts. Perinatol.*, **192**, 77–88

5. Cullinan, J. A., Fleischer, A. C., Kepple, D. M. and Aenoco, A. L. (1995). Sonohysterography: a technique for endometrial evaluation. *Radiographics*, **15**, 501–14
6. Randolph, J. R., Ying, Y. K., Maier, D. B., Schmidt, C. L. and Riddick, D. H. (1986). Comparison of real-time ultrasonography, hysterosalpingography and laparotomy/hysteroscopy in the evaluation of uterine abnormalities and tubal patency. *Fertil. Steril.*, **46**, 828–32
7. Fedele, L., Bianchi, S., Dorta, M., Brioschi, D., Zanotti, F., Vercellini, P. (1991). Transvaginal ultrasonography versus hysteroscopy in the diagnosis of uterine submucous myomas. *Obstet. Gynecol.*, **77**, 745–8
8. Kurjak, A. and Kupesic, S. (1994). Benign uterine conditions. In Kurjak, A. (ed.) *An Atlas*

of *Transvaginal Color Doppler*, pp. 247–317. (Carnforth, UK: Parthenon Publishing)

9. Deligdish, L. and Loewenthal, M. (1970). Endometrial changes associated with myomata of the uterus. *J. Clin. Pathol.*, **23**, 676

10. Farrer-Brown, G., Beilby, J. O. and Tarbit, M. H. (1971). Venous changes in the endometrium of myomatous uteri. *Obstet. Gynecol.*, **38**, 743

11. Winkel, A. C. (1993). Diagnosis and treatment of uterine pathology. In Carr, B. R. and Blackwell, R. E. (eds.) *Textbook of Reproductive Medicine*, pp. 481–505. (Norwalk: Appleton and Lange)

12. Kurjak, A., Kupesic, S. and Miric, D. (1992). The assessment of benign uterine tumor vascularization by transvaginal color Doppler. *Ultrasound Med. Biol.*, **18**, 645–9

13. Brosens, J. J., de Souza, N. M., Barker, F. G., Paraschos, T. and Winston, R. M. (1995). Endovaginal ultrasonography in the diagnosis of adenomyosis uteri: identifying the predictive characteristics. *Br. J. Obstet. Gynaecol.*, **102**, 471

14. Asherman, J. G. (1948). Amenorrhea traumatica (atretica). *J. Obstet. Gynaecol. Br. Emp.*, **55**, 23

15. Dodson, M. (1995). The endometrium. In Dodson, M. (ed.) *Transvaginal Ultrasound*, pp. 73–103. (New York: Churchill Livingstone)

16. Schlaff, W. D. and Hurst, B. S. (1995). Preoperative sonographic measurement of endometrial pattern predicts outcome of surgical repair in patients with severe Asherman's syndrome. *Fertil. Steril.*, **63**, 410–13

17. Gonen, Y. and Casper, R. F. (1990). Prediction of implantation by the sonographic appearance of the endometrium during controlled ovarian stimulation for *in vitro* fertilization. *J. In Vitro Fertil. Embryo Transfer*, **7**, 146–52

18. Dickey, R. P., Olar, T. T., Curole, D. N., Taylor, S. N. and Rye, P. H. (1992). Endometrial pattern and thickness associated with pregnancy outcome after assisted reproduction technologies. *Hum Reprod.*, **7**, 418–21

19. Sher, G., Herbert, C., Massarani, G. and Jacobs, M. H. (1991). Assessment of the late proliferative phase endometrium by ultrasonography in patients undergoing IVF-ET. *Hum. Reprod.*, **6**, 232–7

20. Glissant, A., de Mouzon, J. and Frydman, R. (1985). Ultrasound study of the endometrium during IVF cycles. *Fertil. Steril.*, **44**, 786–90

21. Smith, B., Porter, R., Ahuja, K. and Craft, I. (1984). Ultrasonic assessment of endometrial changes in stimulated cycles in an *in vitro* fertilization and embryo transfer program. *J. In Vitro Fertil. Embryo Transfer*, **1**, 233–8

22. Rabinowitz, R., Laufer, N., Lewin, A., Navot, D., Bar, I., Margalioth, E.J. and Schenker, J.J. (1986). The value of ultrasonographic endometrial measurement in the prediction of pregnancy following *in vitro* fertilization. *Fertil. Steril.*, **45**, 824–8

23. Welker, B. G., Dembruch, U., Diedrich, K., Al-Hasani, S. and Krebs, D. (1989). TVS of the endometrium during oocyte pick-up in stimulated cycles for IVF. *J. Ultrasound Med.*, **1**, 233–8

24. Thickman, D., Arger, P., Turek, R., Biasco, L., Mintz, M. and Coleman, B. (1986). Sonographic assessment of the endometrium in patients undergoing *in vitro* fertilization. *J. Ultrasound Med.*, **5**, 197–210

25. Kepic, T., Applebaum, M. and Valle, J. (1992). Preovulatory follicular size, endometrial appearance, and estradiol levels in both conception and non-conception cycles: a retrospective study. Presented at the *40th Annual Clinical Meeting of the American College of Obstetricians and Gynecologists*, April, Abstr. 20

26. Fleischer, A. C., Herbert, C. M., Sacks, G. A., Wentz, A. C., Entman, S. S. and James, A. E. Jr (1986). Sonography of the endometrium during conception and non-conception cycles of *in vitro* fertilization and embryo transfer. *Fertil. Steril.*, **46**, 442–7

27. Fleischer, A. C., Herbert, C. M., Sacks, G. A., Wentz, A. C. and Entman, S. S. (1986). Nonconception cycles of IVF-ET. *Fertil. Steril.*, **46**, 442–6

28. Li, T. C., Dockery, P. and Cooke, I. D. (1991). Endometrial development in the luteal phase of women with various types of infertility: comparison with women of normal fertility. *Hum. Reprod.*, **6**, 325–30

29. Sterzik, K., Grab, D., Sasse, V., Hutter, W., Rosenbusch, B. and Terinde, R. (1989). Doppler sonographic findings and their correlation with implantation in an *in vitro* fertilization program. *Fertil. Steril.*, **52**, 825–8

30. Steer, C. V., Campbell, S., Tan, S. L., Crayford, T., Mills, C., Mason, B. A. and Collins, W. P. (1992). The use of transvaginal color flow imaging after *in vitro* fertilization to identify optimum uterine conditions before embryo transfer. *Fertil. Steril.*, **57**, 372–6

31. Bassil, S., Magritte, J. P., Roth, J., Nisolle, M., Donnez, J. and Gordts, S. (1995). Uterine vascularity during stimulation and its correlation with implantation in *in vitro* fertilization. *Hum. Reprod.*, **6**, 1497–1501

32. Applebaum, M. (1995). The menstrual cycle, menopause, ovulation induction, and *in vitro* fertilization. In Copel, J. A. and Reed, K. L. (eds.) *Doppler Ultrasound in Obstetrics and Gynecology*, pp. 71–86. (New York: Raven Press Ltd.)

33. Kupesic, S. and Kurjak, A. (1993). Uterine and ovarian perfusion during the periovulatory period assessed by transvaginal color Doppler. *Fertil. Steril.*, **60**, 439–43

34. Aksel, S., Saracoglu, O. F., Yeoman, R. R. and Wiebe, R. H. (1986). Effects of clomiphene citrate on cytosolic estradiol and progesterone

receptor concentrations in secretory endometrium. *Am. J. Obstet. Gynecol.*, **155**, 1219–23

35. Wolman, I., Sagi, J., Pauzner, D., Yove, I., Seidman, D. S. and David, M. P. (1994). Transabdominal ultrasonographic evaluation of endometrial thickness in clomiphene citrate-stimulated cycles in relation to conception. *J. Clin. Ultrasound*, **22**, 109–12

36. Check, J. H., Dieterich, C. and Lurie, D. (1995). The effect of consecutive cycles of clomiphene citrate therapy on endometrial thickness and echo pattern. *Obstet. Gynecol.*, **86**, 341–5

37. Yagel, S., Ben-Chetrit, A., Anteby, E., Zacut, D., Hochner-Celnikier, D. and Ron, M. (1992). The effect of ethinyl estradiol on endometrial thickness and uterine volume during ovulation induction by clomiphene citrate. *Fertil. Steril.*, **57**, 33–6

38. Zaidi, J., Campbell, S., Pittrof, R. and Tan, S. L. (1995). Endometrial thickness, morphology, vascular penetration and velocimetry in predicting implantation in an *in vitro* fertilization program. *Ultrasound Obstet. Gynecol.*, **6**, 191–8

39. Noyes, R. W., Hertig, A. T. and Rock, J. (1950). Dating the endometrial biopsy. *Fertil. Steril.*, **1**, 3–25

40. Dawood, Y. M. (1994). Corpus luteum insufficiency. *Curr. Opin. Obstet. Gynecol.*, **6**, 121–7

41. Doherty, C. M., Silver, B., Binor, Z., Wood Molo, M. and Radwanska, E. (1993). Transvaginal ultrasonography and the assessment of luteal phase endometrium. *Am. J. Obstet. Gynecol.*, **168**, 1702–9

42. Kupesic, S., Kurjak, A., Vujisic, S. and Petrovic, Z. (1997). Luteal phase defect: comparison between Doppler velocimetry, histological and hormonal markers. *Ultrasound Obstet. Gynecol.*, **9**, 105–12

43. Navot, D., Bergh, P. A., Williams, M. A., Garrisi, G. J., Guzman, I., Sander, B. and Grunfeld, L. (1991). Poor oocyte quality rather than implantation failure as a cause of age-related decline in female fertility. *Lancet*, **337**, 1375–7

44. Edwards, R. G., Morcos, S., MacNamee, M., Balamaceda, J. P., Walters, D. E. and Asch, R. (1991). High fecundity of amenorrhoeic women in embryo-transfer programmes. *Lancet*, **338**, 292–4

45. Batista, M., Cartledge, T. P., Zellmer, A. M., Merimo, M. J., Axiotis, C., Bremner, N. J. and Nieman, L. K. (1995). Effects of aging on menstrual cycle hormones and endometrial maturation. *Fertil. Steril.*, **64**, 492–9

46. Kurjak, A. and Kupesic, S. (1995). Ovarian senescence and its significance on uterine and ovarian perfusion. *Fertil. Steril.*, **64**, 532–7

47. Birnholtz, J. (1984). Ultrasonographic visualization of endometrial movements. *Fertil. Steril.*, **41**, 157–8

48. Oike, K., Obata, S., Tagaki, K., Matsuo, K., Ishihan, K. and Kikuchi, S. (1988). Observation of endometrial movements with transvaginal sonography. *J. Ultrasound Med.*, **7**, 899

49. Abramowitz, J. S. and Archer, D. F. (1990). Uterine endometrial peristalsis – a transvaginal ultrasound study. *Fertil. Steril.*, **54**, 451–4

50. De Vries, K., Lyons, F. A., Ballard, G., Levi, C. S. and Lindsay, D. J. (1990). Contractions of the inner third of the myometrium. *Am. J. Obstet. Gynecol.*, **162**, 679–82

51. Lyons, E. A., Ballard, G., Taylor, P. H., Levi, C. S., Zhieng, X. H. and Kredentser, J. V. (1991). Characterization of subendometrial myometrial contractions throughout the menstrual cycle in normal fertile women. *Fertil. Steril.*, **55**, 771–4

52. Oike, K., Ishihara, K. and Kikuchi, S. (1990). A study of the endometrial movement and serum hormonal level in connection with uterine contraction. *Acta Obstet. Gynecol. Jpn.*, **42**, 86–92

53. Beck, V. W. (1988). The cervical factor. In Garcia, C. R., Mastroianni, L., Amelar, R. D. and Dubin, L. (eds.) *Current Therapy of Infertility 3*, pp. 118–21. (Toronto: BC Decker)

Three-dimensional ultrasound contribution in frontal uterus scan study

10

D. Moeglin, B. Benoit, D. de Ziegler and M. Massonneau

PRINCIPLES OF THREE-DIMENSIONAL ULTRASOUND

Three-dimensional ultrasound images are the result of the succession of three steps[1-4]:

(1) Acquisition and storing of consecutive ultrasonic tomograms;

(2) Three-dimensional matrix reconstruction;

(3) Three-dimensional data display.

Acquisition of three-dimensional data

The ultrasound volume is acquired as a series of tomographic images through ultrasonic sweep of a region of interest. This sweep can be a mechanical or a freehand movement.

In freehand acquisition, the operator sweeps the organ in the usual manner. The advantage of this technique is that it offers the operator optimal views and orientations, for example of complex surfaces.

In mechanical acquisition, the third dimension is obtained by mechanical movement (linear or rotational; Figure 1) of the transducer in a precise predefined manner. The advantage of the mechanical scanning approach is that it avoids the problem of scanning gaps that may reduce the image quality. However, it does not offer the flexibility of the freehand method.

A few seconds are required for scanning with any method. Three-dimensional data can be acquired in B-mode, color Doppler and power Doppler.

Limitations

To obtain distinct three-dimensional images, the original tomograms should have good

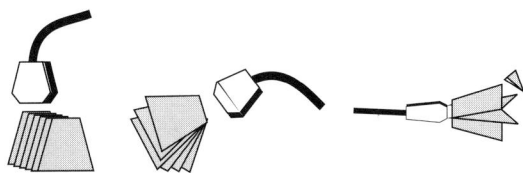

Figure 1 Different mechanical acquisition systems

picture quality and an optimal number of tomographic images. Usually more than 100 tomograms are necessary to constitute a set of three-dimensional data.

Reconstruction

Three-dimensional image reconstruction is the process that permits obtaining a three-dimensional representation from the acquired two-dimensional images.

The reconstruction process has been implemented in two distinct ways. In the first, the series of two-dimensional images are segmented to extract the desired features before the three-dimensional image is reconstructed (for example, in vascular echographic imaging, the lumenogram of a carotid artery). The second approach uses the acquired series of two-dimensional images to build a three-dimensional voxel-based Cartesian volume by placing each acquired two-dimensional image in its correct location in the volume (Figure 2). The gray-scale values of any voxels not sampled by the two-dimensional images are calculated by interpolation between the appropriate images.

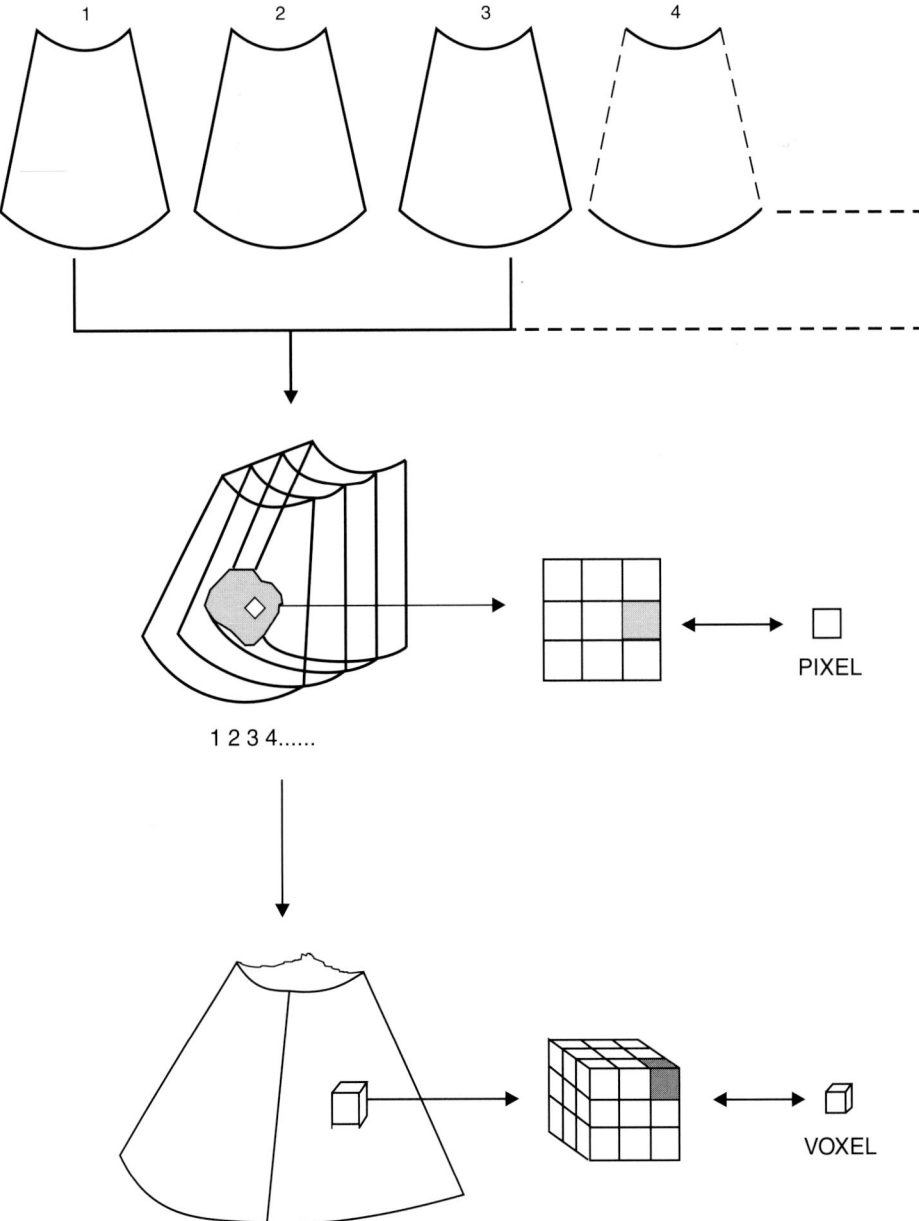

Figure 2 Construction of three-dimensional data sets

Three-dimensional ultrasound image display

There are many techniques for displaying three-dimensional images. These are divided into two classes: multiplanar and volume-based viewing. The optimal choice of the rendering technique is generally determined by the clinical application.

Multiplane viewing

Three perpendicular planes are displayed on the screen simultaneously, with screen cues as to

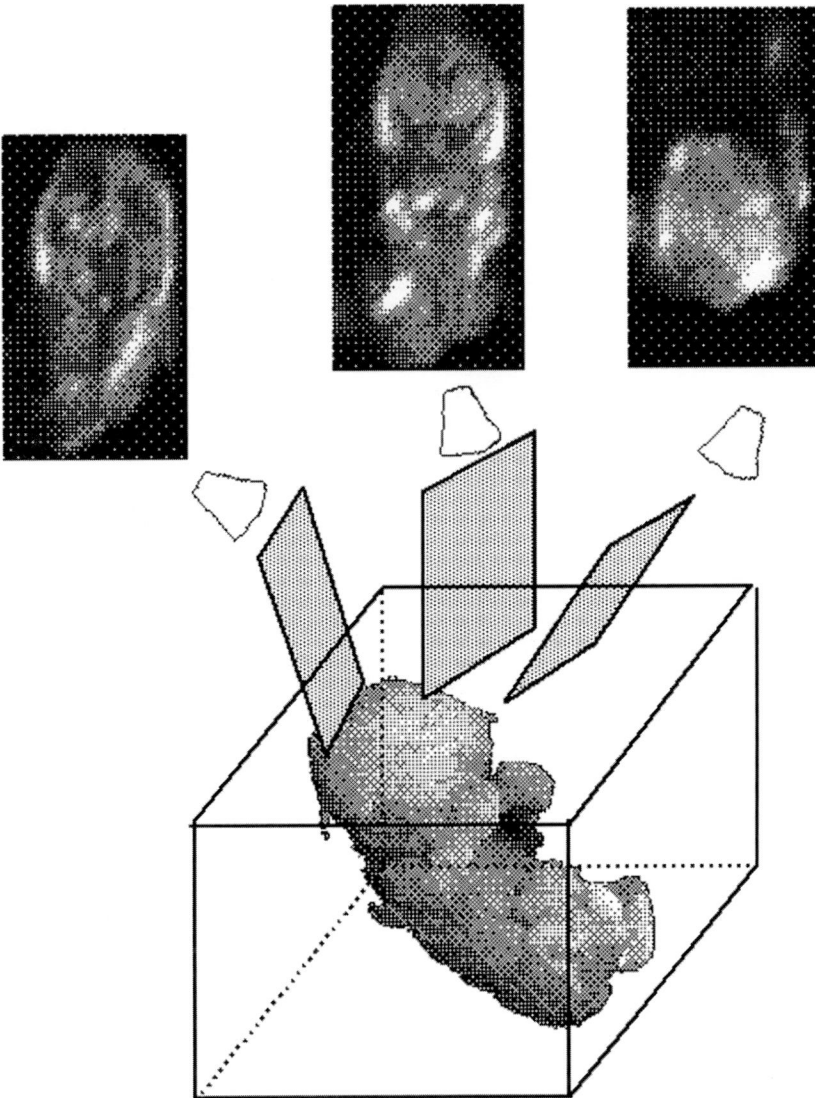

Figure 3 Three-dimensional surface imaging

their relative orientation and intersection. Thus, the operator can visualize a large selection of planes, including the oblique. It is this technique that interested us for the visualization of the frontal cross-sectional plane of the uterus.

Volume-based viewing

With shading, only the surface of the structure, such as the face of a baby or flowing blood, is displayed as an image (Figure 3).

With transparency or X-ray, the anatomy is displayed in a translucent manner. This approach is best suited for studying fetal skeletal images.

MATERIALS AND METHODS

The frontal tomograms of the uterus reported in this present study were obtained by two different methods. The first method is based on

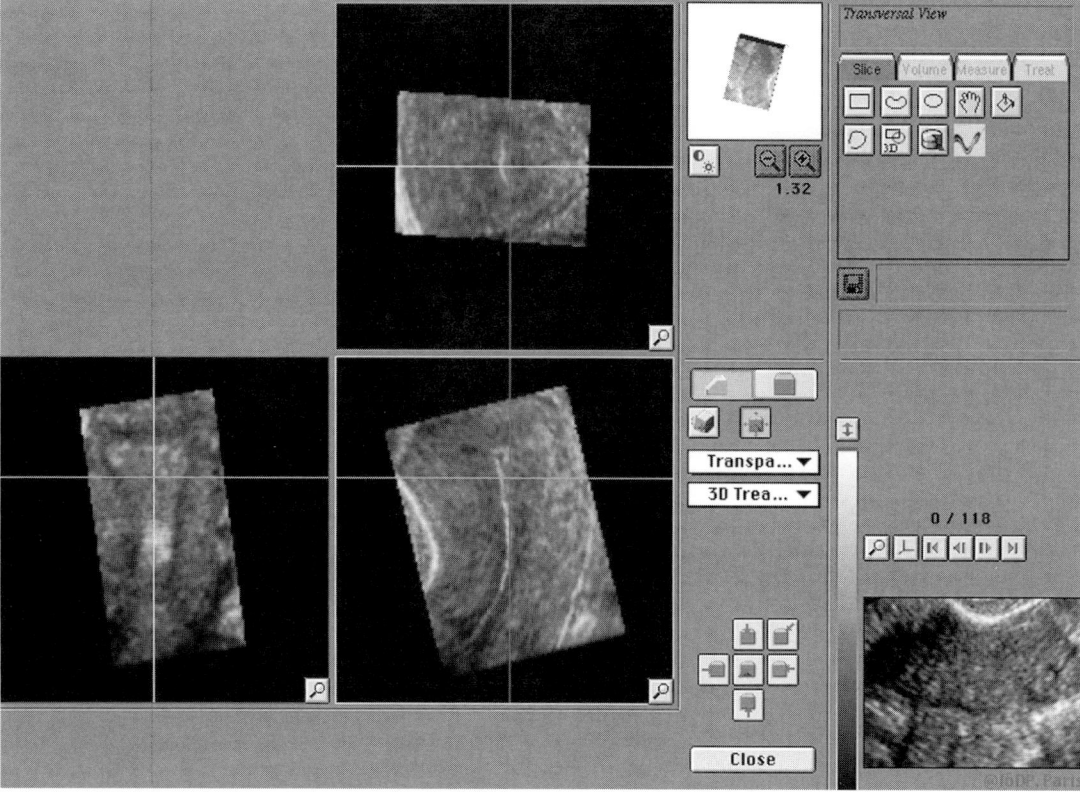

Figure 4 Universal station

an independent system that can be connected to any ultrasound system (imaging station Iô 3.1, provided with a specific module, Gyneco/Obstetric 3D). The second uses a sonograph-integrated system (Combison 530 3D Voluson, Kretz).

Universal station

Ultrasound image acquisition is performed from any kind of sonograph, using any kind of imaging modality (B-mode, color Doppler). For our study, we used a Hitachi EUB 555 ultrasound system. In practice, the video output of the sonograph is connected to the universal station Iô. The station will digitize the images in real time with no loss of quality.

The acquisition of the moving image is obtained from a lateral sweep. The scanning movement starts from right to left on a longitudinal image of the uterus. To optimize the

reconstruction, the scanning translation speed should be regular.

The system permits the acquisition of about 100 images in 5 s. On the Iô station, the three-dimensional matrix is obtained in less than 1 min. This matrix allows then any kind of treatment (Figure 4).

Integrated system

The patient is placed in the procubitus position, and the three-dimensional volume is calculated from a conventional two-dimensional ultrasound scan, obtained after introducing a 7.5-MHz mechanical sectorial endovaginal probe.

An initial longitudinal scan of the uterine axis is obtained with the probe held still, and then the probe is automatically rotated through 360°. The volume obtained is a truncated cone,

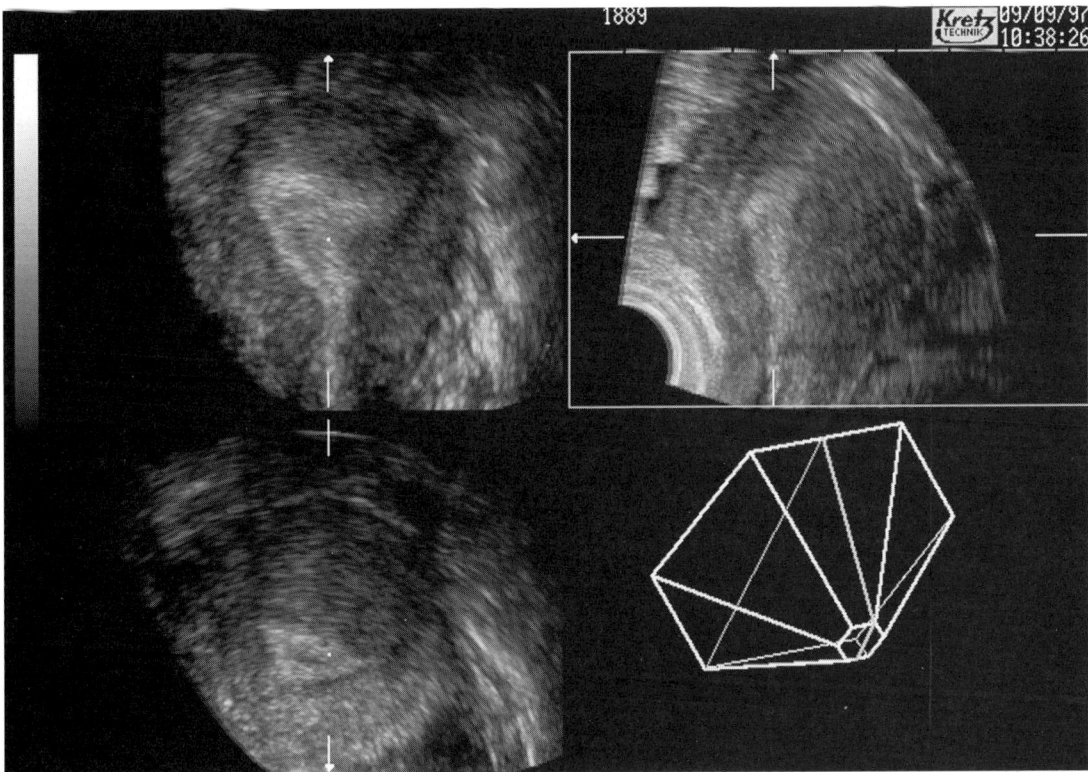

Figure 5 Integrated system

4–6 cm deep, with a vertical angle of 90°. The image acquisition time is about 10 s. The volume thus obtained is saved on a hard disk and takes up about 10 megabytes (MO) of space.

From the reconstituted three-dimensional uterus, visualization of the three orthogonal planes (*xy*, *yz* and *xz*) yields arbitrarily reconstructed sections, which can be used to provide a frontal cross section of the uterus (Figure 5).

VALUE OF THE METHOD AND ITS LIMITATIONS

In the context of assessing infertility and sterility[5], assessment of the uterine cavity – both to check for uterine malformations and to look for intrinsic or extrinsic abnormalities of the cavity – is based on conventional ultrasound, particularly by the endovaginal route and using high-frequency probes.

This detection method exhibits good sensitivity[6], but the analysis of the shape and volume of the uterine cavity is not ideal, and in some cases does not provide an exact diagnosis of the type of uterine malformation suspected[7-9] nor an accurate analysis of the relationship of this cavity with an intrinsic disease process (such as an endometrial polyp) or an extrinsic disease process (such as an intramural myoma). Hysterosalpingography, by making it possible to visualize the uterine cavity, enhances the sensitivity and specificity of the method, but the fact that it involves the use of a contrast medium and requires irradiation leads to a risk of complications.

More recently, some authors[10] have suggested using magnetic resonance imaging (MRI) to evaluate the uterine cavity; however, the high cost of this procedure restricts its use.

Feasibility

Jurkovic and colleagues[11], in a comparative study of two- and three-dimensional

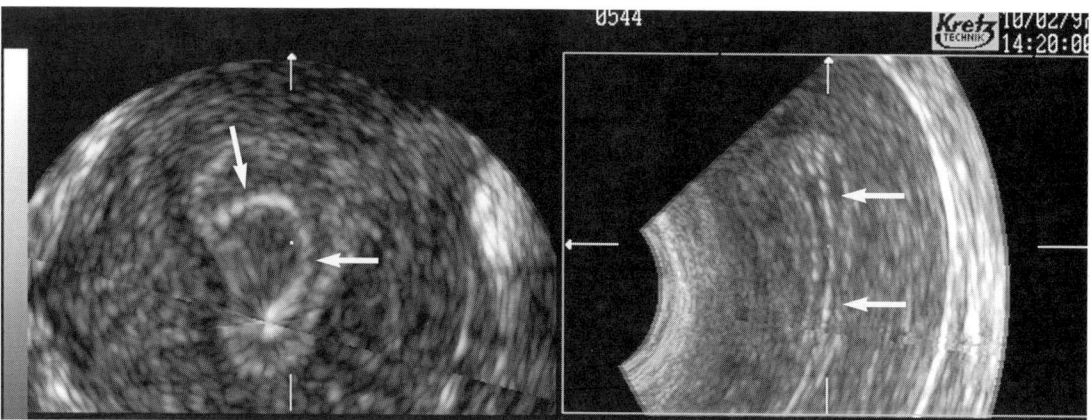

Figure 6   Right: cavity line, longitudinal section. Left: reconstructed frontal artifact

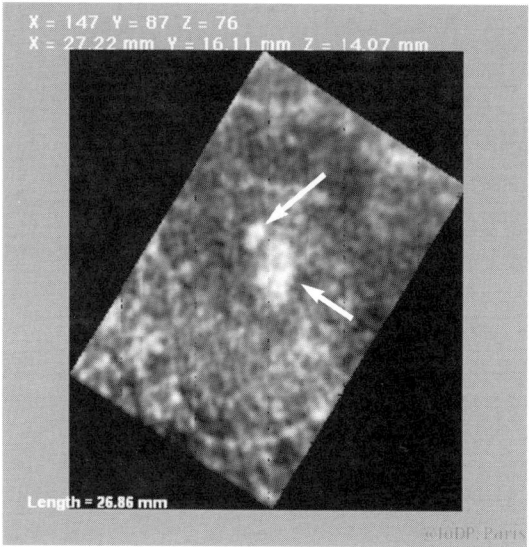

Figure 7   Artifact, cavity line

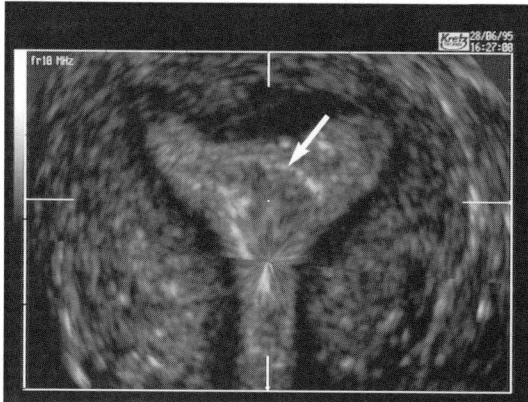

Figure 8   Artifact, cavity line

Artifacts: Misleading images and limitations

During the proliferative phase

ultrasonography versus hysterosalpingography for investigations of the uterine cavity, showed that this new method performs well. Compared to hysterography, its specificity, sensitivity and predictive value all verge on 100%.

A frontal cross section is obtained in 98% of cases, as in our entire experimental group of over 400 patients. Only if the uterus has been seriously deformed as a result of severe myomatosis is it unsuitable for this method.

Kyei-Mensah and co-workers[12] also suggested using three-dimensional imaging to assess the volume of the uterine cavity.

The image of the highly reflective cavity line in the longitudinal section of the uterus may, when the frontal cross section is reconstructed, give rise to false images suggesting the presence of hyper-reflective rounded masses within the cavity; these are in reality simply projections of the boundary of this cavity (Figures 6–9).

Other possible artifactual images consist of areas with low reflectivity, corresponding to the shadow cone behind a structure which prevents the transmission of ultrasound. Figure 10 shows an exaggerated example of a false cross-shaped image resulting from the shadow cone of an intrauterine device. This type of artifact may result when a frontal section is taken behind a structure such as a calcified myoma. These examples highlight, if need be,

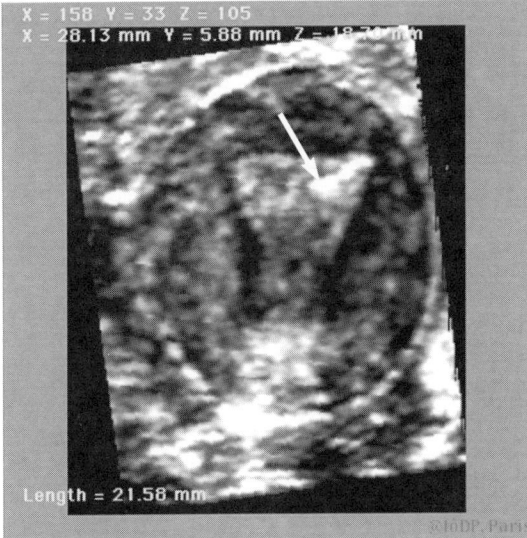

Figure 9   Artifact, cavity line

the value of interpreting the third dimension on the basis of the orthogonal sections, bearing in mind the axis of incidence of the ultrasound beam.

During the secretory phase

The ultrasonographic reflectiveness of the endometrium and its thickness limit the risk of artifacts in the frontal cross section, such as those described above, and this phase of the cycle is therefore the ideal period for carrying out this examination.

During the menstrual phase

Apparent desquamation of the mucosa should not be interpreted as an intrinsic disease.

Global visualization of the uterus

A complete visualization of the cervix, isthmus and endometrial cavity is rarely obtained on a single frontal scan of the uterus. In fact, as a result of the degree of flexibility of the cervix,

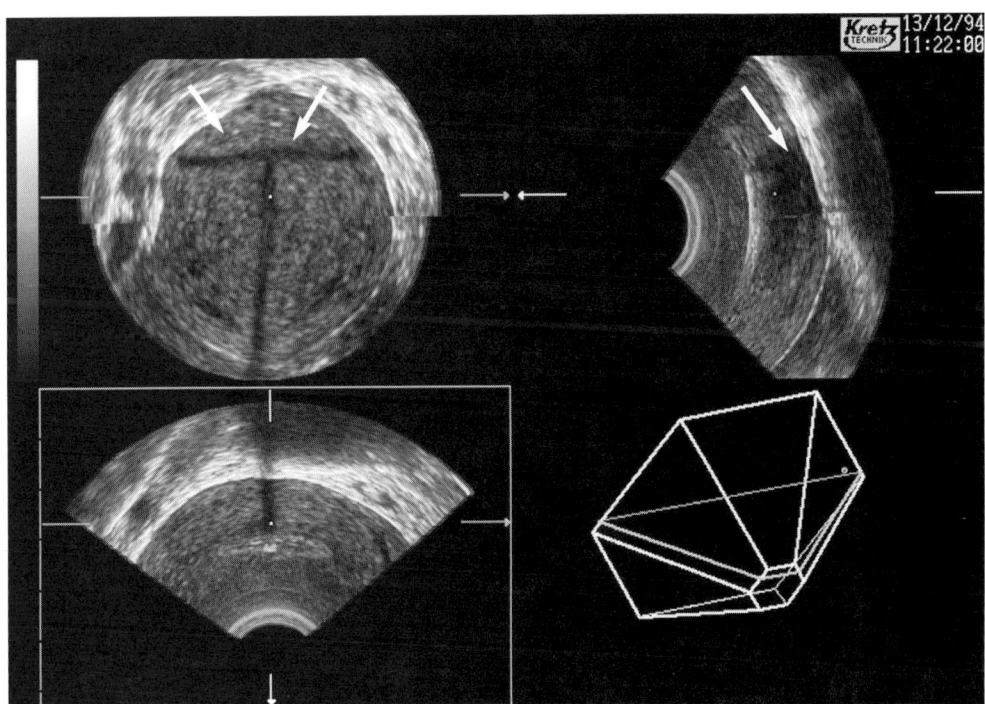

Figure 10   Reconstructed shadow cone in frontal cross section

121

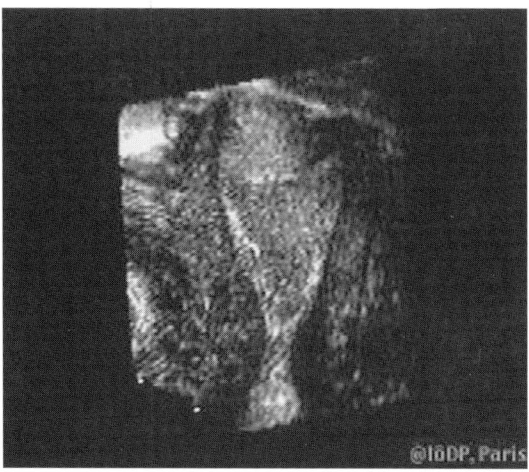

Figure 11 Normal proliferative endometrium (triangular cavity) with visualization of the cervix

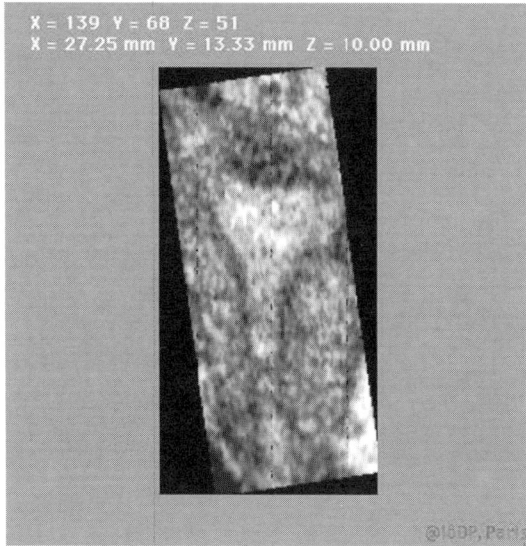

Figure 12 Normal proliferative endometrium (T shaped cavity)

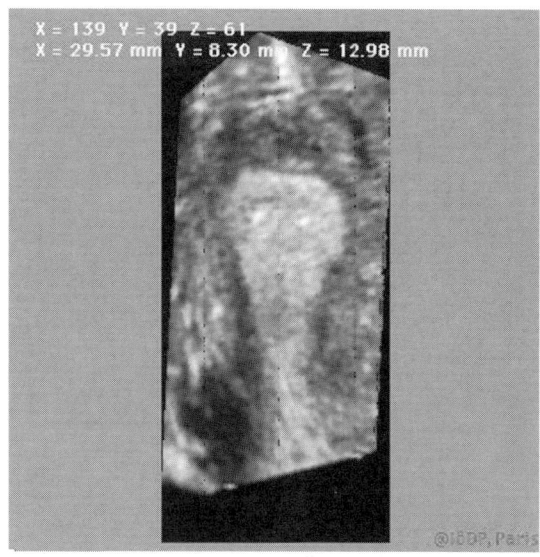

Figure 13 Normal secretory endometrium 'freehand acquisition'

Normal aspects

Proliferative phase

The proliferative phase is particularly suitable for identifying intrinsic disorders of the cavity. The normal appearance is triangular (Figures 11 and 12) which makes it possible to measure the transverse axis of the fundus of the cavity, but also the thickness of the fundic myometrium. The interface with the myometrium can be seen and the contours of this endometrium analyzed.

Secretory phase

A frontal scan during the secretory phase (Figures 13 and 14) is particularly useful for investigating uterine malformations. The ultrasonographic reflectiveness of the endometrium during the second phase of the cycle and the presence of a fundic notch in the cavity or of the entire fundus of the uterus can easily be distinguished.

Ultrasonography during this phase can also be useful in adenomyomatosis and for investigating extrinsic disorders that deform the cavity (myomas).

Measurement of the volume of the cavity is also optimal during this phase[12].

compared to that of the uterine body, it is generally impossible to obtain a frontal scan that simultaneously displays the triangular appearance of the cavity, the isthmus and the endocervix. Consequently, the reconstruction of the frontal section of the endometrium is generally restricted to a cross section from the isthmus to the fundus of the cavity.

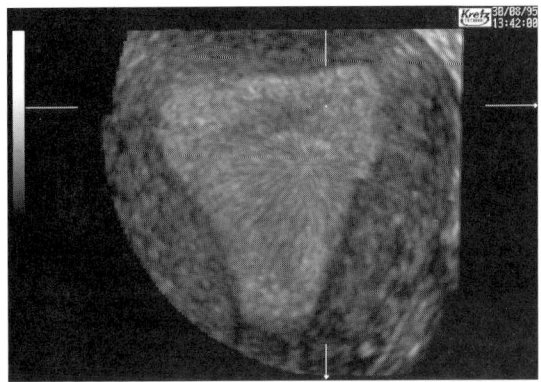

Figure 14 Normal secretory endometrium (mechanical acquisition)

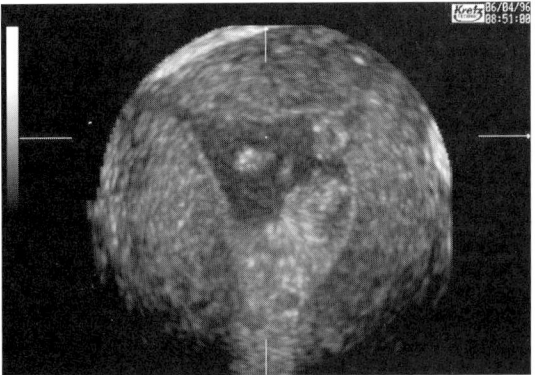

Figure 15 Menstrual phase with desquamation aspects

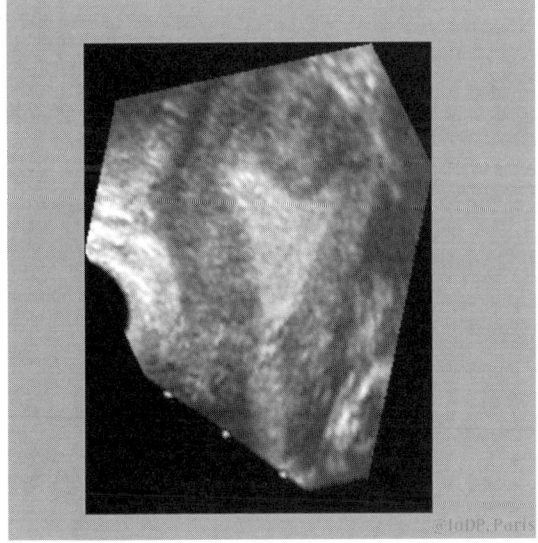

Figure 16 Y-shaped hypoplasia

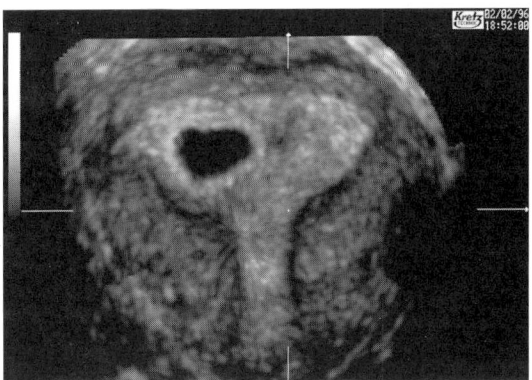

Figure 17 T-shaped hypoplasia (due to diethylstilbestrol) with an early pregnancy in the right cornua

Menstrual phase

Images of desquamation are seen (Figure 15).

Combination with hysterosalpingo-contrast sonography

Use of a contrast medium (saline or an echo-reflective agent: Echovist) can be coupled with ultrasonography[13,14]. Weinraub and co-workers[15] have recently suggested that this method could be combined with three-dimensional ultrasonography; this technique seems to be very promising.

This makes it possible to obtain a better analysis of the uterine cavity in frontal cross section. This aspect is similar to the images obtained in pathological hydrometra (for an example, see Figure 44).

THE FRONTAL UTERUS SCAN IN INFERTILITY

Uterine hypoplasia

Uterine hypoplasia is defined on the basis of a transverse diameter of the fundus of the uterus which is less than 4 cm (a frontal scan makes it possible to measure this accurately). Malformative hypoplasia may be visualized as a Y-shaped cavity (Figure 16; hypoplasia combined with a slightly notched appearance of the fundus of the uterus) or T-shaped hypoplasia, particularly in hypoplasia due to taking diethylstilbestrol (Distilbene)[16], (Figure 17).

These forms of uterine hypoplasia, which can be responsible for late miscarriages or premature childbirth, can be identified just as clearly from three-dimensional frontal scans as by hysterography.

Some authors[8,12,17] also suggest that, in the future, as a result of the contribution of three-dimensional ultrasonography in determining the volume of the cavity, it will be possible to obtain objective measurements and etablish thresholds to define uterine hypoplasia.

Uterine malformations

The classification of Musset and colleagues[18] is used below.

Uterine aplasia

This is an abnormality that develops between the 6th and 9th week of formation.

In true uterus unicornis (Figure 18) frontal ultrasonography reveals a similar aspect to that obtained by hysterography.

In uterus pseudo-unicornis (Figure 19), a cavity that is abnormal in morphological appearance on one side is combined with a rudimentary cornu or horn on the other, within which, as in this example, a pregnancy may develop. The absence of a myometrial layer between these two endometrial images should also be noted.

Hemi-uterus

This results from an embryological disorder that develops between weeks 10 and 13. Paired paramesonephric ducts persist.

A frontal ultrasound scan makes it possible to assess the distance separating the endometrial horns and to see whether there is any inserted myometrial tissue (notched appearance). By definition, if the notch in the fundus of the uterus is greater than 1 cm, the uterus is taken to be bicornuate.

Vascular structures can be seen between the endometrial horns, which rules out the possibility of uterus bilocularis. This visualization offers better differential diagnosis than hysterography. The conventional criteria used

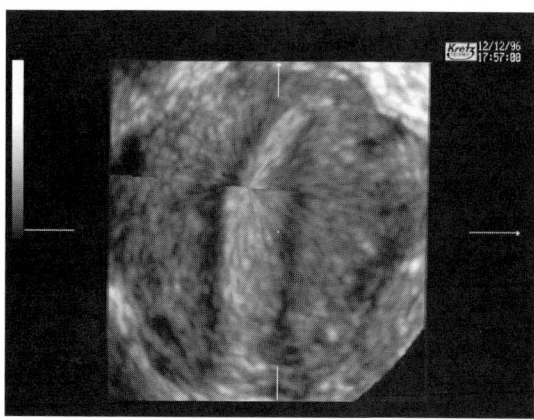

Figure 18   True uterus unicornis

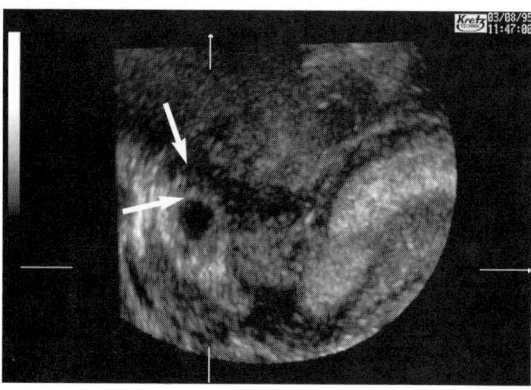

Figure 19   Uterus pseudo-unicornis, with a pregnancy in the rudimentary horn

for hysterographic differential diagnosis between uterus bicornis and uterus bilocularis can also be used. For example, in Figures 23 to 28, a gap can be seen between the two endometrial horns, which is set (a) classical above 60° in uterus bicornis and (b) under 60° in uterus bilocularis. The angle between the axes should be examined, as should the transverse axis of the fundic notch.

Uterus bicornis unicollis is shown in Figure 20. Uterus bicornis bicollis is shown in Figures 21 and 22.

Uterus bilocularis

Uterus bilocularis results from failure of the median partition of the cervix to be resorbed

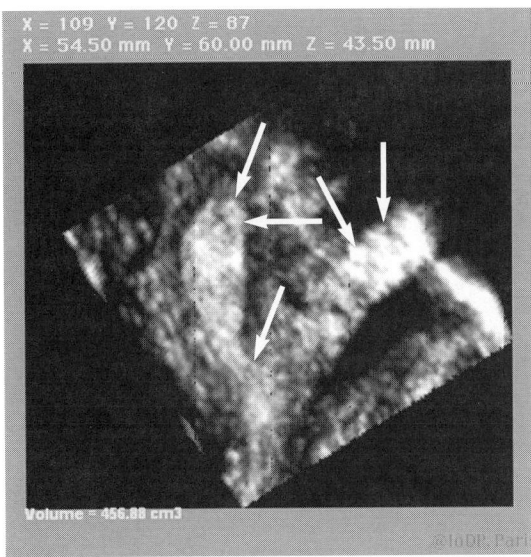

Figure 20   Uterus bicornis unicollis

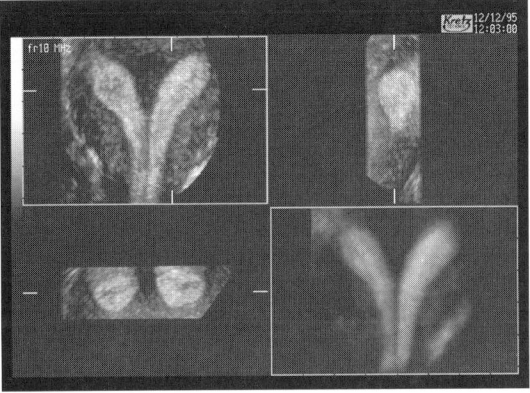

Figure 21   Uterus bicornis bicollis (multiplanar view)

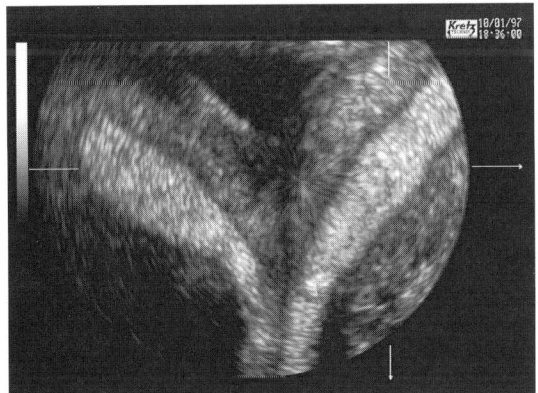

Figure 22   Uterus bicornis bicollis

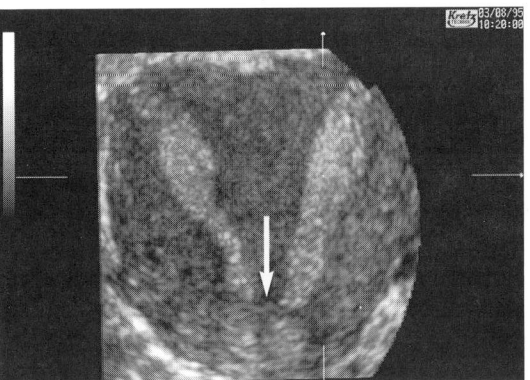

Figure 23   Total uterus bilocularis bicollis

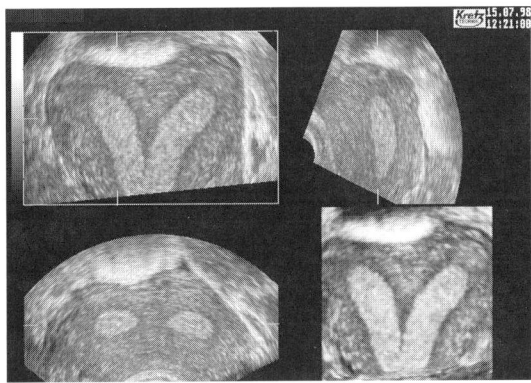

Figure 24   Uterus bilocularis unicollis (multiplanar view)

into the fundus of the cavity (an anomaly that develops after 13 weeks).

On the frontal scan, the presence of a non-vascularized myometrial structure can be seen, confirming the diagnosis and also making it possible to see the extent of the incision in the fundus of the uterus and to measure the depth and breadth of this partition.

Total uterus bilocularis bicollis is shown in Figure 23.

Subtotal uterus bilocularis unicollis is shown in Figures 24 and 25.

Corporeal uterus bilocularis with a base of varying breadth, with or without a notch in the fundus of the cavity, is shown in Figures 26–29.

Uterus with a notched fundus is shown in Figure 30.

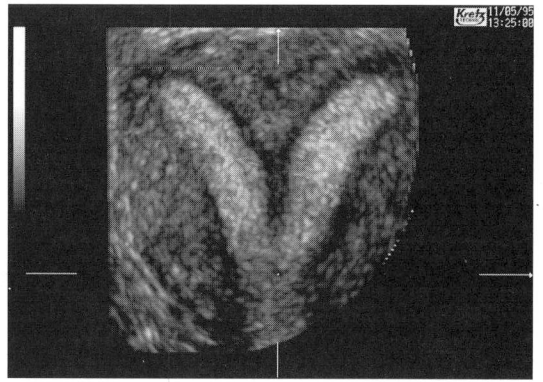

Figure 25 Subtotal uterus bilocularis unicollis

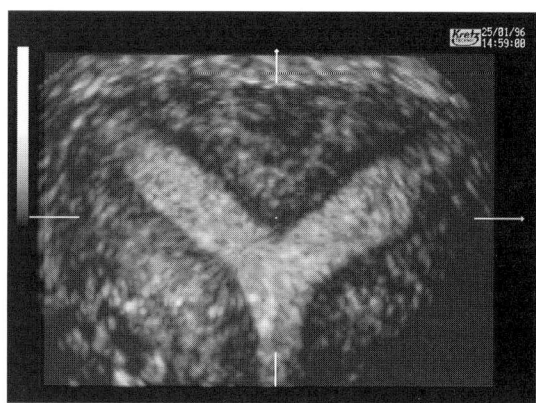

Figure 28 Corporeal uterus bilocularis

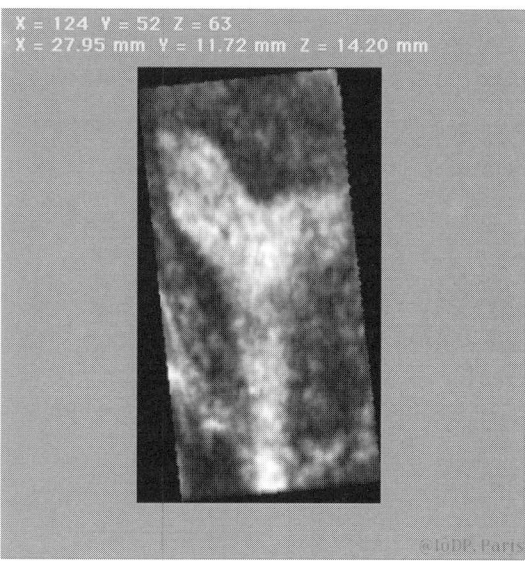

Figure 26 Corporeal uterus bilocularis

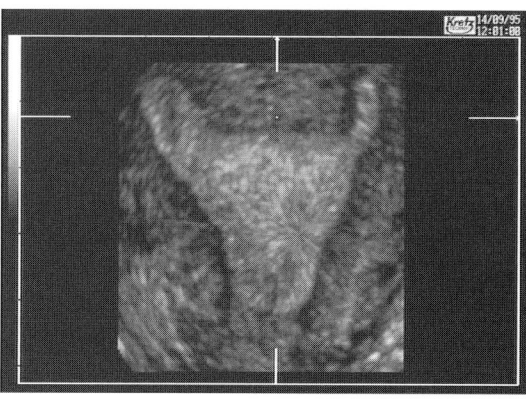

Figure 29 Cow's-horn shape of corporeal uterus bilocularis

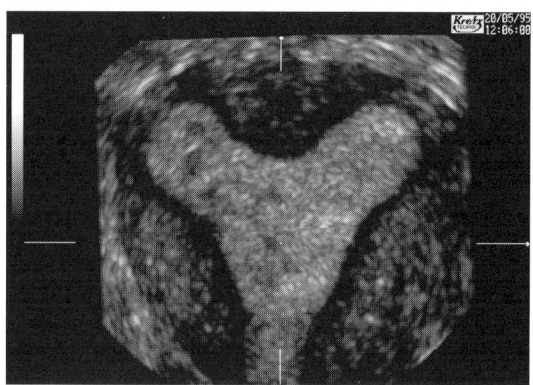

Figure 27 Corporeal uterus bilocularis

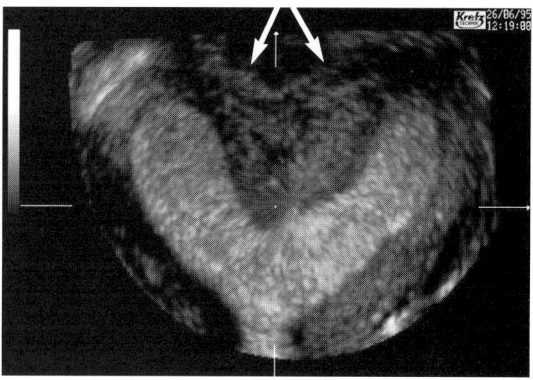

Figure 30 Uterus with a notched fundus

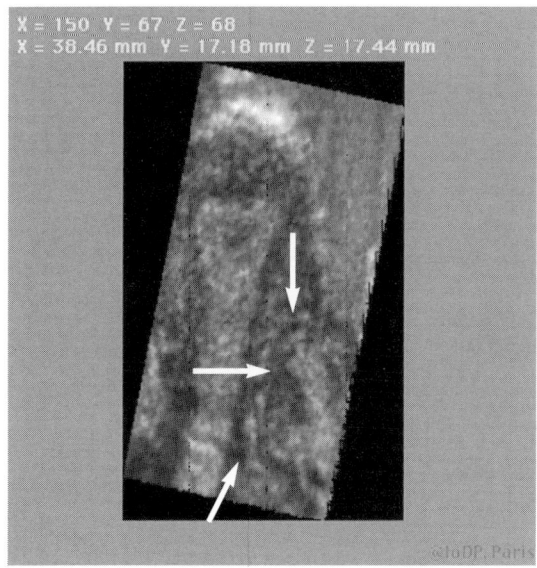

Figure 31 Intramural myoma remote from the cavity

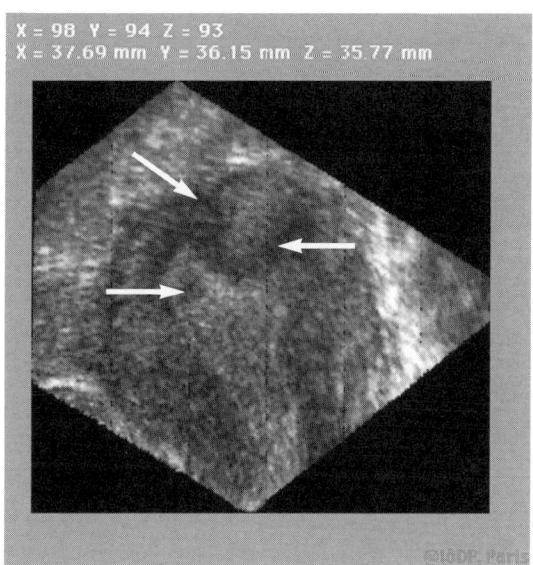

Figure 33 Fundic and submucosal myomas

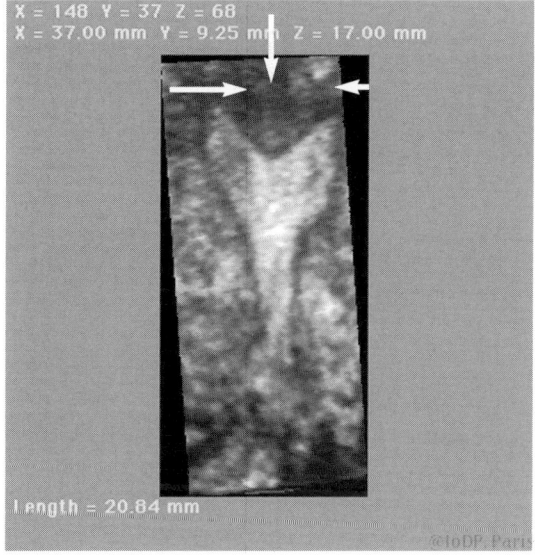

Figure 32 Fundic myoma

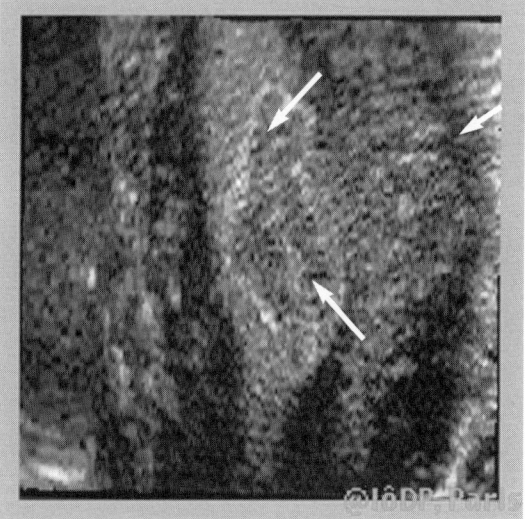

Figure 34 Imprint of an intramural myoma

Uterine fibromas

Intramural (interstitial) myomas are shown in Figures 31–38. On the three-dimensional frontal scan, the topography of these myomas relative to the cavity can be made out, and it is possible to see whether the cavity is misshapen in any way. The scan also shows the position of these myomas relative to interstitial tubular portions. The cavity may be deformed, asymmetrical and/or enlarged.

Sub-mucosal myomas are shown in Figures 39 and 40. These myomas can be clearly identified if their echo-reflectivity is clearly different from that of the endometrium, particularly during the secretory

127

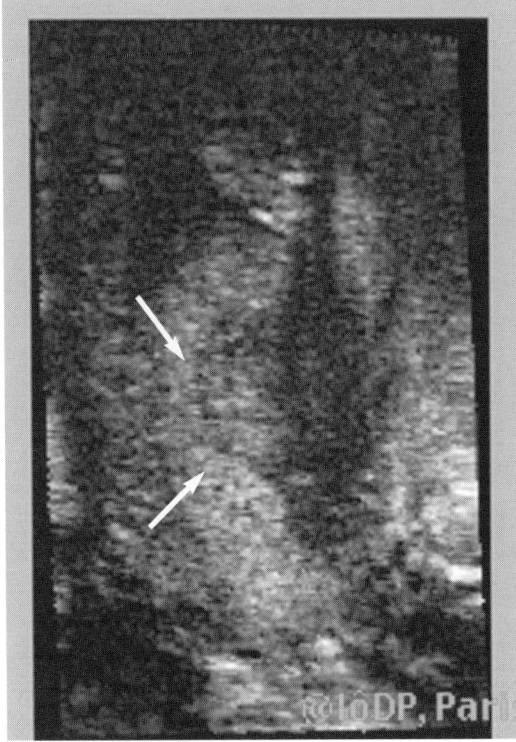

Figure 35   Imprint of an intramural myoma

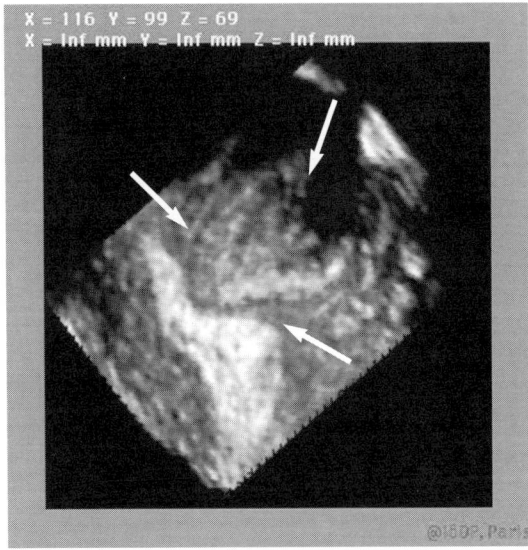

Figure 36   Imprint and deformation due to an intramural myoma

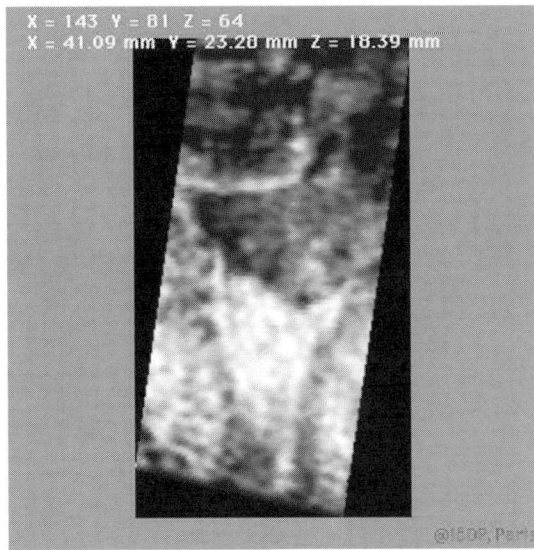

Figure 37   Imprint and deformation due to an intramural myoma

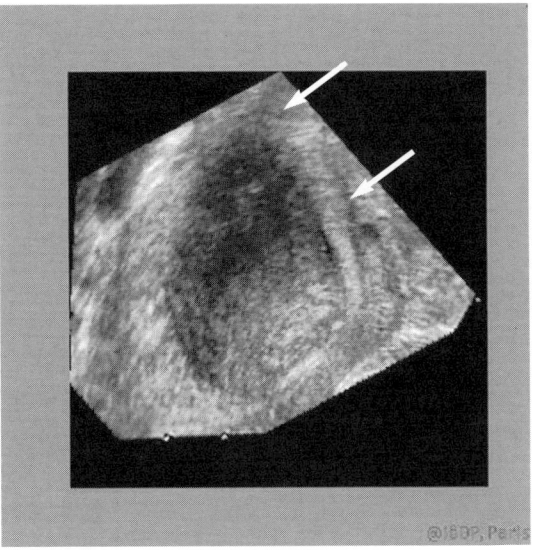

Figure 38   Lamination of the cavity by an intramural myoma

phase. For a more detailed investigation, three-dimensional ultrasonography using a frontal section can be combined with a contrast medium.

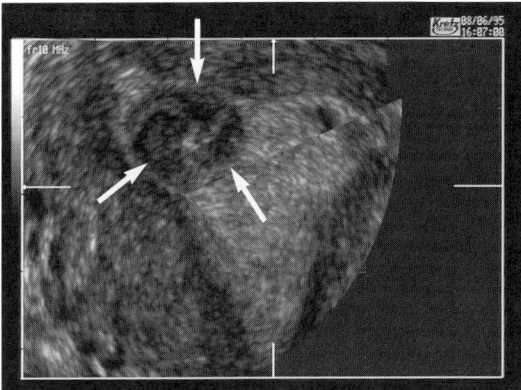

Figure 39 Submucosal myoma

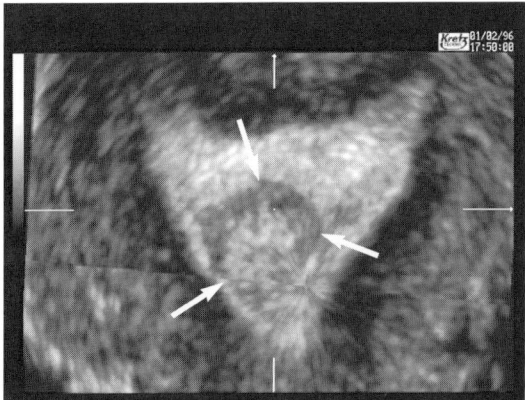

Figure 40 Submucosal myoma

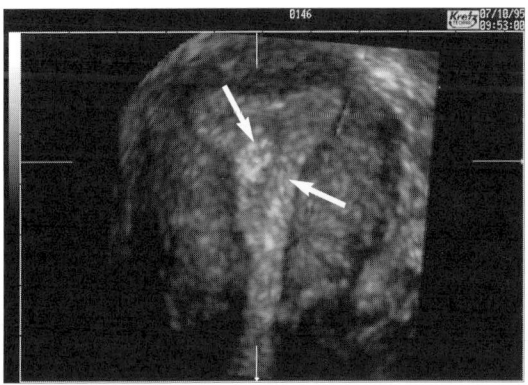

Figure 41 Endometrial polyp (fine implantation)

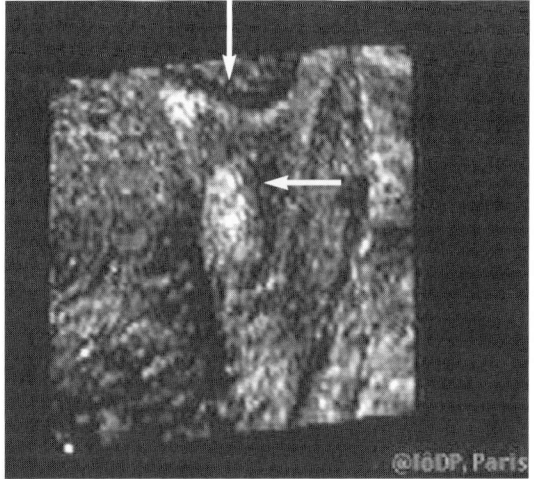

Figure 42 Endometrial polyp (wide implantation)

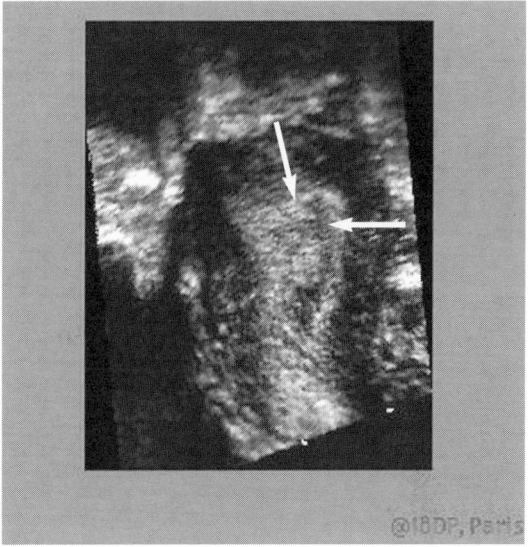

Figure 43 'Polypoid' hyperplasia

Mucosal polyps of the endometrium

These polyps result in an image including an empty space within the cavity in the frontal view (Figures 41–43). In the presence of hydrometra, this aspect is particularly clearly identifiable (in the same way as when a contrast medium is used)[11] (Figure 44).

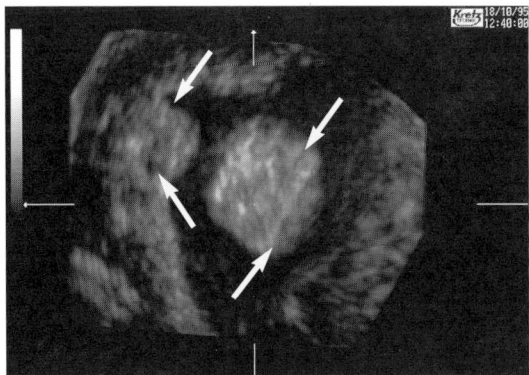

Figure 44 Endometrial polyps and hydrometra

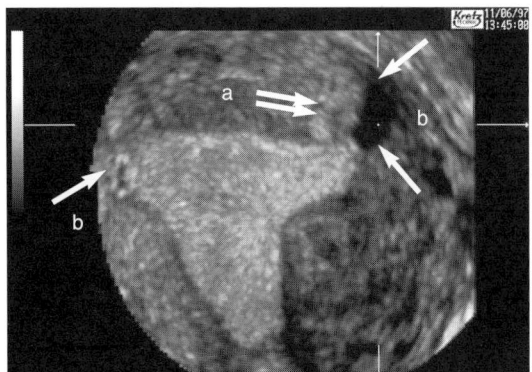

Figure 45 (a) Endometrial area; (b) adenomyotic cyst

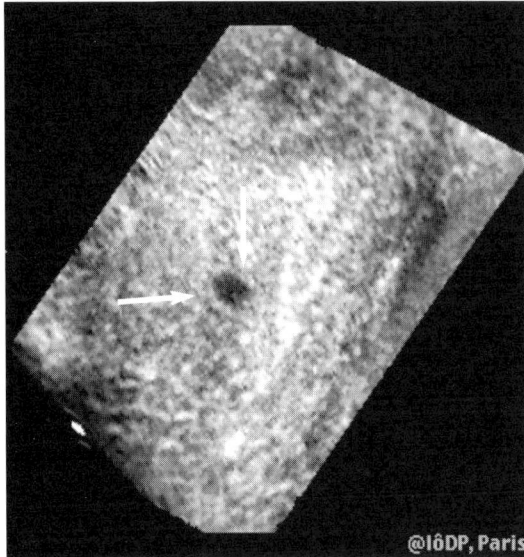

Figure 46 Adenomyotic cyst

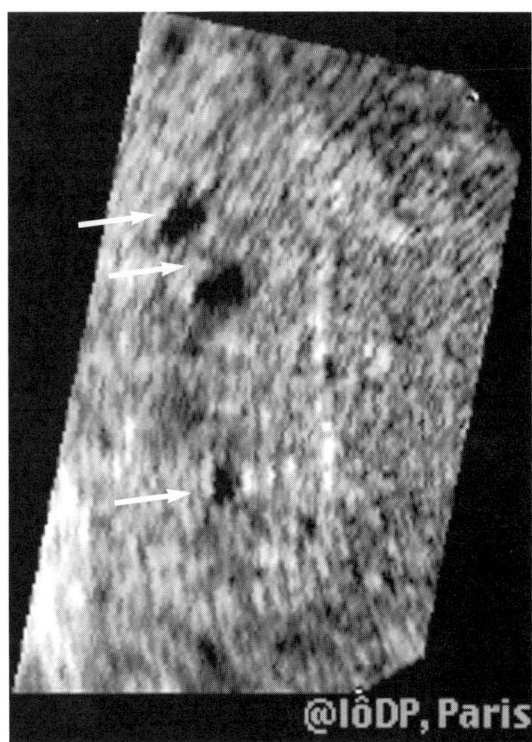

Figure 47 Adenomyotic cyst

For the purposes of differential diagnosis of endometrial polyps, the misleading image discussed in the section on artifacts should be recalled; this can be produced by the boundary of an empty uterus in the proliferative phase (Figure 6).

Others

In adenomyomatosis[19], a frontal scan can be used to identify the presence of an endometrial area in the myometrium with glands and a cytogenic chorion leading to a hyper-reflective aspect (rarely reported aspect, Figure 45a). The diagnosis is usually reached on the basis of liquid structures, owing to the accumulation of endometrial fluid within the myometrium (Figures 45b, 46 and 47). This aspect tends to occur in elderly women (particularly in a context of infertility in women around 40 years of age) who usually tend to be nulliparous.

The irregular appearance of the outline of the cavity in the presence of adjacent liquid structures should be noted, and a frontal scan

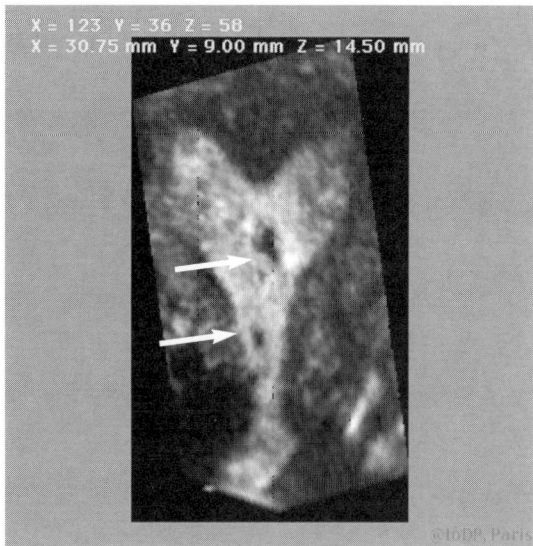

Figure 48 Endometrial cyst

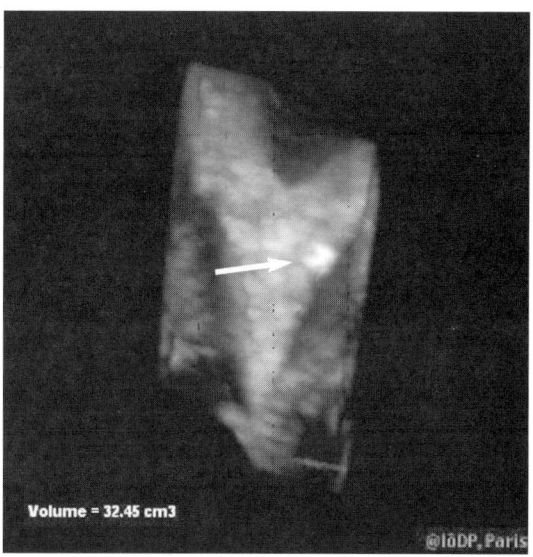

Figure 51 Calcification of the submucosal myoma

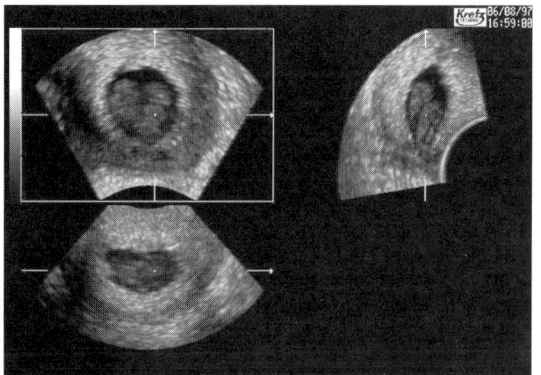

Figure 49 Endocervical retention due to stenosis of the outer orifice of the cervix (multiplanar view)

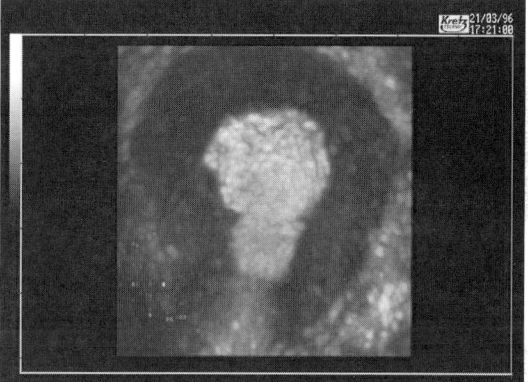

Figure 52 'Cuttle-fish' calcification

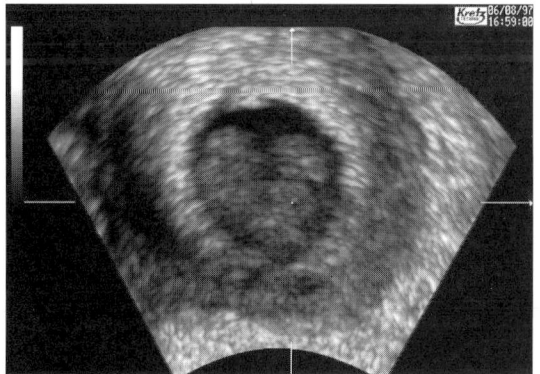

Figure 50 Endocervical retention due to stenosis of the outer orifice of the cervix (magnified coronal view of the cervix)

can be used to determine the depth of insertion into the myometrium. The frontal view makes it possible to reach a differential diagnosis from endometrial glandular cysts, which are not inserted into the myometrium (Figure 48).

Synechiae are not spontaneously visualized by ultrasonography; however, they can be revealed by combining an ultrasound scan with an injection of saline solution into the cavity. Synechiae can also be detected from hydrometra distal to the synechia. In the example shown in Figures 49 and 50, the endocervical retention results from an exocervical synechia.

In endometrial chondromatosis, a frontal scan may reveal endometrial calcifications (which may, for instance, be secondary to the calcification of a submucosal myoma) (Figure 51).

In a context of infertility, global chondromatosis may be observed, as shown in Figure 52, with a 'cuttle-fish'-like aspect of the cavity.

CONCLUSION

The routine use of three-dimensional ultrasonography in the assessment of infertility is still in its very early stages. The feasibility of the procedure and its safety, particularly in contrast to that of hysterography, should soon make it a first-line diagnostic method.

The illustrations of normal aspects and those corresponding to various disorders shown here may therefore constitute a bank of reference images for use in studies involving large numbers of randomized patients. This should make it possible in the future to obtain a more accurate assessment of the accuracy of this technique compared to that of existing techniques.

References

1. Baba, K. and Okai, T. (1997). Basis and principles of three-dimensional ultrasound. In Baba, K. and Jurkovic, D. (eds.) *Three-dimensional Ultrasound in Obstetrics and Gynecology*, pp. 1–19. (Carnforth, UK: Parthenon Publishing)

2. Feichtinger, W. (1993). Transvaginal three-dimensional imaging. *Ultrasound Obstet. Gynecol.*, **3**, 375–8

3. Mansour, S., Massonneau, M. and Pineau, P. (1997). Echographie tridimensionnelle: quelques notions techniques à l'usage du futur opérateur. *J.E.M.U.*, **18**, 299–305

4. Steiner, H., Staudach, A., Spitzer, D. and Schaffer, H. (1994). Three-dimensional ultrasound in obstetrics and gynaecology: technique, possibilities and limitations. *Hum. Reprod.*, **9**, 1773–8

5. Kessler, I. and Lancet, M. (1986). Hysterography and hysteroscopy: a comparison. *Fertil. Steril.*, **46**, 709

6. Nicolini, U., Belloti, M., Bonazzi, B., Zamberletti, D. and Candiani, G. B. (1987). Can ultrasound be used to screen uterine malformations? *Fertil. Steril.*, **47**, 89–93

7. Valdes, C., Malini, S. and Malinak, L. R. (1984). Ultrasound evaluation of female genital tract anomalies: a review of 64 cases. *Am. J. Obstet. Gynecol.*, **149**, 285–9

8. Fedele, L., Ferrazzi, E., Dorta, M., Vercellini, P. and Canadiani, G. B. (1988). Ultrasonography in the differential diagnosis of 'double' uteri. *Fertil. Steril.*, **48**, 361–4

9. Randolph, J. R., Ying, Y. K., Maier, D. B., Schmidt, C. L. and Riddick, D. H. (1986). Comparison of real-time ultrasonography, hysterosalpingography, and laparoscopy/hysteroscopy in the evaluation of uterine abnormalities and tubal patency. *Fertil. Steril.*, **46**, 828–32

10. Pellerito, J. S., McCarthy, S. M., Doyle, M. B., Glickman, M. G. and DeCherney, A. H. (1992). Diagnosis of uterine anomalies: relative accuracy of MR imaging, endovaginal sonography and hysterosalpingography. *Radiology*, **183**, 795–800

11. Jurkovic, D., Geipel, A., Gruboeck, K., Jauniaux, E., Natucci, M. and Campbell, S. (1995). Three-dimensional ultrasound for the assessment of uterine anatomy and detection of congenital anomalies: a comparison with hysterosalpingography and two-dimensional sonography. *Ultrasound Obstet. Gynecol.*, **5**, 233–7

12. Kyei-Mensah, A., Zaidi, J., Pittrof, R., Shaker, A., Campbell, S. and Tan, S. L. (1995). Transvaginal three dimensional ultrasound: accuracy and reliability of ovarian and endometrial volume measurements. *Hum. Reprod.*, **10**, 109

13. Maroulis, G. B., Parsons, A. K. and Yeko, T. H. (1992). Hydroynecography: a new technique enables vaginal sonography to visualize pelvic adhesions and other pelvis structures. *Fertil. Steril.*, **58**, 1073–5

14. De Ziegler, D. and Frydman, R. (1992). Progrès de l'echographie gynecologique: sondes endo uterines et echographie vaginale avec augmentation de contraste. *Contracept. Fertil. Sex.*, **20**, 776–48

15. Weinraub, Z., Maymo, R., Shulman, J. and Bukovski, J. (1996). Three dimensional saline contrast hysterosonography and surface rendering of uterine cavity pathology. *Ultrasound Obstet. Gynecol.*, **8**, 277–82

16. Kaufmann, R. H., Adam, E., Binder, G. L. and Gerthoffer, E. (1980). Upper genital tract changes associated with exposure *in utero* to diethylstilboestrol. *Am. J. Obstet. Gynecol.*, **37**, 299–308

17. Balen, F. G., Allen, C. M., Gardener, J. E., Siddle, N. C. and Lees, W. R. (1993). 3-dimensional reconstruction of ultrasound images of the uterine cavity. *Br. J. Radiol.*, **66**, 588–91

18. Musset, R. *et al.* (1967). Nécessité d'une classification globale des malformations utérines. Les malformations urinaires associées. Intérêt de certaines particularités à la lumière de 141 cas. *Gynécol. Obstét.*, **66**, 145–66

19. Douay, N., Ardaens, Y., Bethouart, M., Gauthier, A., Collier, F. and Ardaens, K. (1992). What can be expected from transvaginal ultrasonography in adenomiosis presumption? *Contracept. Fertil. Sex.*, **20**, 1058–65

Uterine perfusion in fertile and infertile patients

11

S. Kupesic and A. Kurjak

ANGIOGENESIS IN THE UTERUS

The majority of the blood supply to the uterus is from the uterine arteries, with only slight additional contributions from the ovarian arteries. The uterine arteries give rise to the arcuate arteries (Figure 1), which are oriented circumferentially in the outer third of the myometrium. These vessels give rise to the radial arteries, which, after crossing the myometrium–endometrium border, further branch and give rise to the basal arteries and the spiral arteries. The basal arteries, which are relatively short, terminate in a capillary bed that serves the stratum basalis of the endometrium. The spiral arteries, on the other hand, project further into the endometrium and terminate in a vast capillary network that serves the stratum functionalis of the endometrium.

Interestingly, only the spiral arteries undergo substantial anatomical changes during the menstrual cycle[1]. At the time of menstruation, probably as a result of decreasing estrogen and progesterone levels, the spiral arteries constrict, producing local hypoxia, ischemia, and eventually cell death within the stratum functionalis. The distal portion of the arteriolar system, and the capillary and venous beds, are then shed with the functionalis. The basal arteries, which are insensitive to decreasing estrogen and progesterone titers[2], are relatively unaffected and serve to maintain the integrity of the stratum basalis throughout the menstrual cycle. As the endometrium thickens three- to five-fold during the next menstrual cycle, the remnants of the spiral arteries in the basalis must undergo substantial growth and give rise to a completely new capillary bed in order to maintain the integrity of the rapidly

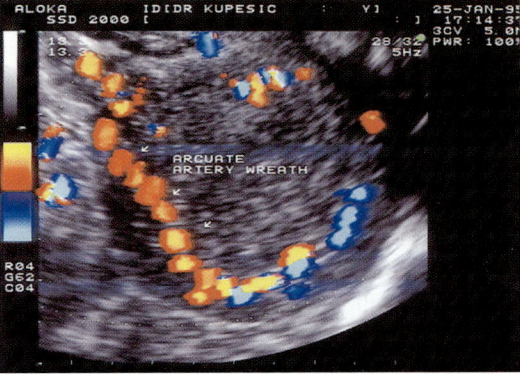

Figure 1 A transvaginal ultrasound scan of the uterus demonstrating an arcuate artery network encircling the uterus

growing stroma. This process is initiated by the growth of new capillaries from the existing vasculature in the basalis[2]. These capillaries eventually differentiate into arteries and arterioles as the elastic and vascular smooth muscle components develop around the new capillaries[3]. Uterine angiogenesis during the proliferative and secretory phases provides an existing vascular supply for the trophoblast to invade if fertilization of the ovum occurs[4].

Following fertilization, the first stage of implantation is the adhesion of the blastocyst to the endometrial epithelium. This is followed by the penetration of the trophoblast through the epithelial lining. With further invasion of the trophoblast, maternal capillaries are encountered, surrounded, and induced to undergo profound physiological and architectural changes[5]. One of the first changes is an increase in vascular permeability at the site of implantation[6]. This is followed by metabolic activation of the endothelium in preparation for angiogenesis, and then vascular remodeling[6]. The subsequent remodeling of the maternal vasculature facilitates placentation.

UTERINE PERFUSION CHANGES DURING THE MENSTRUAL CYCLE

More than any other available technique, transvaginal color Doppler affords detailed delineation of the uterus, and its myometrium, endometrium and vessels[7–10]. It is well known that uterine perfusion is largely dependent on the patient age, the phase of the menstrual cycle, and other specific conditions (e.g. pregnancy, tumor)[11]. In this chapter we analyze these factors in detail.

There are complex relationships between the concentration of the ovarian hormones in peripheral venous plasma and uterine artery blood flow parameters[12–15]. In most women, there is a small amount of end-diastolic flow in the uterine arteries in the proliferative phase (Figure 2). The resistance index (RI) hovers around 0.88 ± 0.04 until day 13 of the 28-day menstrual cycle. Steer and co-workers[14] reported that diastolic flow in the uterine arteries disappears during the day of ovulation. Goswamy and Steptoe[12] found an increasing resistance index and an increasing systolic/diastolic ratio during the postovulatory drop in the serum estradiol concentration. Increased uterine artery impedance was reported 3 days after the peak in luteinizing hormone (LH), and Scholtes and colleagues[16] recorded the highest value for the pulsatility index (PI) in the uterine arteries on cycle day 16. These findings may be explained by increased uterine contractility[17] and compression of the vessels traversing the uterine wall, which decrease their diameter and consequently cause higher resistance to flow. During the normal menstrual cycle, there is a sharp increase in end-diastolic velocities between the proliferative and secretory phases[8]. It is particularly interesting that the lowest blood flow impedance occurs during the time of peak luteal function (resistance index 0.84 ± 0.04), during which implantation is most likely to occur (Figure 3). It is logical that blood supply to the uterus

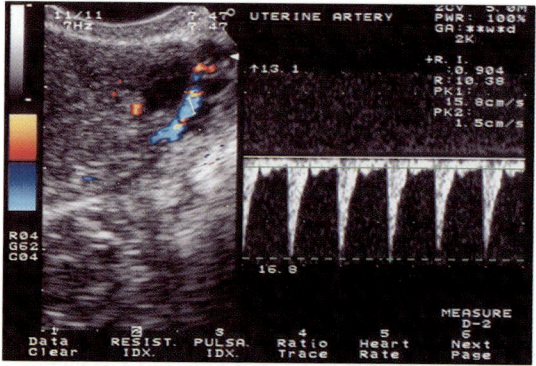

Figure 2 The uterine artery is demonstrated laterally from the cervix at the level of the cervicocorporeal junction. The blood flow velocity from the uterine artery in the proliferative phase is characterized by a small amount of end-diastolic flow and high impedance to blood flow (resistance index 0.90)

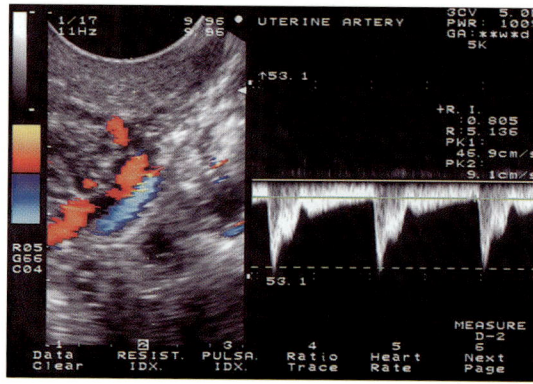

Figure 3 Blood flow velocity waveforms extracted from the uterine artery in the secretory phase are characterized by increased velocity and decreased resistance index (0.81)

should be high in the late luteal phase, as has been reported by Kurjak and associates[8], Goswamy and associates[12,13], Steer and associates[14], and Battaglia and colleagues[18]. The persistently lower RI in the luteal phase suggests that the relaxation effects on the uterine arteries persist until the onset of menstruation. Zaidi and colleagues[19] observed that there is a circadian rhythm in uterine artery blood flow during the periovulatory period which appears to be independent from hormonal changes.

Similar circulatory changes to those observed in the main uterine arteries have

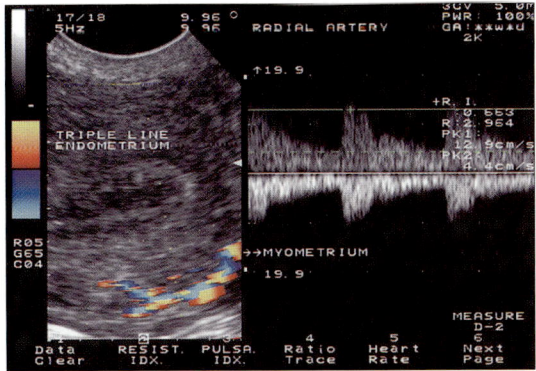

Figure 4 Blood flow velocity waveforms of the radial arteries. Note the position of the gate on the left panel (within the myometrium) for sampling flow velocity waveforms. Lower velocity and lower impedance (resistance index 0.69) blood flow signals are obtained from the examined vessels

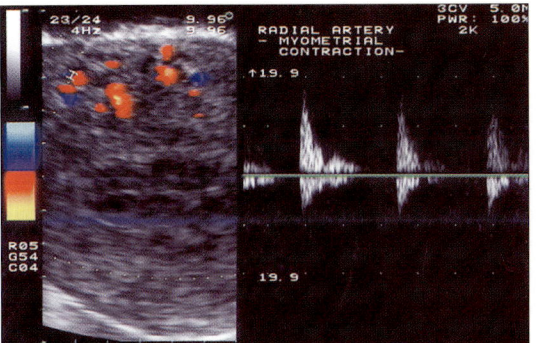

Figure 5 Blood flow velocity waveforms extracted from the radial arteries during the periovulatory phase. The interruption of the diastolic flow is a transitory effect of the myometrial contractions

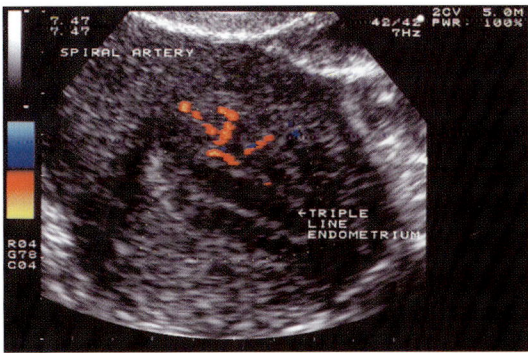

Figure 6 Color signals obtained from the spiral arteries on the periphery of the triple-line endometrium

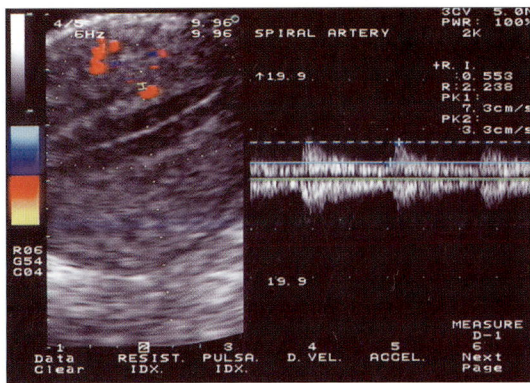

Figure 7 Blood flow velocity waveforms of the spiral arteries during the periovulatory period. A decreased resistance index (0.55) and an increased flow velocity occur during the day of ovulation

been seen in the minute arteries (radial and spiral) with the introduction of transvaginal color and pulsed Doppler[20] (Figure 4). Our results show an increase of the RI in the myometrial vessels after ovulation, during the postovulatory drop in the serum estradiol concentration (Figure 5).

Increased uterine contractility has been shown to coincide with decreased endometrial blood flow[17]. It is well known that the endometrium has an exceptional capacity to undergo changes in structure and function during the menstrual cycle. The histological changes include striking development of the blood vessels (Figure 6). The spiral arteries become more developed during the menstrual cycle. The increased endometrial vascularity is highly dependent upon the uterine, arcuate and radial artery blood flow. Blood flow velocity waveform changes in the spiral arteries during normal ovulatory cycles are characterized by lower velocity ($p < 0.05$) and lower impedance to blood flow ($p < 0.05$) than are those observed in the uterine arteries, with larger diameter[21] (Figure 7). It seems that features of endometrial blood flow may be used to predict the implantation success rate and to reveal unexplained infertility problems more precisely than evaluation of the main uterine artery alone.

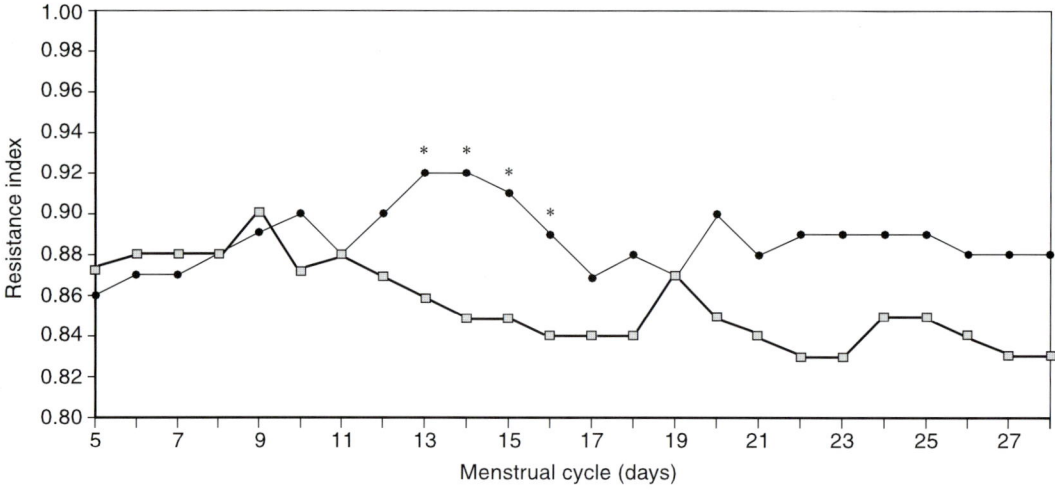

Figure 8 Uterine artery blood flow changes in anovulatory (–•–) and fertile (–□–) patients during the menstrual cycle. $^*p < 0.05$

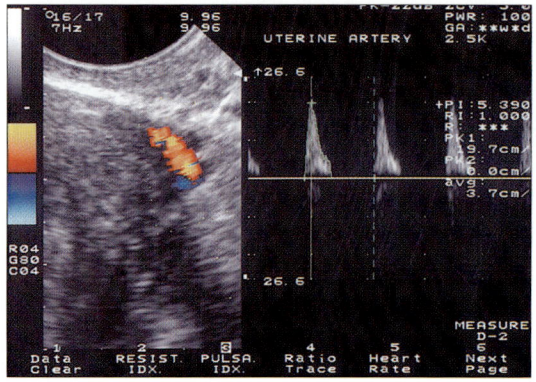

Figure 9 Absent diastolic flow is noted in both uterine arteries of a primary infertile patient

UTERINE PERFUSION IN INFERTILE PATIENTS

The expanding experience with transvaginal color and pulsed Doppler sonography has established this technique as an additional tool in the management of infertile patients. In anovulatory cycles, a continuous increase of the uterine artery RI has been detected[8] (Figure 8). Moreover, in some infertile patients, end-diastolic flow is absent[13] (Figure 9). There are not enough data to speculate whether absent diastolic flow is associated with infertility and poor reproductive performance.

The uterine artery blood flow could be used to predict a hostile uterine environment prior to embryo transfer. Steer and colleagues[14] calculated the probability of pregnancy by using PI values obtained from the uterine artery on the day of embryo transfer. With the use of these measurements, the highest probability of becoming pregnant was obtained in those patients with medium values of uterine artery PI. A mean PI of more than 3.0 before the transfer can predict up to 35% of failures to become pregnant. Tsai and colleagues[22] evaluated the prognostic value of uterine perfusion on the day of human chorionic gonadotropin (hCG) administration in patients who were undergoing intrauterine insemination. They calculated the PI of the ascending branch of the uterine arteries on the day of administration of hCG, and compared the uterine artery vascular resistance to the outcome of intrauterine insemination. No pregnancy occurred when the pulsatility index of the ascending branch of the uterine arteries was more than 3. The fecundity rate was 18% when the PI was less than 2, and was 19.8% when the PI was between 2 and 3. Their data suggest that the measurement of uterine perfusion on the day of hCG administration may have predictive value regarding fecundity in patients undergoing intrauterine insemination. Zaidi and associates[23] tried to assess whether measurement of the uterine artery blood flow impedance on the day of hCG administration can predict pregnancy and implantation rates in patients undergoing *in vitro* fertilization (IVF) procedures. They investigated 135 patients undergoing 139 IVF cycles. Their study suggests that the measurement of the uterine artery pulsatility index can predict the subsequent implantation rate, since the highest pregnancy rates (34.7%) occurred when the uterine artery PI was between 2 and 3. Furthermore, the administration of hCG should be deferred until the uterine artery PI falls to < 3, which may result in improved implantation rates. However, more studies are necessary to establish the precise relationship between uterine artery perfusion and the probability of pregnancy. Those women with poor uterine perfusion could be advised to have their embryos cryopreserved for transfer at a later date.

An improvement of the uterine blood flow may be achieved by administration of estradiol[24] and perhaps even progesterone[25]. One of the major problems associated with current practice in *in vitro* fertilization is the necessity to use multiple embryo transfer to increase the pregnancy rate. This leads to an increased incidence of multiple pregnancy. This may contribute to increased obstetric risk and poorer perinatal outcome, when compared to singleton pregnancies. It is well known that the probability of pregnancy is strongly related to embryo quality and uterine receptivity. Instead of doing endometrial biopsy, which may cause trauma and bleeding at the implantation site, uterine receptivity should be assessed by color Doppler ultrasound[26]. Zaidi and colleagues[27] evaluated 96 women undergoing *in vitro* fertilization treatment on the day of hCG administration by transvaginal color Doppler. They assessed endometrial thickness, endometrial morphology, presence or absence of subendometrial or intraendometrial color flow, and intraendometrial vascular penetration on the day of hCG administration, and related the results to pregnancy rates. The overall pregnancy rate was 32.3% and there was no

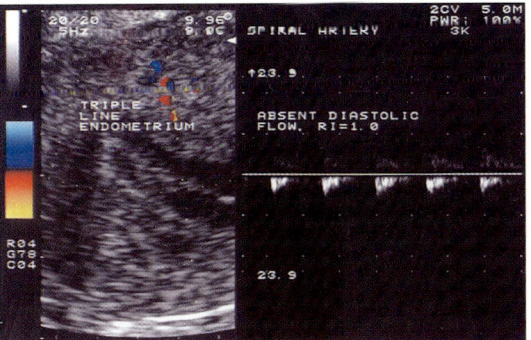

Figure 10 Blood flow velocity waveforms of the spiral arteries obtained from a triple-line endometrium. The absence of diastolic flow is a sign of poor endometrial perfusion and correlates with poor endometrial receptivity

significant difference between the pregnant and non-pregnant groups with regard to endometrial thickness, subendometrial peak systolic blood flow velocity and subendometrial index. However, the absence of subendometrial blood flow was always related to failure of implantation. Transvaginal color and pulsed Doppler examination is easily repeatable, rapid, simple to perform and may predict the likelihood of implantation, minimizing the risk of multiple pregnancy. Studies of uterine blood flow might become a non-invasive assay of uterine receptivity, giving us more information on the pathophysiology of infertility, especially in the group of patients with unexplained causes.

UTERINE PERFUSION IN SPONTANEOUS AND INDUCED OVARIAN CYCLES WITH CONFIRMED OVULATION

Kupesic and Kurjak[20] measured the flow velocity of the uterine, radial and spiral arteries during the periovulatory period in spontaneous and induced ovarian cycles with confirmed ovulation. They studied daily measurements of 78 patients attending an infertility clinic because of male factor infertility.

In spontaneous cycles, the uterine flow velocity had a PI of 3.16, 2 days before ovulation, and this started to decrease the day before ovulation (PI 2.22). In stimulated cycles, these changes did not occur, and the mean PI of 3.06 remained at that level during the peri-ovulatory period. Clear flow velocity wave-forms were obtained from the endometrium and myometrium at around the time of ovula-tion. The pulsatility indices of radial and spiral arteries showed significantly higher values in stimulated than in spontaneous cycles.

Clomiphene citrate is known to deplete estrogen receptors in estrogen-sensitive tissues, influencing endometrial growth and pattern[28]. There was a strong correlation between endo-metrial thickness and flow velocities. However, this did not apply to the group of patients stimulated with clomiphene citrate/human menopausal gonadotropin (hMG) who had normal endometrial growth, where the authors demonstrated the absence of diastolic flow in spiral arteries in 55.6% of patients (Figure 10). However, no difference in endometrial thick-ness and perfusion was observed between hMG-stimulated patients and those in sponta-neous cycles. Indeed, spiral artery blood flow changes may be used as an accurate predictor of implantation success rate in treatment with IVF and embryo transfer. Those women with poor uterine perfusion in their current treat-ment cycles could be advised to have their embryos cryopreserved and transferred either in a spontaneous cycle or after correction of the endometrial perfusion by appropriate treatment.

References

1. Torry, R. J. and Rongish, B. J. (1992). Angio-genesis in the uterus: potential regulation and relation to tumor angiogenesis. *Am. J. Reprod. Immunol.*, **27**, 171–9
2. Kaiserman-Abramof, I. R. and Padykula, H. A. (1989). Angiogenesis in the postovulatory primate endometrium: the coiled arteriolar system. *Anat. Rec.*, **224**, 479–89
3. Ramsey, E. M. and Donner, M. E. (1980). *Placental Vasculature and Circulation*, pp. 1–52. (Philadelphia, PA: Saunders)
4. Khong, T. Y., De Wolf, F., Robertson, W. B. and Brosens, I. (1986). Inadequate maternal vas-cular response to placentation in pregnancies complicated by pre-eclampsia and by small-for-gestational age infants. *Br. J. Obstet. Gynaecol.*, **93**, 1049–59
5. Ramsey, E. M. and Donner, M. V. (1988). Pla-cental vasculature and circulation in primates. In Kaufmann, P. and Miller, R.K. (eds.) *Trophoblast Research. Vol. 3: Placental Vascularization and Blood Flow*, pp. 217–33. (New York: Plenum Press)
6. Christofferson, R. and Nilsson, B. O. (1988). Morphology of the endometrial microvascula-ture during early placentation in the rat. *Cell Tissue Res.*, **253**, 209–20
7. Kurjak, A. and Kupesic-Urek, S. (1992). Nor-mal and abnormal uterine perfusion. In Jaffe, R. and Warsof, L. S. (eds.) *Color Doppler Imaging in Obstetrics and Gynecology*, pp. 255–63. (New York: McGraw Hill)
8. Kurjak, A., Kupesic-Urek, S., Schulman, H. and Zalud, I. (1991). Transvaginal color flow Doppler in the assessment of ovarian and uterine blood flow in infertile women. *Fertil. Steril.*, **56**, 870–3
9. Du Bose, T. J., Hill, L. W. and Henningan, J. W. Jr (1985). Sonography of arcuate uterine blood vessels. *J. Ultrasound Med.*, **4**, 229–33
10. Jurkovic, D., Jauniaux, E., Kurjak, A. and Campbell, S. (1991). Transvaginal color Doppler assessment of the uteroplacental circulation in early pregnancy. *Obstet. Gynecol.*, **77**, 365–9
11. Long, M. G., Boultbee, J. E., Hanson, M. E. and Begent, J. H. R. (1989). Doppler time velocity waveform studies of the uterine artery and uterus. *Br. J. Obstet Gynaecol.*, **96**, 588–93
12. Goswamy, R. K. and Steptoe, P. C. (1988). Doppler ultrasound studies of the uterine artery in spontaneous ovarian cycles. *Hum. Reprod.*, **3**, 721–3
13. Goswamy, R. K., Williams, G. and Steptoe, P. C. (1988). Decreased uterine perfusion – a cause of infertility. *Hum. Reprod.*, **3**, 955–8
14. Steer, C. V., Mills, C. V. and Campbell, S. (1991). Vaginal color Doppler assessment on the day of embryo transfer accurately predicts patients in an *in vitro* fertilization program with suboptimal uterine perfusion who fail to become pregnant. *Ultrasound Obstet. Gynecol.*, **1**, 79–82
15. Bourne, T. H., Jurkovic, D., Waterstone, J., Campbell, S. and Collins, W. P. (1991). Intrafol-licular blood flow during human ovulation. *Ultrasound Obstet. Gynecol.*, **1**, 53–7
16. Scholtes, M. C. W., Wladimiroff, J. W., van Rijen, H. J. M. and Hop, W. C. J. (1989). Uterine and

ovarian flow velocity waveforms in the normal menstrual cycle: a transvaginal study. *Fertil. Steril.*, **52**, 981–5

17. Haukson, A., Akerlund, M. and Melin, P. (1988). Uterine blood flow and myometrial activity at menstruation, and the action of vasopressin and a synthetic antagonist. *Br. J. Obstet. Gynaecol.*, **95**, 898–904

18. Battaglia, C., Larocca, E., Lanzani, A., Valentini, M. and Genanzzani, A. R. (1990). Doppler ultrasound studies of the uterine arteries in spontaneous and IVF cycles. *Gynecol. Endocrinol.*, **4**, 245–50

19. Zaidi, J., Jurkovic, D., Campbell, S., Pitroff, R., McGregor, A. and Tan, S. L. (1995). Description of circadian rhythm in uterine artery blood flow during the peri-ovulatory period. *Hum. Reprod.*, **10**, 1642–6

20. Kupesic, S. and Kurjak, A. (1993). Uterine and ovarian perfusion during the periovulatory period assessed by transvaginal color Doppler. *Fertil. Steril.*, **60**, 439–43

21. Kupesic, S., Kurjak, A. and Stilinovic, K. (1994). The assessment of female infertility. In Kurjak, A. (ed.) *An Atlas of Transvaginal Color Doppler*, pp. 171–99. (Carnforth, UK: Parthenon Publishing)

22. Tsai, Y. C., Chang, J. C., Tai, M. J., Kung, F. T., Yang, L. C. and Chang, S. Y. (1996). Relationship of uterine perfusion to outcome of intrauterine insemination. *J. Ultrasound Med.*, **15**, 633–6

23. Zaidi, J., Pitroff, R., Shaker, A., Kyei-Mensah, A., Campbell, S. and Tan, S. L. (1996). Assessment of uterine artery blood flow on the day of human chorionic gonadotropin administration by transvaginal color Doppler ultrasound in an *in vitro* fertilization program. *Fertil. Steril.*, **5**, 377–81

24. Ford, S. P., Reynolds, R. P. and Farley, D. B. (1984). Interaction of ovarian steroids and periarterial alpha-1-adrenergic receptors in altering uterine blood flow during the estrous cycle of gilts. *Am. J. Obstet. Gynecol.*, **150**, 480–4

25. de Ziegler, D., Bessis, R. and Frydman, R. (1991). Vascular resistance of uterine arteries: physiological effects of estradiol and progesterone. *Fertil. Steril.*, **55**, 775–8

26. Kupesic, S., Kurjak, A., Vujisic, S. and Petrovic, Z. (1997). Luteal phase defect: comparison between Doppler velocimetry, histological and hormonal markers. *Ultrasound Obstet. Gynecol.*, **9**, 105–112

27. Zaidi, J., Campbell, S., Pitroff, R. and Tan, S. L. (1995). Endometrial thickness, morphology, vascular penetration and velocimetry in predicting implantation in an *in vitro* fertilization program. *Ultrasound Obstet. Gynecol.*, **6**, 191–8

28. Glissant, A., de Mouzon, J. and Frydman, R. (1985). Ultrasound study of the endometrium during *in vitro* fertilization cycles. *Fertil. Steril.*, **44**, 786–90

Is it possible to improve uterine blood flow in infertile women?

12

B. Cacciatore

Transvaginal Doppler sonography has allowed us to study the uterine and ovarian blood flow pattern, providing us with new insights into uterine physiology. Uterine impedance to blood flow varies during the spontaneous or hormonally stimulated menstrual cycle, mostly as a result of the cyclic changes in circulating ovarian hormones, but also following a circadian rhythm[1-4]. In a spontaneous menstrual cycle, uterine impedance to flow decreases constantly while approaching the end of the cycle, being lowest at the mid-luteal phase, indicating an increase of uterine perfusion coincident with the time of implantation. At this time, the uterine artery pulsatility index (PI) is generally below 3.0 and the resistance index (RI) below 0.90. In anovulatory cycles these changes have not been found[5,6], and the mid-luteal phase uterine artery PI is above 3.0 in 20–40% of these subjects. Such high pulsatility in the uterine artery Doppler velocity waveform has been found to be associated with a significantly reduced chance of implantation in *in vitro* fertilization and embryo transfer (IVF–ET)[7,8] as well as in natural cycles in which frozen–thawed embryos are replaced[9]. These findings imply that vascular impedance is a determinant of the successful implantation and development of a fertilized ovum, but the mechanism of action is still unclear.

Estradiol is a vasodilator *in vitro* and *in vivo*[10], and plays a key role in the regulation of uterine vascular impedance. Hypoestrogenism is accompanied by a significant rise in uterine pulsatility, reversible by 17β-estradiol replacement[11,12]. However, 17β-estradiol may not be involved in the increased uterine impedance to flow seen in some infertile women, who maintain high uterine blood flow impedance even with the high 17β-estradiol concentrations produced by ovarian stimulation[13]. These women respond poorly to assisted reproductive technology and require treatment *ad hoc* to improve receptivity. They account for only a fraction of those suffering from infertility, but they pose a problem of management. Should the embryo transfer be postponed until later in the same treatment cycle, or even a subsequent one? Is there any pharmacological possibility to improve uterine blood flow?

DOES UTERINE IMPEDANCE TO FLOW CHANGE DURING THE LUTEAL PHASE?

In women with elevated uterine impedance to flow, postponing embryo transfer for a few days to achieve better uterine perfusion would assume a spontaneous improvement in uterine impedance during the luteal phase. Although uterine artery pulsatility has been described to fluctuate through the normal menstrual cycle, this issue has not been studied in infertile women during treatment cycles. Therefore, we decided to evaluate uterine artery impedance to flow prospectively in infertile women at the early, mid- and late luteal phase, to see whether there were significant changes in PI and, more important, whether there were more favorable conditions for implantation, i.e. a PI below 3.

We recruited 20 volunteers: women suffering from unexplained infertility and participating in our IVF program. They were studied in an IVF–ET cycle stimulated with gonadotropin releasing hormone (GnRH)-analog, human menopausal gonadotropin (hMG) and human

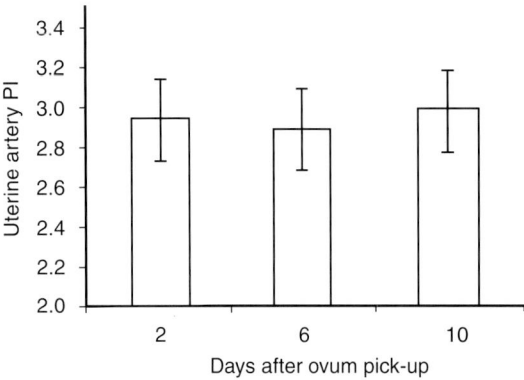

Figure 1 Uterine artery pulsatility index (PI; mean ± SD) after ovum pick-up in 20 infertile women

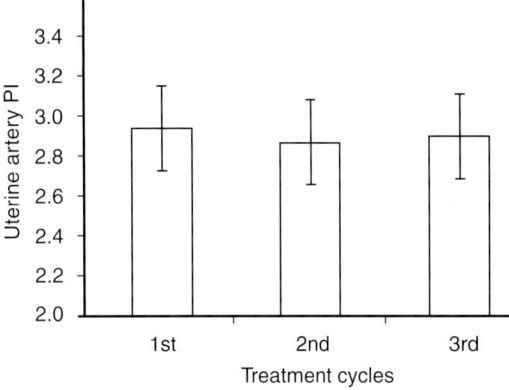

Figure 2 Uterine artery pulsatility index (PI; mean ± SD) at the time of embryo transfer in three consecutive cycles with *in vitro* fertilization–embryo transfer or with frozen–thawed embryos (n = 22)

chorionic gonadotropin (hCG). Transvaginal color Doppler was performed 2, 6 and 10 days after ovum pick-up, and the PI from the main branch of the uterine artery was measured by a single investigator, between 10.00 and 12.00 to avoid circadian variations. At day + 2, the mean PI was 2.9 ± 0.5 and it was over 3 in eight (40%) women. Subsequent examinations (Figure 1) showed no significant changes in mean uterine PI (ANOVA for repeated measurements), nor were these changes in the number of women in whom the PI was above 3 (seven at the mid-luteal phase and eight at the late luteal phase). Four of these women

conceived a normal intrauterine pregnancy as a result of the treatment cycles, and all of these had a PI below 3 at the time of embryo transfer.

These results indicate that, among infertile women with elevated uterine impedance to flow, uterine pulsatility remains rather stable in the same treatment cycle, and therefore it may not be useful to postpone embryo transfer for 1 or more days, since the chance that uterine perfusion will improve later during the luteal phase appears very small.

DOES UTERINE IMPEDANCE TO FLOW VARY BETWEEN DIFFERENT TREATMENT CYCLES?

Another possibility to overcome the problem of an elevated impedance to flow at the time of embryo transfer would be to cancel the cycle and try again in a subsequent one. This would presume that uterine impedance to flow might be better in another treatment cycle. Since this interesting issue has also not yet been addressed, we retrospectively searched among all infertile women who had participated in our IVF–ET program for those in whom the uterine artery PI had been assessed in more than one treatment cycle. We identified 22 women who had undergone evaluation of uterine artery impedance to flow three times at the time of embryo transfer, either in spontaneous cycles in which a frozen–thawed embryo had been transferred (n = 10), or in IVF–ET cycles (n = 12). The time between different treatment cycles varied between 2 and 6 months for the spontaneous cycles and between 4 and 12 months for the IVF–ET cycles. In each patient the different cycles were comparable with regard to hormonal profiles (serum levels of 17β-estradiol and progesterone) and treatment protocol (GnRH-analog, hMG, hCG for IVF–ET cycles; spontaneous menstrual cycles for frozen–thawed embryos). A slight fluctuation in mean PI was found (Figure 2), which, however, did not reach statistical significance. The changes remained nonsignificant when cycles from IVF–ET and frozen–thawed embryos were pooled. The proportion of women whose uterine artery PI was over 3 also did not change. These new data therefore imply that, in a single infertile woman, uterine artery impedance to flow varies little in different treatment cycles with a similar hormonal milieu.

CAN WE IMPROVE UTERINE IMPEDANCE TO FLOW PHARMACOLOGICALLY?

In pregnancy, uterine vascular tone may be regulated by nitric oxide (NO)[14], a very potent vasodilator primarily produced by vascular endothelium to act as a physiological regulator of blood flow and pressure in the cardiovascular circulation[11]. Intravenous[15] or transdermal[16] administration of glycerol trinitrate (GTN), an NO donor, reduced the uterine vascular impedance in normal and pre-eclamptic pregnant women. The synthase for NO has also been found in the stroma of endometrial glandular epithelium and in myometrial vessels[17], suggesting a role for NO in the paracrine control of the uterine circulation in nonpregnant women.

It is therefore possible that GTN administration might improve the uterine impedance to flow in infertile women. To this end, we prospectively studied 15 infertile women with increased impedance to flow (uterine PI > 3). The cause of infertility was tubal occlusion in nine women, endometriosis in four and unexplained in three. These women were examined first during a spontaneous menstrual cycle and then in a subsequent cycle in which a patch of GTN 10 mg/24 h was applied daily for the entire cycle. The uterine artery PI was assessed as described above by transvaginal Doppler sonography at four times: cycle days 4–6, 11–13, 19–21 and 24–26.

GTN administration led to a significant ($p < 0.01$) fall in mean uterine artery PI at each examination point (Figure 3). The uterine artery RI dropped in 13 of the 15 (87%) women and remained substantially unchanged in two women (14%). On average, the uterine artery PI was 19% lower in the GTN cycle than in the baseline cycle at cycle days 4–6, 25% at

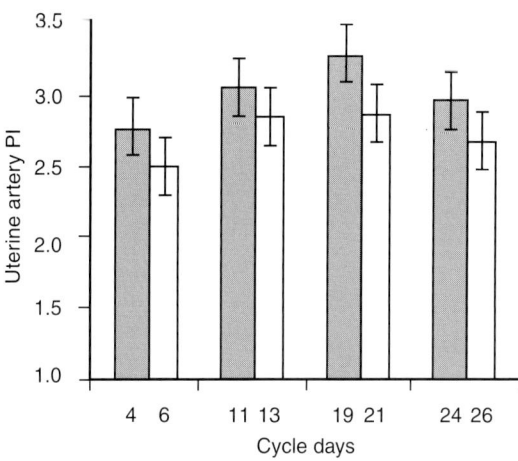

Figure 3 Uterine artery pulsatility index (PI; mean ± SE) in a normal cycle (shaded bars) and during administration of a patch of glycerol trinitrate 10 mg/24 h (open bars). The reduction in PI was highly significant at each examination point (Friedman's test)

cycle days 11–13, 20% at cycle days 19–21 and 19% at cycle days 24–26. As a result of this fall, GTN reduced the number of women who had a PI above 3 at cycle days 19–21 from 15 to only five (33%, $p < 0.01$).

GTN is rapidly oxygenated in the bloodstream; transdermal administration as a single patch keeps circulating concentrations stable for up to 24 h, without remarkable side-effects[16]. It is noteworthy that GTN administration significantly reduced the uterine pulsatility (PI < $3^{2,3}$) around the time of implantation (cycle days 19–21), increasing the chance of implantation in the vast majority of women. NO released by GTN may have reduced the impedance to flow in uterine vessels directly by relaxing endometrial and myometrial vascular smooth muscle cells[17]. It is therefore possible that the fall in uterine impedance was caused by vasodilatory effects on uterine vessels or by a reduction of uterine muscular tone, or synergistically by both mechanisms. GTN treatment did not prevent ovulation in any of our patients. Further studies will address whether administration of GTN for shorter periods of time or at different dosages will change its effect on uterine and ovarian impedance to flow.

CONCLUSION

High impedance to flow in the uterine arteries appears to be a constant feature in a number of infertile women, and therefore may require pharmacological help. Our initial experience would suggest that the use of nitric oxide donors, such as glycerol trinitrate, may improve uterine blood flow. Prospective studies in treatment cycles will have to demonstrate whether the fall in pulsatility achieved is beneficial to uterine receptivity in infertile women, with Doppler evidence of impaired uterine perfusion and poor response to assisted reproductive technologies.

References

1. Goswamy, R. K. and Steptoe, P. C. (1988). Doppler ultrasound studies of the uterine arteries in spontaneous ovarian cycles. *Hum. Reprod.*, **3**, 721–6
2. Steer, C. V., Campbell, S., Pompiglione, J. S., Kingsland, C. R. C., Mason, B. A. and Collins, W. P. (1990). Transvaginal colour flow imaging of the uterine arteries during the ovarian and menstrual cycle. *Hum. Reprod.*, **5**, 391–5
3. Tan, S. L., Zaidi, J., Campbell, S., Doyle, P. and Collins, W. (1996). Blood flow changes in the ovarian and uterine arteries during the normal menstrual cycle. *Am. J. Obstet. Gynecol.*, **175**, 625–31
4. Zaidi, J., Jurkovic, D., Campbell, S., Okokon, E. and Tan, S. L. (1995). Circadian variation in uterine artery blood flow indices during the follicular phase of the menstrual cycle. *Ultrasound Obstet. Gynecol.*, **5**, 406–10
5. Kupesic, S. and Kurjak, A. (1993). Uterine and ovarian perfusion during the periovulatory period assessed by transvaginal color Doppler. *Fertil. Steril.*, **60**, 439–43
6. Steer, C. V., Tan, S. L., Mason, B. A. and Campbell, S. (1994). Midluteal-phase vaginal color Doppler assessment of uterine artery impedence in a subfertile population. *Fertil. Steril.*, **61**, 53–8
7. Coulam, C. B., Bustillo, M., Soenksen, D. M. and Britten, S. (1994). Ultrasonographic predictors of implantation after assisted reproduction. *Fertil. Steril.*, **62**, 1004–10
8. Cacciatore, B., Simberg, N., Fusaro, P. and Tiitinen, A. (1996). Transvaginal Doppler study of uterine artery blood flow in *in vitro* fertilization and embryo transfer cycles. *Fertil. Steril.*, **66**, 130–4
9. Tekay, A., Martikainen, H. and Jouppila, P. (1996). Comparison of uterine blood flow characteristics between spontaneous and stimulated cycles before embryo transfer. *Hum. Reprod.*, **11**, 364–8
10. White, M. M., Zamudio, S., Stevens, T., Tyler, R., Lindefeld, J., Leslie, K. *et al.* (1996). Estrogen, progesterone and vascular reactivity: potential cellular mechanisms. *Endocrine. Rev.*, **16**, 739–51
11. De Ziegler, D., Bessis, R. and Frydman, R. (1991). Vascular resistance of uterine arteries: physiological effects of estradiol and progesterone. *Fertil. Steril.*, **55**, 775–9
12. Hillard, T. C., Bourne, T. H., Whitehead, M. I., Crayford, T. B., Collins, W. P. and Campbell, S. (1992). Differential effects of transdermal estradiol and sequential progestogens on impedance to flow within the uterine arteries of postmenopausal women. *Fertil. Steril.*, **58**, 959–63
13. Cacciatore, B. and Tiitinen, A. (1996). Does ovarian hyperstimulation affect uterine artery impedance? *J. Assist. Reprod. Genet.*, **13**, 15–18
14. Myatt, L., Brewer, A. and Brockman, D. E. (1991). The action of nitric oxide in the perfused human fetal–placental circulation. *Am. J. Obstet. Gynecol.*, **164**, 687–92
15. Ramsay, B., De Belder, A., Campbell, S., Moncada, S. and Martin, J. F. (1994). A nitric oxide donor improves uterine artery diastolic blood flow in normal and early pregnancy and in women at high risk of preeclampsia. *Eur. J. Clin. Invest.*, **24**, 76–8
16. Cacciatore, B., Halmesmaki, E., Teramo, K. and Ylikorkala, O. (1998). Transdermal nitroglycerin administration reduces uterine impedance to flow in pregnancy complicated by preeclampsia. *Am. J. Obstet. Gynecol.*, in press
17. Telfer, J. F., Lyall, F., Norman, J. E. and Cameron, J. T. (1995). Identification of nitric oxide synthase in human uterus. *Hum. Reprod.*, **10**, 19–23

Ultrasound and Doppler assessment of uterine anomalies

13

S. Kupesic and A. Kurjak

INTRODUCTION

Congenital uterine malformations are variable in frequency and are usually estimated to occur in 3–4% of the general population, although less than one-half of these have clinical symptoms[1-3]. Uterine anomalies can be organized into the following categories: unicornuate uterus, uterus didelphus, bicornuate uterus and septate uterus. Unicornuate uterus is due to a failure of development in one Mullerian duct. A rudimentary horn may be present and implantation in this horn is followed by a very high rate of pregnancy wastage or tubal pregnancies. This anomaly can be precisely diagnosed using three-dimensional ultrasound (Figure 1). Uterus didelphus is due to a lack of fusion of the two Mullerian ducts. This results in duplication of the corpus and cervix. These patients usually have no difficulties with menstruation and coitus. Pregnancy in this anomaly is associated with an increased risk of malpresentations and premature labor. Partial lack of fusion of the

two Mullerian ducts produces a single cervix with a varying degree of separation in the two uterine horns. This anomaly is called 'bicornuate uterus', and has a high rate of early abortion, preterm labor and breech presentations (Figure 2). Partial lack of resorption of the midline septum between the two Mullerian ducts results in defects that range from a partial midline septum to a significant midline division of the endometrial cavity. A total failure in resorption results in a longitudinal vaginal septum, a so-called 'double vagina'.

UTERINE ANOMALIES: COMPLICATIONS AND DIAGNOSIS

The frequency of symptomatic malformations is greatest for septate uterus (close to 50%), compared with other malformations[3,4]. During the first trimester of pregnancy, the risk of spontaneous abortion in this group is between 28 and 45%, while during the second trimester

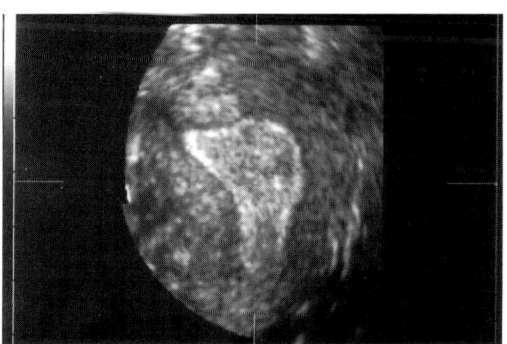

Figure 1 Three-dimensional ultrasound scan demonstrating a unicornuate uterus. Note the absence of the left horn

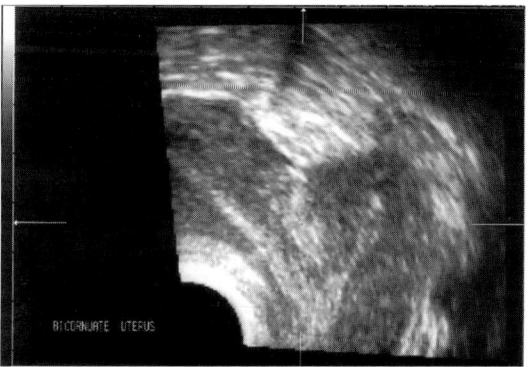

Figure 2 Three-dimensional ultrasound scan of a bicornuate uterus. Note the clear separation of the two horns and the concave shape of the fundus

the frequency of late spontaneous abortion is approximately 5%[3]. Premature deliveries, abnormal fetal presentations, irregular uterine activity and dystocia at delivery are likely to prevail in cases of septate uterus[5]. Poor vascularization of the septum has been proposed as a potential cause of miscarriages[4]. An electron microscopy study by Fedele and colleagues[6] indicated a decrease in the sensitivity of the endometrium covering the septa of malformed uteri to preovulatory changes. This could play a role in the pathogenesis of primary infertility in patients with septate uterus.

It is clear that an unfavorable obstetric prognosis can be transformed by surgical correction of the intrauterine septum. Formerly, removal of the septum was performed by transabdominal metroplasty[7]. Hysteroscopic treatment is currently proposed as the procedure of choice for the management of this disorder. This simple and effective treatment has the obvious advantage that the uterus is not weakened by a myometrial scar. Cararach and colleagues[8] and Goldenberg and associates[9] reported pregnancy rates of 75 and 88.7%, respectively, after operative hysteroscopy. The simplicity and effectiveness of hysteroscopy mean that an early and correct diagnosis of the uterine anomaly is preferable. When used as a screening test for detection of congenital uterine anomalies transvaginal ultrasound had a sensitivity of almost 100%[10,11]. However, a clear distinction between some types of abnormalities is impossible and is operator dependent[12,13].

X-ray hysterosalpingography (HSG) is an invasive test which requires the use of a contrast medium and exposure to radiation. Although HSG provides a good outline of the uterine cavity, the visualization of minor anomalies and a clear distinction between different types of lateral fusion disorders are sometimes impossible. More recently, hysterosonography has been introduced[14]. In these patients transvaginal ultrasound is carried out after distension of the uterine cavity by instillation of a saline solution. This simple and minimally invasive approach allows anatomical images of the endometrium and myometrium,

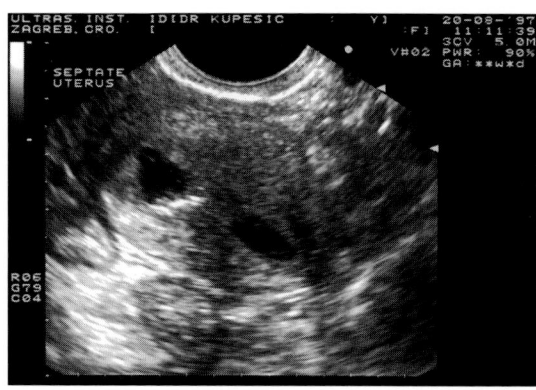

Figure 3 A septate uterus imaged using hysterosonography. Note the two separated endometrial echoes divided by a thick septum

accurate depiction of the septate uterus and even measurement of the thickness and height of the septum[15] (Figure 3).

Although some reports have indicated a high diagnostic accuracy of magnetic resonance imaging[16,17] and three-dimensional ultrasound[18] in the diagnosis of congenital uterine anomalies, these techniques are rarely used routinely for this indication. In patients scheduled for corrective surgery the evaluation is usually completed by another invasive procedure – CO_2 diagnostic hysteroscopy[19].

ULTRASOUND IMAGING IN THE DIAGNOSIS AND TREATMENT OF SEPTATE UTERUS

Our studies attempted to evaluate the combined use of transvaginal ultrasound, transvaginal color and pulsed Doppler sonography, hysterosonography and three-dimensional ultrasound in the preoperative diagnosis of septate uterus[20,21]. In the first study we analyzed obstetric and perinatal complications of septate uterus, and assessed the reproductive outcome after the hysteroscopic treatment[20]. A total of 420 infertile patients undergoing operative hysteroscopy were included in this study. Table 1 summarizes the intraoperative findings. The final diagnosis of the uterine disorder was confirmed by hysteroscopy, and 278 patients had intrauterine septum corrected surgically. Forty-three of the patients with

Table 1 Intraoperative findings in 420 infertile patients undergoing hysteroscopy

Hysteroscopic finding	n
Submucous leiomyoma	46
Endometrial polyp	35*
Intrauterine synechiae	19*
Septate uterus	278
Arcuate uterus	28
Bicornuate uterus	16†
Total	422

*One patient with endometrial polyp and one with intrauterine synechiae had intrauterine septum; †diagnosis made by combined use of laparoscopy and hysteroscopy. From reference 20, with permission

septate uterus had a history of repeated spontaneous abortion, 71 had one spontaneous abortion (56 in the first trimester, 15 during the second trimester), 82 had primary sterility and 20 had premature delivery, including six with breech and two with transverse presentation. A positive history of ectopic pregnancy was noticed in 76 patients.

Each patient underwent transvaginal ultrasound and transvaginal color Doppler examination during the luteal phase of their cycle. A systematic examination of the uterine position, size and morphological characteristics was performed. With the use of B-mode transvaginal sonography, the morphology of the uterus was carefully explored, with emphasis on the endometrial lining in both sagittal and transverse sections. The septum was visualized as an echogenic portion separating the uterine cavity into two parts. Once B-mode examination was completed by an experienced sonographer, transvaginal color Doppler examination was performed by another skilled operator who was unaware of the previous findings.

Color and pulsed Doppler were superimposed to visualize intraseptal and myometrial vascularity. Flow velocity waveforms were obtained from all the interrogated vessels. For each recording, at least five waveform signals of good quality were obtained. During each procedure the resistance index (RI) was automatically calculated. The RI was calculated from the maximum frequency envelope as the peak systolic velocity minus the end-diastolic

velocity, divided by the peak systolic velocity. Instillation of isotonic saline (hysterosonography) was carried out on a gynecological examination table. In 76 patients the uterine cervix was exposed with a speculum disinfected with iodine solution. A catheter with an external diameter of 1.6 mm and an internal diameter of 1.1 mm was slowly introduced into the cervix. The balloon was insufflated with 1.5 to 2 ml of sterile saline to avoid outflow of the fluid. A syringe containing 20 ml isotonic saline solution was attached to the catheter and fluid was slowly injected. For distension of the uterine cavity about 10 to 20 ml of the contrast solution was required. The speculum was then withdrawn and the endovaginal probe introduced. Transverse and sagittal sections were carefully explored, and the septum was visualized as an echogenic portion separating the uterine cavity into two parts.

Eighty-six women undergoing hysteroscopy were examined by three-dimensional ultrasound. They all had a transvaginal scan and color and pulsed Doppler evaluation prior to the three-dimensional examination. Twelve of these patients underwent the additional examination of instillation of isotonic saline into the uterine cavity. The results of the previous diagnostic tests were not available to the ultrasonographer. Three perpendicular planes of the uterus were simultaneously displayed on the screen, allowing a detailed analysis of the uterine morphology. Frontal reformatted sections were particularly useful for detection of the uterine abnormalities.

Table 2 summarizes the sensitivity, specificity and positive and negative predictive values of transvaginal sonography, transvaginal color and pulsed Doppler ultrasound, hysterosalpingography and three-dimensional ultrasound for the diagnosis of the septate uterus[21]. In 264 cases septate uterus was suspected by transvaginal ultrasonography, whereas 14 patients were reported to have normal findings and were expressed as representing false-negative results. Therefore, the sensitivity of transvaginal sonography in the diagnosis of septate uterus was 95.21%. Transvaginal color and pulsed Doppler sonography enabled the

Table 2 Sensitivity, specificity, positive predictive value (PPV) and negative predictive value (NPV) of transvaginal sonography, transvaginal color Doppler, hysterosonography and three-dimensional ultrasound for the diagnosis of septate uterus in 420 patients with a history of infertility and recurrent abortions

Imaging modality	Sensitivity (%)	Specificity (%)	PPV (%)	NPV (%)
Transvaginal sonography	95.21	92.21	95.86	91.03
Transvaginal color Doppler	99.29	97.93	98.3	98.61
Hysterosonography	98.18	100.00	100.00	95.46
Three-dimensional ultrasound	98.38	100.00	100.00	96.00

From reference 21, with permission

diagnosis of septate uterus in 276 cases, reaching a sensitivity of 99.28%. In one patient with endometrial polyp and one with intrauterine synechiae, septate uteri were not correctly diagnosed. The reliability of color and pulsed Doppler examination was reduced if other intracavitary structures (such as intrauterine synechiae, endometrial polyp or submucous leiomyoma) were present. Color and pulsed Doppler studies of the septal area revealed vascularity in 198 (71.22%) patients (Figure 4). The RI values obtained from the septum ranged from 0.68 to 1.0 (mean RI, 0.84 ± 0.16) (Figure 5). Eighteen patients demonstrated absence of diastolic blood flow, while in the rest a continuous diastolic flow was present.

Hysterosonography, which was carried out in 76 patients, reached 100% specificity and positive predictive value. In one patient with extensive intrauterine synechiae, hysterosonography did not detect a intrauterine septum, although it was successful in diagnosing septate uterus in the remaining 54 patients.

Good quality three-dimensional images were obtained in 86 patients (Figure 6). The sensitivity and specificity of three-dimensional ultrasonography were 93.38% and 100%, respectively. A false-negative result in one patient was caused by a fundal fibroid distorting the uterine cavity. Three-dimensional ultrasonography therefore correctly detected septate uterus in 61 patients. Interestingly, in our study septate uterus was not mistaken for bicornuate uterus when transvaginal color Doppler sonography, hysterosonography, and three-dimensional ultrasonography were performed. However, in one patient with

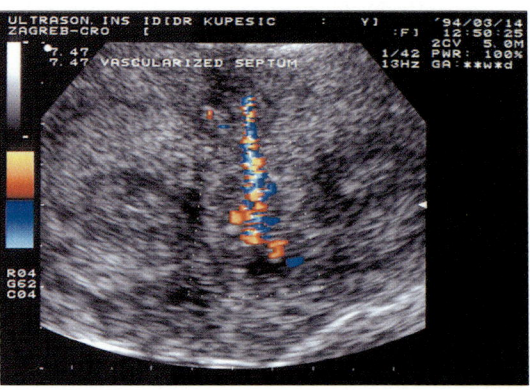

Figure 4 A transvaginal ultrasound scan demonstrating a septate uterus. Note the two separate endometria in the proliferative phase of the menstrual cycle. Color Doppler exposes small myometrial vessels within the uterine septum

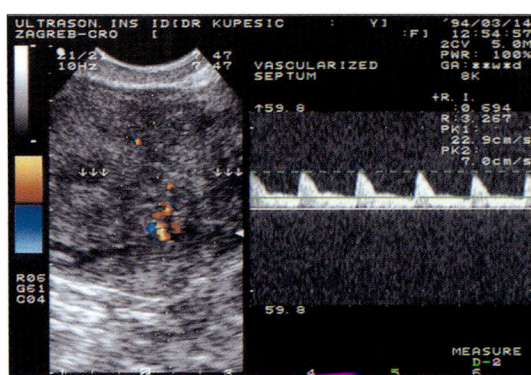

Figure 5 In the same patient as in Figure 4, color signals explored by pulsed Doppler waveform analysis show moderate-to-high resistance to blood flow (resistance index 0.69) typical of radial arteries

bicornuate uterus transvaginal ultrasonography misinterpreted septate uterus[11].

A total of 188 patients underwent X-ray HSG within 12 months prior to our examination[20].

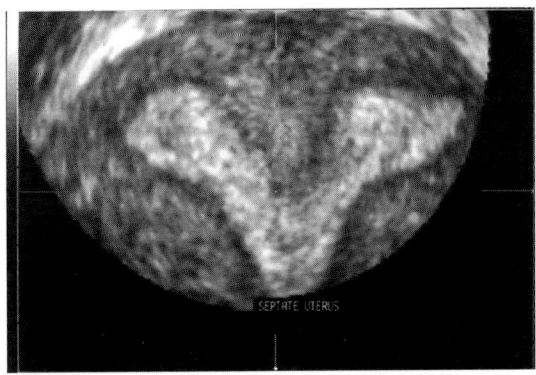

Figure 6 A three-dimensional ultrasound scan of a septate uterus which is characterized by a normal outer uterine contour and a thick septum extending into the uterine cavity

X-ray HSG made a diagnosis of septate uterus in 49 patients according to the criteria of Reuter[15]. A septate uterus was suspected if the angle between the two cavities was < 75°, while a bicornuate uterus was suspected for angles > 105°. In 15 cases (7.98%) hysterosalpingography indicated a deformed uterine cavity, but congenital anomaly of the uterus was not suspected. The sensitivity of X-ray HSG in the diagnosis of septate uterus was only 26.06%.

We also attempted to evaluate the obstetric complications in a population of 278 patients with septate uterus and to compare them with the general population during the period 1992 to 1996[20]. Early abortions appeared at a rate of 114/278 (41.01%), compared to a rate of 15% for the general population. Late abortions and premature deliveries appeared at a rate of 35/278 (12.59%), as compared to a rate of 7% for normal pregnancies. Intrauterine growth retardation appeared in two (8.7%) pregnancies with septate uterus, compared with 6% among the general population. Intrauterine fetal death occurred in one (4.35%) patient, compared with 0.5% in the general population. Abruptio placenta was found in one (4.35%) patient with septate uterus, as well as placenta previa (4.35%). Breech presentation was found in six (26.09%) pregnancies complicated by intrauterine septum, while transverse presentation

occurred in two (8.70%) patients. Since abnormal fetal presentation was significantly more frequent in patients with septate uterus, a remarkably high rate of Cesarean section (34.78%) occurred, compared with 12% in the general population. Cervical incompetance during pregnancy appeared in nine (25.71%) women with intrauterine septum. Extrauterine pregnancy appeared in 76 patients (27.34%), which was a two-times higher incidence than in the general population (13.3%). Bilateral ectopic pregnancy was noticed in seven patients with septate uterus.

We assessed the reproductive outcome in 116 patients (32 with primary sterility, 16 with one spontaneous abortion, 12 with premature deliveries and 26 with recurrent abortions) following operative hysteroscopy for an intrauterine septum. The prospective follow-up period was 24 months for each patient. The pregnancy rate in the study group was 50.86%: 44 patients (74.58%) had term deliveries, 11 (18.64%) had first-trimester abortion and four (6.78%) reported preterm delivery. Other patients (*n* = 162) were followed in the same manner, but the follow-up period was less than 24 months and the results are therefore not reported in this study.

NEW DEVELOPMENTS

Until now at least two procedures have been used for detection of congenital uterine anomalies. Gynecologists should be aware that long diagnostic evaluation delays treatment, and increases the cost, patient discomfort and risk associated with each of the diagnostic procedures[15]. Therefore, quick and reliable diagnosis is important in patients with septate uterus, since surgical correction should be recommended. Fedele and colleagues[6] recently indicated that intrauterine septum may be a cause of primary infertility. They demonstrated significant ultrastructural alterations in septal endometrium compared with endometrium from the lateral uterine wall in samples obtained during the preovulatory phase. The ultrastructural alterations included a reduced number of glandular ostia distributed irregularly, ciliated cells with incomplete ciliogenesis, and a reduced ciliated-to-non-ciliated ratio. The ultrastructural morphological alterations were indicative of irregular differentiation and estrogenic maturation of septal endometrial mucosa. Since the hormonal levels of the patients enrolled in this study were normal for the cycle phase, the most convincing hypothesis was that endometrial mucosa covering the septum was poorly responsive to estrogens, probably due to poor vascularization of the septal connective tissue.

March[22] stated that the septum is composed of a fibroelastic tissue, while Fayez[23] believed that in the septum there are fewer muscle fibers and more connective tissue. However, our study did not confirm this statement. Color and pulsed Doppler sonography revealed septal vascularity in 71.22% of the patients, suggesting that most of the septa comprised myometrial vessels[20].

Dabrashrafi and colleagues[24] performed a histologic study of the uterine septa from 16 patients undergoing abdominal metroplasty. Four biopsy specimens were taken from the uterus in each case: from the septum near the serosal layer, at the midpoint of the septum, at the level of the tip of the septum and from the left posterior aspect of the uterus away from the septum. The analysis confirmed that most of the uterine septa were composed of the muscle tissue, muscle interfacing and vessels with a muscle wall, which is contradictory to the classic view on the histologic features of the uterine septum.

Less connective tissue in the septum can be the reason for poor decidualization and placentation in the area of implantation[23,24]. Increased amounts of muscle tissue and muscle interlacing in the septum can cause an abortion by the higher and unco-ordinated contractility of these muscles.

In a recent study we found no correlation between septal height and occurrence of obstetric complications ($p > 0.05$)[25]. Abortions and late pregnancy complications occurred with the same rate in patients with small septa that were dividing less than one-third of the uterine cavity and those with division of

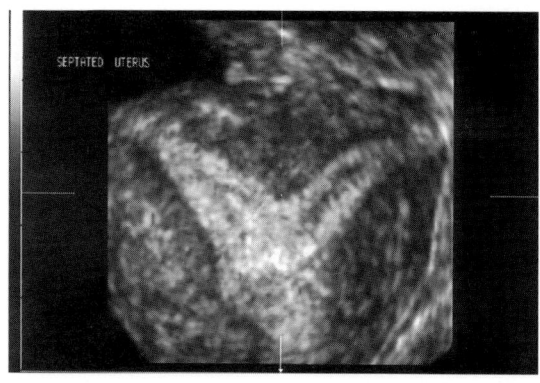

Figure 7 A three-dimensional ultrasound scan of a septate uterus. A thick septum divides the uterine cavity. The extent of the defect is clearly visualized

more than two-thirds of the uterine cavity. The same result was observed in relation to septal thickness: obstetric complications were found in the same proportion of patients with thin and patients with thick septa ($p > 0.05$). Indeed, pregnancy loss correlated significantly with septal vascularity. Patients with vascularized septa had a significantly higher incidence of early pregnancy failure and late pregnancy complications than those with avascularized septa ($p < 0.05$).

By using transvaginal ultrasound it is possible to perform a precise assessment of the uterine morphology, including the endometrial lining and the outer shape of the uterine muscle. The color Doppler technique allows simultaneous visualization of morphology and the vascular network, giving full information on the type of anomaly and the extent of the defect. The visualization of the myometrial portion is further enhanced by detection of the myometrial vessels by the color Doppler technique. Furthermore, Doppler imaging can detect deficient intraseptal vascularity and/or inadequate endometrial development in patients with septate uteri[26,27].

Three-dimensional ultrasound enables planar reformatted sections through the uterus, which allow precise evaluation of the fundal indentation and the length of the septum (Figure 7). Based on our experience, this technique may give a wrong impression of an arcuate uterus in patients with fundal location of a leiomyoma. In these cases the uterine cavity has a concave shape, while fundal indentation is more shallow. Furthermore, shadowing caused by uterine fibroids, irregular endometrial lining and a decreased volume of the uterine cavity (in cases of intrauterine adhesions) are obvious limitations of three-dimensional ultrasound.

Our study clearly proved that obstetric complications are more frequent among patients with septate uterus than among other women[20]. Furthermore, it demonstrated that ectopic pregnancy occurs at a rate (27.34%) in these patients which is twice that in controls (13.3%). A possible etiology for this finding is menstrual reflux, commonly present in patients with uterine anomalies, the sequelae of which may interfere with passage of the fertilized egg into the uterine cavity. Our study clearly demonstrated the benefit of removing the intrauterine septum in patients suffering from infertility and recurrent pregnancy wastage[20]. Furthermore, it is expected that the cumulative pregnancy rate will be even higher, since some of the primary infertile patients who are involved in *in vitro* fertilization programs due to male factor infertility await the procedure.

Conventionally it has been agreed not to intervene until the first obstetric accidents have occurred, because a great proportion of septate uteri have no obstetric pathology[3]. However, hypofecundity in this group of patients and good results achieved by endoscopic surgical treatment obligate us to propose hysteroscopy as soon as we diagnose septate uterus, even prior to any pregnancy[20,25,26]. It seems that septal incision eliminates an unsuitable site of implantation, through revascularization of the connective uterine fundal tissue or elimination of the unfavorable uterine contractions[6]. Since both of these events can be detected by color and pulsed Doppler ultrasound, this technique can be efficiently used for detection of congenital uterine malformations and follow-up of the patients undergoing hysteroscopy.

References

1. Ashton, D., Amin, H. K., Richart, R. M. and Neuwirth, R. S. (1988). The incidence of asymptomatic uterine anomalies in women undergoing transcervical tubal sterilization. *Obstet. Gynecol.*, **72**, 28–30
2. Sorensen, S. (1988). Estimated prevalence of mulerian anomalies. *Acta Obstet. Gynecol. Scand.*, **67**, 441–5
3. Gaucherand, P., Awada, A., Rudigoz, R. C. and Dargent, D. (1994). Obstetrical prognosis of septate uterus: a plea for treatment of the septum. *Eur. J. Obstet. Gynecol. Reprod. Biol.*, **54**, 109–12
4. Fedele, L., Arcaini, L., Parazzini, F., Vercellini, P. and Nola, G. D. (1993). Metroplastic hysteroscopy and fertility. *Fertil. Steril.*, **59**, 768–70
5. Heinonen, P. K., Saarikoski, S. and Pystynen, P. (1982). Reproductive performance of women with uterine anomalies. An evaluation of 182 cases. *Acta Obstet. Gynecol. Scand.*, **61**, 157–62
6. Fedele, L., Bianchi, S., Marchini, M., Franchi, D., Tozzi, L. and Dorta, M. (1996). Ultrastructural aspects of endometrium in infertile women with septate uterus. *Fertil. Steril.*, **65**, 750–2
7. McShane, P. M., Reilly, R. J. and Schiff, L. (1983). Pregnancy outcome following Tompkins metroplasty. *Fertil. Steril.*, **40**, 190–4
8. Cararach, M., Penella, J., Ubeda, J. and Labastida, R. (1994). Hysteroscopic incision of the septate uterus: scissors versus resectoscope. *Hum. Reprod.*, **9**, 87–9
9. Goldenberg, M., Sivan, E. and Sharabi, Z. (1995). Reproductive outcome following hysteroscopic management of intrauterine septum and adhesions. *Hum. Reprod.*, **10**, 2663–5
10. Valdes, C., Malini, S. and Malinak, L. R. (1984). Ultrasound evaluation of female genital tract anomalies: a review of 64 cases. *Am. J. Obstet. Gynecol.*, **149**, 285–90
11. Nicolini, U., Bellotti, B., Bonazzi, D., Zamberleti, G. and Battista, C. (1987). Can

ultrasound be used to screen uterine malformation? *Fertil. Steril.*, **47**, 89–93

12. Reuter, K. L., Daly, D. C. and Cohen, S. M. (1989). Septate versus bicornuate uteri: errors in imaging diagnosis. *Radiology*, **172**, 749–52

13. Randolph, J., Ying, Y., Maier, D., Schmidt, C. and Riddick, D. (1986). Comparison of real-time ultrasonography, hysterosalpingography, and laparoscopy/hysteroscopy in the evaluation of uterine abnormalities and tubal patency. *Fertil. Steril.*, **5**, 828–32

14. Richman, T. S., Viscomi, G. N., Cherney, A. D. and Polan, A. (1984). Fallopian tubal patency assessment by ultrasound following fluid injection. *Radiology*, **152**, 507–10

15. Salle, B., Sergeant, P., Galcherand, P., Guimont, I., De Saint Hilaire, P. and Rudigoz, R. C. (1996). Transvaginal hysterosonographic evaluation of septate uteri: a preliminary report. *Hum. Reprod.*, **11**, 1004–7

16. Marshall, C., Mintz, D. I., Thickman, D., Gussman, H. and Kressel, Y. (1987). Magnetic resonance evaluation of uterine anomalies. *Radiology*, **148**, 287–9

17. Carrington, B. M., Hricak, M. and Naruddin, R. N. (1990). Mullerian duct anomalies: magnetic resonance evaluation. *Radiology*, **170**, 715–20

18. Jurkovic, D., Giepel, A., Gurboeck, K., Jauniaux, E., Natucci, M. and Campbell, S. (1995). Three-dimensional ultrasound for the assessment of uterine anatomy and detection of congenital anomalies: a comparison with hysterosalpingography and two-dimensional sonography. *Ultrasound Obstet. Gynecol.*, **5**, 233–7

19. Taylor, P. J. and Cumming, D. C. (1979). Hysteroscopy in 100 patients. *Fertil. Steril.*, **31**, 301–4

20. Kupesic, S. and Kurjak, A. (1998). Diagnosis and treatment outcome of the septate uterus. *Croat. Med. J.*, **39**, 185–90

21. Kupesic, S. and Kurjak, A. (1993). Uterine and ovarian perfusion during the periovulatory period assessed by transvaginal color Doppler. *Fertil. Steril.*, **3**, 439–43

22. March, C. M. (1983). Hysteroscopy as an aid to diagnosis in female infertility. *Clin. Obstet. Gynecol.*, **26**, 302–12

23. Fayez, J. A. (1986). Comparison between abdominal and hysteroscopic metroplasty. *Obstet. Gynecol.*, **68**, 399–403

24. Dabrashrafi, H., Bahadori, M., Mohammad, K., Alavi, M., Moghadami-Tabrizi, N. and Zandinejad, R. (1995). Septate uterus: new idea on the histologic features of the septum in this abnormal uterus. *Am. J. Obstet. Gynecol.*, **172**, 105–7

25. Kupesic, S. and Kurjak, A. (1998). Comparison of B-mode, color Doppler, three-dimensional ultrasound and hysterosonography in detection of septate uteri. *J. Ultrasound Med.*, **17**, 631–6

26. Keltz, M. D., Olive, D. L., Kim, A. H. and Arici, A. (1997). Sonohysterography for screening in recurrent pregnancy loss. *Fertil. Steril.*, **67**, 670–4

Selection of candidates for *in vitro* fertilization based on color Doppler findings

14

S. L. Tan and M. M. Biljan

INTRODUCTION

Since the introduction of *in vitro* fertilization (IVF) almost 20 years ago, the field of assisted reproduction has vastly expanded, and has helped hundreds of thousands of couples to conceive a much desired baby. In the last decade, results have greatly improved to the extent that in the best IVF programs today, the results of treatment compare favorably with spontaneous conception in the natural menstrual cycle[1]. At the McGill Reproductive Center, for instance, of 150 IVF cycles performed in the latter part of 1996 in women with a median age of 37 years (range 25–45 years), 143 patients achieved fertilization and 96.4% of patients underwent embryo transfer. The overall pregnancy rate per cycle commenced was 29.9%, and in the group of women aged 34 years and younger the pregnancy rate was 40.0%. The introduction of intracytoplasmatic sperm injection (ICSI)[2] has revolutionized the treatment of severe male factor infertility which was previously considered to be amenable only to treatment with donor sperm. It has been shown that even in men with azoospermia, sperm can be successfully retrieved from the spermatocele[3], epididymis[4] and testis[5], which can then be used to achieve relatively high pregnancy rates. Nevertheless, despite these advances in assisted reproduction therapy, there still remain a number of important unresolved problems. In this review article we will address three intriguing problems in which the use of color Doppler ultrasound could prove valuable: prediction of the response of patients to ovarian stimulation in assisted

conception; assessment of oocyte quality based on peri-follicular flow; and parameters influencing implantation following embryo transfer.

PREDICTION OF PATIENT RESPONSE TO OVULATION STIMULATION

Ovarian stimulation for assisted reproduction is used in virtually all assisted reproduction programs because, in general, if more oocytes are collected, more embryos are produced, and the transfer of several embryos results in higher pregnancy rates. In the last 13 years, the use of gonadotropin-releasing hormone (GnRH) agonists being initiated in the mid-luteal or early follicular phase, in conjunction with gonadotropins, has emerged as the favored form of ovarian stimulation for assisted conception. This regimen, the so-called long protocol, improves follicular response and fertilization and implantation rates, leading to a net increase in pregnancy rate[6]. Determining the starting dose of gonadotropins, however, is still sometimes difficult, especially in patients undergoing a first cycle of assisted conception. Traditionally, the starting dose prescribed is often based on the patient age. Owing to the high variability between patients, however, age is not an absolutely reliable marker of ovarian response. Some women will have diminished ovarian function in their twenties, while others maintain their ovarian function until their late forties. These two groups are not distinguishable by any standard gynecological parameters, as both continue to have normal menstrual cycles with no obvious hormonal dysfunction. It has been suggested that several other hormonal and ultrasonic parameters could offer additional information regarding ovarian response.

Hormonal predictors

Following an initial report by Muasher and colleagues[7], a number of studies have confirmed a link between the basal level of follicle-stimulating hormone (FSH) and ovarian responsiveness following stimulation for assisted conception. In a large prospective study including 1478 cycles, Scott and colleagues[8] reported that the basal FSH level predicts the patient response independently of the patient age and can be used as an additional parameter for doing so. In an effort to increase the accuracy of basal FSH measurements, Navot and colleagues[9] suggested monitoring FSH levels following administration of clomiphene citrate from day 5 to day 9 of the menstrual cycle. The basis of this testing would be to demonstrate that, in women with normal ovarian reserve, FSH levels should decline to the normal range by cycle day 10. Several groups have shown a direct correlation between abnormal FSH levels and the chances of cycle cancellation in assisted conception cycles[10-12]. Recently, several groups have also demonstrated the possible prognostic value of basal estradiol measurement in predicting ovarian response. Smotrich and colleagues[13], in a prospective study of 225 patients undergoing IVF treatment, reported that a serum estradiol level > 80 pg/ml taken on day 3 of the menstrual cycle is predictive of poor ovarian response and treatment outcome, independently of age and FSH level.

Although potentially promising, hormonal tests have several important shortcomings. Primarily, intercycle variability is high, and the use of different assays in different centers increases the variability of results obtained and makes it more difficult to compare results. Moreover, while hormonal tests may indicate diminished ovarian responsiveness, no hormonal test provides precise information related to the optimal dose of gonadotropins required to achieve satisfactory stimulation.

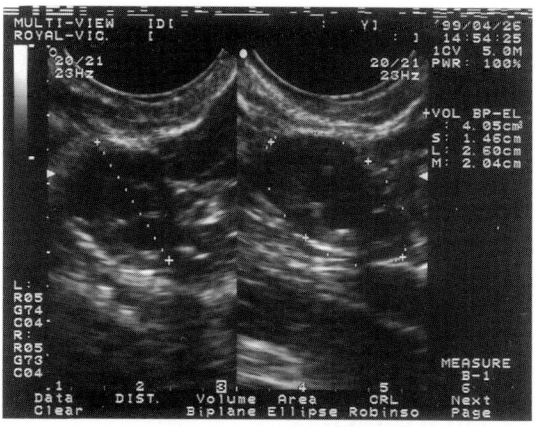

Figure 1 Assessment of the ovarian volume

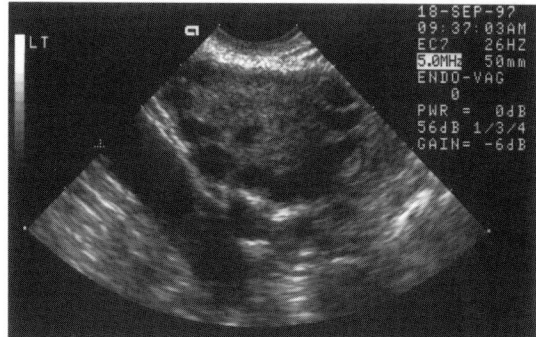

Figure 2 Ultrasound appearance of the polycystic ovary

Ultrasonic predictors

In the last several years a number of groups have tried to correlate certain morphological and Doppler features on baseline ultrasound with subsequent response to ovulation stimulation. In a retrospective study, Syrop and colleagues[14] examined ultrasonic images of 188 patients undergoing assisted conception. Estimation of ovarian volume was based on two ultrasonic images taken in saggital and coronal planes (Figure 1). Patients who had part of an ovary removed were excluded from the study. The results demonstrated a correlation between total ovarian volume and peak estradiol concentrations, number of eggs retrieved, number of embryos obtained, and clinical pregnancy rate. The major criticism of this study is the failure to exclude patients with polycystic ovarian syndrome (PCOS). It is reasonable to believe that the majority of patients with large

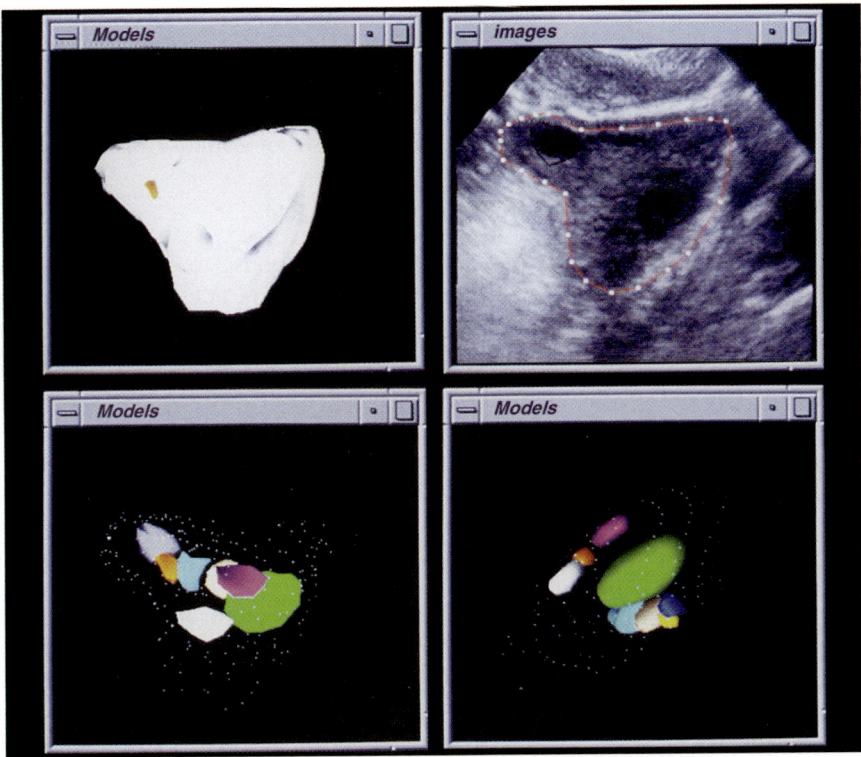

Figure 3 Three-dimensional reconstruction of the ovary

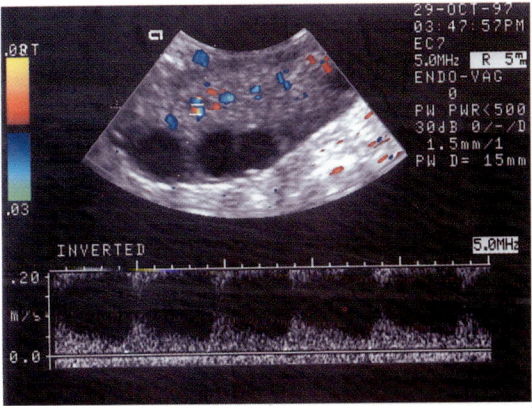

Figure 4 Assessment of the intraovarian blood flow

ovaries were in fact patients with PCOS who, as we have previously shown[15], normally exhibit an exaggerated response to ovarian stimulation (Figure 2). A group from Finland[16] studied the predictive value of ovarian volume and the number of small follicles (2–5 mm in diameter) seen at the time of the baseline ultrasound scan on ovarian response. They divided 166 patients studied into three groups according to the number of small follicles: inactive (< 5 follicles), normal (5–15), and polycystic (> 15). The authors confirmed previous observations showing that patients with smaller ovaries and fewer small follicles on the initial ultrasound scan developed less follicles than patients with PCOS. They also concluded that the number of small follicles at the beginning of the cycle may be more representative of the actual functional ovarian reserve than the patient age. We have previously demonstrated that young age and the presence of polycystic ovaries are risk factors for developing ovarian hyperstimulation syndrome (OHSS)[17]. In a separate study using three-dimensional ultrasound, Danninger and colleagues[18] found that, even after excluding patients with PCOS, there was a relationship between the volume of ovaries and the likelihood of developing OHSS. They reported that women with larger ovaries developed more follicles, had more embryos for transfer, had a higher clinical pregnancy rate, and had a higher risk of developing OHSS. We conclude that a baseline ultrasound scan to assess whether there are polycystic ovaries (enlarged ovaries with multiple small cysts scattered around their periphery and highly echogenic stroma) is useful in predicting subsequent ovarian response. We have recently reported the development of a new three-dimensional ultrasound technology which enables more accurate measurement of ovarian volume[19] (Figure 3). The use of this method of ovarian volume measurement might increase the predictive value of this test.

Color Doppler

Until recently, there had been no attempts to use color Doppler ultrasound in the assessment of ovarian reserve. To investigate this, we performed a study on 105 patients, 26 of whom had ultrasonic features of PCOS, undergoing IVF treatment[20]. In our study, both ovarian morphology and blood flow were assessed during the early follicular phase of the IVF cycle (Figure 4). We defined a poor ovarian response as the development of six or less follicles, which represented the 10% of patients who exhibited the worst response. This study showed a positive independent relationship between the ovarian stromal peak systolic blood flow velocity at the time of baseline ultrasound scan, and the subsequent follicular response. There was no relationship found between ovarian stromal pulsatility index (PI) (an index of resistance to blood flow) and follicular response. It is, therefore, likely that women with greater ovarian stromal peak systolic blood flow velocity have increased intraovarian perfusion. Thus, in response to the same dose of gonadotropin administration, a larger amount is delivered to the target cells. Interestingly, we have found that women with polycystic ovaries have a higher ovarian stromal blood flow velocity not only at the baseline scan[21] but also during the entire menstrual cycle[22]. Color Doppler ultrasound, therefore, offers valuable information regarding the dose of

gonadotropin required for successful ovarian stimulation in assisted conception. Further studies are required to establish a precise relationship between peak velocities and the optimum doses of gonadotropins to be used.

SUMMARY

Ovarian response to stimulation is paramount to the success of IVF treatment. Determination of the initial dose of gonadotropins based solely upon the chronological age of the patient is imprecise and frequently leads to expensive and frustrating under or over-stimulation. Measurement of hormonal levels, such as serum FSH or estradiol concentrations, or the use of more elaborate provocative hormonal tests, is likely to identify only a limited number of patients who are unlikely to respond to a standard dose of medication. The performance of a baseline ultrasound scan to assess whether there are polycystic ovaries, and the use of color Doppler sonography to assess stromal perfusion, improves the selection of the appropriate dose of gonadotropins required for ovarian stimulation.

FOLLICULAR CHARACTERISTICS ASSESSMENT IN PREDICTING OOCYTE QUALITY

Follicular size

Since the beginning of IVF treatment, measurement of the follicular size and the volume of follicular fluid have been recognized as possible predictors of oocyte quality. Edwards[23], using a human chorionic gonadotropin (hCG) and human menopausal gonadotropin (hMG) stimulation protocol, reported a higher rate of oocyte recovery for large-size follicles (46% recovery for follicles < 1 cm in diameter, 69% for follicles 1.0 to 1.75 cm and 73% for follicles > 1.75 cm in diameter). Moreover, they showed that smaller follicles contained mature oocytes only in 20% of cases, a percentage that rose to 46% of cases with larger follicles. In a much larger group of patients, Simonetti and colleagues[24] found that not only were collection and fertilization rates of oocytes retrieved from the cohort of small follicles lower, but the chances of miscarriage were also increased in patients who had oocytes obtained from smaller follicles. In a small study performed on patients undergoing a flare regimen as a part of their IVF treatment, Clark and colleagues[25] found that delaying the administration of hCG by 1 day led to a significantly lower pregnancy rate. They concluded that extending the follicular phase when the short protocol of GnRH agonist is used may lead to a reduction in oocyte quality as a result of follicular aging. These results were not reflected in other studies performed thereafter. In a recent retrospective study on more than 6000 follicles from 1109 patients undergoing IVF, Wittmaack and colleagues[26] investigated the effect of follicular size on collection, fertilization and pregnancy rates. They found relatively constant oocyte recovery in follicles measuring between 12.5 mm and 24 mm in diameter. Oocyte recovery rates were significantly decreased only in very small and large follicles. The study also showed a continuous increase in fertilization and cleavage rates with increasing follicular size. Only when follicular size exceeded 24 mm was a small decrease in fertilization rate noted. On the basis of these data, it was concluded that a larger number of mature eggs will be retrieved if smaller follicles in a cohort are allowed to reach at least 12 mm in diameter. The authors therefore challenged the policy adopted by many centers where hCG is given when three follicles reach 18 mm, suggesting that oocyte collection should be delayed until the majority of follicles reach maturity.

To determine if there is an optimum time for the administration of hCG when the long protocol of GnRH agonist is used in an IVF program, we performed a randomized controlled trial involving 247 patients[27]. In this study the first group of patients had hCG administered on the day when the largest follicle reached 18 mm in diameter, two other follicles were larger than 14 mm and the levels of serum estradiol were appropriate for the number of follicles. Patients in the other two groups had hCG administered 1 and 2 days

later. The results of this study showed that patients who had hCG injection delayed for up to 2 days had higher serum estradiol levels and a larger number of follicles greater than 14 mm in diameter on the day of hCG administration. However, the number of oocytes collected and embryos cleaved were comparable among the three groups studied and there were no significant differences in the pregnancy rates observed. It would appear that optimal oocyte recovery and fertilization rates can be obtained from follicles between 14 and 24 mm in diameter. Oocyte recovery starts to decrease after the follicles exceed 24 mm in diameter.

Clearly the usefulness of ultrasound depends on precise measurements. It has been shown previously that transvaginal ultrasound measurement of follicular dimensions has a lower intraobserver and interobserver variability, when compared with transabdominal measurement. The superiority of transvaginal images is the result of the ability of a transvaginal probe to be inserted very close to the ovary. This permits the use of higher ultrasound frequencies and minimizes artifactual echoes caused by multiple reflections from intervening tissues. Recently it became possible to estimate follicular volume by using three-dimensional ultrasound. This system provides an additional view of the coronal or C-plane which is parallel to the transducer face. The computer-generated scan is displayed in three perpendicular planes. Translation or rotation can be carried out in one plane while maintaining the perpendicular orientation of all three so that serial translation will result in an ultrasound tomogram from which volumetric data can be captured[28]. To evaluate the possible advantages of this new technique over traditional transvaginal follicular measurement, we have recently performed a prospective study on 25 patients undergoing IVF treatment[29]. Patients had both two and three-dimensional estimation of follicular volume performed immediately prior to oocyte collection. The estimated volumes were compared with volumes obtained at the time of collection. Results of this study showed that the upper and lower limits of agreement encompassing

95% of measurements were wider for two-dimensional ultrasound over the range of volumes measured. When three-dimensional ultrasound was used, all measurements were within 1 ml of the true volume. On the other hand, conventional two-dimensional ultrasound produced limits of agreement that were up to 3.5 ml above or 2.5 ml below the true volume within the most important clinical range. Errors of measurement were relatively larger in smaller follicles where the precise measurement of volume is more important. The reliability of the standard two-dimensional ultrasound technique for follicular volume measurement is influenced by the shape and number of the follicles. There may be technical difficulty in measuring the diameters of the follicle when its shape is distorted because of compression by adjacent follicles. Accuracy of three-dimensional measurement is unaffected by follicular shape and therefore its superiority over traditional scanning is likely to be greatest in patients who have multiple follicles. Although still at the research stage, three-dimensional scanning could in future lead to more accurate follicular measurements and more precise determination of oocyte maturity.

Color Doppler

Although the diameter of the follicle is a relatively good predictor of oocyte maturity it is not a perfect indicator of oocyte quality. Despite optimal follicular size and no impairment of semen quality, more than 20% of oocytes fail to fertilize[26]. It would, therefore, be beneficial to have an additional test of oocyte quality available before hCG administration. A number of early studies in natural ovulatory cycles have demonstrated a relationship between hormonal levels and blood flow velocities in ovarian arteries[30–34], as well as increased flow in ovaries containing a follicle or corpus luteum[35,36]. To elucidate the precise changes in intra-ovarian and uterine circulation relative to the time of ovulation, we recently performed a prospective observational study which included seven healthy individuals[22]. In this study patients had 6-hourly hormonal and Doppler ultrasound assessments around the time of ovulation. We observed a rapid rise in blood flow velocity in the peri-follicular and ovarian stromal blood vessels at the time of the luteinizing hormone (LH) surge. These changes may be a result of neo-angiogenesis occurring during late follicular development. A marked increase in the peak systolic blood flow velocity around the follicle, in the presence of a relatively constant pulsatility index, could be a sign of follicle maturity and herald impending ovulation. Recently, several groups have tried to utilize those findings and have used color Doppler ultrasound to determine oocyte quality in stimulated cycles. In a study performed on 52 patients undergoing IVF treatment, Balakier and Stronell[37] reported a strong correlation between follicular dimensions and peak systolic blood flow velocity. In both small and large follicles, administration of hCG resulted in a rapid increase in peak velocities. The authors, however, failed to show any correlation between peri-follicular blood flow velocity and pregnancy rates, and concluded that the velocity of peri-follicular blood flow is unlikely to be a major factor determining the quality of oocytes. In a similarly designed study in women undergoing IVF treatment, it was reported that the maximum peak systolic velocity in both ovaries before oocyte recovery was comparable in women who subsequently became pregnant when compared with those who did not[38]. A major flaw in both these studies was the fact that the researchers did not track the outcome of oocytes obtained from each follicle. Therefore, peak velocities from all follicles in each patient were pooled together for analysis. In an attempt to improve the sensitivity of intra-ovarian Doppler scanning, Oyesanya and colleagues[39] investigated the predictive value of different indices of peri-follicular flow for oocyte collection rates. They failed to correlate either peri-follicular impedance or peak systolic velocities with collection rates. However, they found that the semi-quantitative peri-follicular vascularity index, defined as the ratio of the total number of follicles to the number of follicles with demonstrable pulsatile vascularity, was highly correlated with oocyte recovery

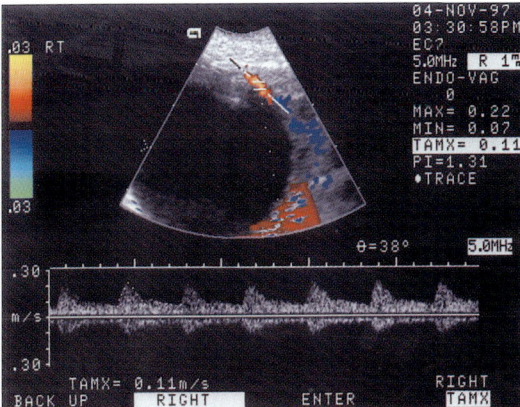

Figure 5 Assessment of the peri-follicular blood flow

and concluded that higher oocyte recovery rates could be achieved if peri-follicular flow is assessed prior to the administration of hCG. It was, however, not clear from this study whether peri-follicular flow provided information independent of follicular size. In two recent studies, Nargund and colleagues[40,41] studied the relationship between follicular blood flow and the production of morphologically normal embryos. These authors investigated individual follicles, oocytes and pre-implantation embryos, rather than pooling data. Interestingly, by using this approach, a very strong relationship between peak systolic velocities, collection rates, embryo development and implantation rates was found. From this study it appeared that harvesting oocytes from follicles with a peak systolic velocity of $\geqslant 10$ cm/s (Figure 5) is significantly more likely to result in obtaining grade I embryos, which in turn are more likely to implant. These findings were supported recently by another study in which follicles were divided arbitrarily according to the percentage of vascularized surface[42]. Oocytes obtained from highly vascularized follicles were of a higher quality, and were more likely to fertilize and result in pregnancy. From the available data, it appears that assessment of peri-follicular vascular perfusion could lead to a better selection of oocytes and ultimately a higher pregnancy rate. However, it is difficult to envision its practical value in patients who have abundant follicles. In this particular group of

patients, it would be very time-consuming to measure the vascularity of each individual follicle. Moreover, due to the large number of follicles, it may be difficult to determine the exact vascularization of each single follicle. In women who develop relatively few follicles, however, peri-follicular blood flow measurements may prove to be very useful.

IMPLANTATION

A major problem associated with current IVF practice is the necessity of transferring multiple embryos in order to increase the pregnancy rate. This becomes problematic as it leads to an increased incidence of multiple pregnancy. This in turn contributes to an increased obstetrical risk and diminished perinatal outcome, when compared with singleton pregnancies. Uterine receptivity is a crucial element in achieving implantation. It is dependent upon the development of a normal endometrium, which is suitable for implantation and the maintenance of pregnancy. Interestingly, uterine receptivity does not seem to be significantly affected by the age of the patient, as evidenced by the high implantation rates seen with oocyte donation[37], even in postmenopausal women[43]. An additional factor which plays an important role in implantation is embryo quality. Differentiation between these two factors is not always obvious in an individual patient. A mathematical analysis by Walters and colleagues[44] estimated the relative contribution to conception of embryo quality and uterine receptivity to be 31 and 64%, respectively. This estimate agrees with the coefficient of uterine receptivity, determined as 0.43, based upon a statistical model. The role of uterine receptivity is likely to be more important in cases where excellent embryos are replaced, such as in young patients or in oocyte donation patients where the donor is of a young age. Unfortunately, there is no universally accepted test of uterine receptivity. Recently a number of investigators have tried to correlate different hormonal and ultrasonic parameters with uterine receptivity. Here we will critically assess some of these approaches.

To achieve successful implantation it is important to have appropriate endometrial maturation. To achieve this endometrial growth and differentiation, the proliferative phase must be followed by timely secretory changes during the luteal phase with stromal decidualization. This sequence of events is probably regulated by locally produced growth factors and is altered by the hormonal environment. The interaction of different elements and the importance of factors such as various endometrial proteins, and uterine and ovarian perfusion, is still not fully understood. Until these factors are fully elucidated, our knowledge of human implantation and our ability to predict it reliably will remain somewhat limited.

The traditional method of assessing endometrial receptivity involves histological dating of the endometrium[45]. The value of this invasive test is, however, rather restricted in assisted conception cycles due to its relatively low predictive value, and due to concern over performing a biopsy during the treatment cycle itself because of the associated bleeding.

Recently several groups have reported the potential value of assessing the endometrial epithelial surface by scanning electron microscopy (SEM). By using this technique they have described apical protrusions, called pinopods, which were noted to develop and regress during a short period during the mid-luteal phase spanning 4 to 7 days following hCG administration[46]. Initial pinopod development begins in the region of the glandular orifices, with substantially fewer occurring outside this region. It is postulated that the appearance of pinopods marks the duration of the endometrial implantation window. In a recent study on 40 patients undergoing oocyte donation, Reddy and colleagues[47] performed endometrial biopsy in the pretreatment assessment cycle. They reported an 83% pregnancy rate in patients who developed pinopods and no pregnancies in patients who had absence of pinopods on endometrial biopsy. This technique of predicting implantation may prove promising if confirmed by other studies.

Serum levels of reproductive hormones appear to be of relatively little value in predicting endometrial maturation. Although there is a correlation between endometrial thickness and serum estrogen levels in both natural[48] and stimulated cycles[49], estrogen levels alone express the activity of granulosa cells and not the maturity of the endometrium. The maturity of the endometrium probably depends upon estrogen receptor development, which is genetically coded for each individual and, therefore, similar levels of estrogen can initiate different levels of endometrial maturity in different individuals. This discrepancy has been shown in both natural[48] and assisted conception[50] cycles.

From the above, it is clear that histological and hormonal assessment are not reliable predictors of endometrial status. Pinopod assessment, although promising, is expensive and experimental. It is therefore important to find alternative, non-invasive ways of assessing uterine receptivity. Turnbull and colleagues[51] have demonstrated the potential value of magnetic resonance imaging (MRI) in distinguishing conceptional and non-conceptional cycles. However, owing to its high cost, MRI is unlikely to be incorporated into daily infertility practice. In the last few years, ultrasound has been proposed as an alternative tool in the assessment of endometrial receptivity. Here we will review existing data concerning its value in predicting endometrial maturation and the likelihood of conception.

Ultrasound prediction of endometrial maturation

Two anatomical parameters have been suggested for the evaluation of the endometrium by ultrasound: endometrial thickness and endometrial pattern.

Endometrial thickness is defined as the maximal distance between the echogenic interfaces of the myometrium and the endometrium, measured in the plane through the central longitudinal axis of the uterus (Figure 6). It is an easily measurable ultrasonic parameter, and it represents a bioassay of estrogenic activity. Endometrial thickness is unrelated to endometrial pattern[52]. In natural cycles, on

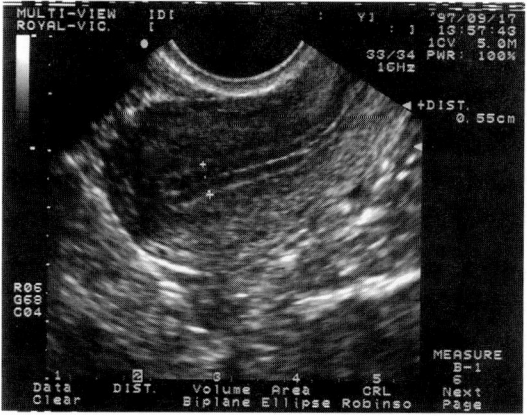

Figure 6 Appearance of multilayered endometrium

the day of ovulation, the endometrium has been reported to be significantly thicker in conceptual cycles[53]. Dynamic change in endometrial thickness in assisted conception cycles was first described by Rabinowitz and colleagues[50]. They reported an approximate daily growth of 0.5 mm at the time of oocyte collection. The growth continued, albeit at a slower pace of 0.1 mm per day, in the luteal phase. In conception cycles, a rapid increase in endometrial thickness was noted 11 days following embryo transfer, reaching a significantly greater thickness compared with non-conception cycles 17 days post-embryo transfer. Using transvaginal scanning, Gonen and colleagues[52] suggested that endometrial thickness, on the day before oocyte recovery, was significantly greater in pregnant than in non-pregnant women, and postulated that it may predict the likelihood of implantation. However, Glissant and co-workers[53], Fleischer and colleagues[54], and Welker and co-workers[55] found that measurement of endometrial thickness had no predictive value for pregnancy. Moreover, Li and colleagues[56] reported no correlation between endometrial thickness, measured by abdominal ultrasound, and histological dating of the endometrium. In their study of endometrial thickness, Dickey and colleagues[57] found an increased rate of early miscarriage in a group of patients with very thin (< 6 mm) or thick (> 13 mm) endometrium.

Krampl and Feichtinger[58], however, found no correlation between endometrial thickness and the likelihood of miscarriage. Imoedemhe and colleagues[59] compared the endometrial thickness in three groups of patients who were prescribed three different ovulation induction regimens. They found that the endometrial thickness in all three groups of patients was similar and comparable to that observed in a group of spontaneously ovulating, fertile control patients, despite significantly higher serum estradiol concentrations in all the hyperstimulated cycles. Their findings suggest that there is a maximum endometrial response, inducible by estrogen, which is virtually achieved in the normal menstrual cycle. Recently, Freidler and colleagues[60] reviewed 2665 assisted conception cycles from 25 reports. Eight reports found that the difference in the mean endometrial thickness of conception and non-conception cycles was statistically significant, while 17 reports found no significant difference. They concluded that results from various trials are conflicting and that insufficient data exist describing a linear correlation between endometrial thickness and the probability of conception. The main advantage of measuring endometrial thickness lies in its high negative predictive value in cases where there is minimal endometrial thickness. Gonen and colleagues[61] reported an absence of pregnancies in donor insemination cycles where the endometrium thickness did not reach at least 6 mm. Similarly, in a group of oocyte recipients, no pregnancies were reported in women who had an endometrial thickness of less then 5 mm, whereas several pregnancies occurred in patients with an endometrium thinner than 7.5 mm[62]. Finally, in IVF cycles, Khalifa and colleagues reported a minimal endometrial thickness of 7 mm to be compatible with pregnancy[63].

In summary, the question of a correlation between endometrial thickness and the likelihood of conception, in the context of assisted conception, remains a contentious issue. However, a very thin endometrium (below 7 mm) (Figure 7) seems to be accepted as a reliable sign of sub-optimal implantation potential.

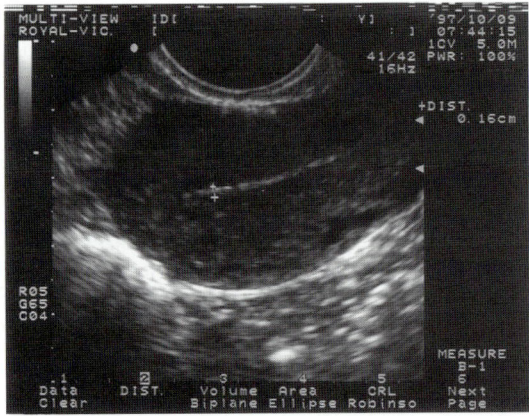

Figure 7 Appearance of thin endometrium

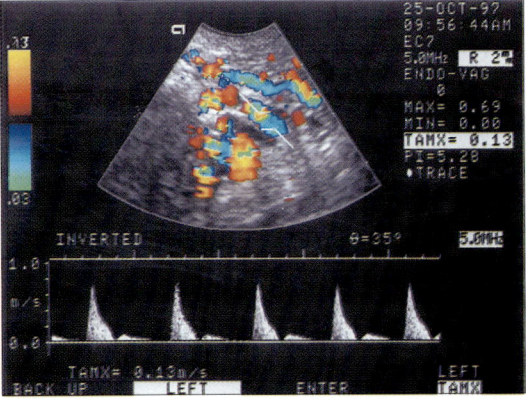

Figure 8 High blood flow impedence in the uterine artery

Endometrial pattern is defined as the relative echogenicity of the endometrium and the adjacent myometrium as demonstrated on a longitudinal ultrasound scan. In principle, the central echogenic line represents the uterine cavity; the outer lines represent the basal layer of the endometrium, or the interface between the endometrium and myometrium. The relatively hypo-echogenic regions between two outer lines and the central line may represent the functional layer of endometrium[64]. Classification of the types of appearance of the endometrium has been simplified over time. The first classification proposed four patterns describing a gradual change from a fully echogenic endometrium (Grade A) to a distinct echogenic black region surrounding the midline[65]. Nowadays, intermediate patterns are often discarded and the endometrium is simply described as multilayered (Figure 6) or non-multilayered[66]. In a prospective study, Serafini and colleagues[67] found the multilayered pattern to be more predictive of implantation than any other parameter measured. Sher and colleagues[66] correlated a non-multilayered echo pattern with advanced age and the presence of uterine abnormalities. In the literature, of 13 studies which examined the value of endometrial pattern in predicting pregnancy, only four failed to confirm its predictive value. It is, however, important to emphasize that a poor endometrial pattern does not exclude pregnancy. Many authors have demonstrated that pregnancies can occur in patients with a non-multilayered pattern of endometrium, albeit at a lower frequency[57,67]. The endometrial pattern does not appear to be influenced by the type of ovarian stimulation and it is of prognostic value in both fresh IVF as well as frozen embryo transfer cycles.

DOPPLER STUDIES OF UTERINE ARTERIES

Steer and colleagues[68] were the first to use transvaginal color Doppler to study the uterine arteries in 23 normally cycling women. Daily measurements of the PI of both uterine arteries were made. They noted that the lowest uterine artery PI was found 9 days after the LH peak, which is consistent with maximum uterine perfusion at the time of peak luteal function and expected implantation. Steer and colleagues also showed that the uterine artery impedance was different in the mid-luteal phase in women with subfertility compared with those with normal fertility[69].

What are the clinical implications for infertility treatment of these findings? Sterzik and colleagues[70] reported that the resistance index measured on the day of embryo transfer was significantly lower in patients who subsequently became pregnant as compared with those who failed to achieve pregnancy. Steer and colleagues have used transvaginal color Doppler to study the uterine arterial blood flow in 82 women undergoing IVF on the day of embryo transfer[71]. The PI was calculated and the patients were grouped according to whether the PI was low (1–1.99), medium (2–2.99) or high (3.0+) There were no pregnancies in the high PI group and the PI was significantly lower in the women who become pregnant as compared with those who did not. However, although measurement of uterine artery blood flow impedance on the day of embryo transfer may be able to predict pregnancy, it would be more useful to detect flow abnormalities earlier in the cycle. To investigate this Zaidi and associates recently measured uterine artery PI in 135 women undergoing IVF on the day of hCG injection[72]. They found significantly lower implantation rates in women with uterine artery PI > 3.0 (Figure 8). The ability to predict implantation before the administration of hCG allows the clinician the option to delay giving hCG until the uterine artery PI improves. An alternative approach would be to try to improve uterine perfusion by the administration of glyceryl trinitrate (GTN). In a preliminary study, Cacciatore and colleagues reported that in a group of patients with increased uterine artery PI, a 20% increase in uterine blood flow occurred following the administration of GTN throughout the normal menstrual cycle[73]. It has been suggested that administration of GTN may increase pregnancy rates in women with poor uterine perfusion. However, no randomized studies have been performed to address this issue.

SUMMARY

In the last decade, results of IVF treatment have greatly improved to the extent that, in the best IVF programs today, the results of treatment compare favorably with spontaneous conception in the natural menstrual cycle[1]. Nevertheless, despite these advances in assisted reproduction therapy, there still remain a number of important unresolved problems. In this review article we addressed three intriguing problems: prediction of the response of patients to ovarian stimulation in assisted conception; assessment of oocyte quality based on peri-follicular flow; and parameters influencing implantation following embryo transfer. We believe that in the above three areas, the use of color Doppler ultrasound has emerged as an important diagnostic technique.

References

1. Tan, S. L., Royston, P., Campbell, S., Jacobs, H. S., Betts, J., Mason, B. and Edwards, R. G. (1992). Cumulative conception and livebirth rates after *in vitro* fertilisation. *Lancet*, **339**, 1390–4

2. van Steirteghem, A. C., Liu, J., Joris, H., Nagy, Z., Janssenswillen, C., Tournaye, H., Derde, M. P., van Asche, E. and Devroy, P. (1993). Higher success rate by intracytoplasmic sperm injection than by subzonal insemination. Report of a second series of 300 consecutive treatment cycles. *Fertil. Steril.*, **8**, 1055–60

3. Craft, I. L., Khalifa, Y., Boulos, A., Pelekanos, M., Foster, C. and Tsirigotis, M. (1995). Factors influencing the outcome of *in vitro* fertilization with percutaneous aspirated epididymal spermatozoa and intracytoplasmic sperm injection in azoospermic men. *Hum. Reprod.*, **10**, 1791–4

4. Girardi, S. K. and Schlegel, P. N. (1996). Microsurgical epididymal sperm aspiration: review of techniques, preoperative considerations, and results. [Review]. *J. Androl.*, **17**, 5–9

5. Devroey, P., Liu, J., Nagy, Z., Goossens, A., Tournaye, H., Camus, M., van Steirteghem, A. and Silber, S. (1995). Pregnancies after testicular sperm extraction and intracytoplasmic sperm injection in non-obstructive azoospermia. *Hum. Reprod.*, **10**, 1457–60

6. Tan, S. L., Maconochie, N., Doyle, P., Campbell, S., Balen, A., Bekir, J., Brinsden, P., Edwards, R. G. and Jacobs, H. S. (1994). Cumulative conception and live-birth rates after *in vitro* fertilization with and without the use of long, short, and ultrashort regimens of the gonadotropin-releasing hormone agonist buserelin. *Am. J. Obstet. Gynecol.*, **171**, 513–20

7. Muasher, S. J., Oehninger, S., Simonetti, S., Matta, J., Ellis, L. M., Liu, H. C., Jones, G. S. and Rosenwaks, Z. (1988). The value of basal and/or stimulated serum gonadotropin levels in prediction of stimulation response and *in vitro* fertilization outcome. *Fertil. Steril.*, **50**, 298–307

8. Scott, R. T., Toner, J. P., Muasher, S. J., Oehninger, S., Robinson, S. and Rosenwaks, Z. (1989). Follicle-stimulating hormone levels on cycle day 3 are predictive of *in vitro* fertilization outcome. *Fertil. Steril.*, **51**, 651–4

9. Navot, D., Rosenwaks, Z. and Margalioth, E. J. (1987). Prognostic assessment of female fecundity. *Lancet*, **2**, 645–7

10. Scott, R. T., Leonardi, M. R., Hofmann, G. E., Illions, E. H., Neal, G. S. and Navot, D. (1993). A prospective evaluation of clomiphene citrate challenge test screening of the general infertility population. *Obstet. Gynecol.*, **82**, 539–44

11. Tanbo, T., Dale, P. O., Lunde, O., Norman, N. and Abyholm, T. (1992). Prediction of response to controlled ovarian hyperstimulation: a comparison of basal and clomiphene citrate-stimulated follicle-stimulating hormone levels. *Fertil. Steril.*, **57**, 819–24

12. Loumaye, E., Billion, J. M., Mine, J. M., Psalti, I., Pensis, M. and Thomas, K. (1990). Prediction of individual response to controlled ovarian hyperstimulation by means of a clomiphene citrate challenge test. *Fertil. Steril.*, **53**, 295–301

13. Smotrich, D. B., Widra, E. A., Gindoff, P. R., Levy, M. J., Hall, J. L. and Stillman, R. J. (1995). Prognostic value of day 3 estradiol on *in vitro* fertilization outcome. *Fertil. Steril.*, **64**, 1136–40

14. Syrop, C. H., Willhoite, A. and van Voorhis, B. J. (1995). Ovarian volume: a novel outcome predictor for assisted reproduction. *Fertil. Steril.*, **64**, 1167–71

15. MacDougall, M. J., Tan, S. L., Balen, A. and Jacobs, H. S. (1993). A controlled study comparing patients with and without polycystic ovaries undergoing *in vitro* fertilization. *Hum. Reprod.*, **8**, 233–7

16. Tomas, C., Nuojua-Huttunen, S. and Martikainen, H. (1997). Pretreatment transvaginal ultrasound examination predicts ovarian responsiveness to gonadotropins in *in vitro* fertilization. *Hum. Reprod.*, **12**, 220–3

17. MacDougall, M. J., Tan, S. L. and Jacobs, H. S. (1992). *In vitro* fertilization and the ovarian hyperstimulation syndrome. *Hum. Reprod.*, **7**, 597–600

18. Danninger, B., Brunner, M., Obruca, A. and Feichtinger, W. (1996). Prediction of ovarian hyperstimulation syndrome of baseline ovarian volume prior to stimulation. *Hum. Reprod.*, **11**, 1597–9

19. Kyei-Mensah, A., Maconochie, N., Zaidi, J., Pittrof, R., Campbell, S. and Tan, S. L. (1996). Transvaginal three-dimensional ultrasound: reproducibility of ovarian and endometrial volume measurements. *Fertil. Steril.*, **66**, 718–22

20. Zaidi, J., Barber, J., Kyei-Mensah, A., Bekir, J., Campbell, S. and Tan, S. L. (1996). Relationship of ovarian stromal blood flow at the baseline ultrasound scan to subsequent follicular response in an *in vitro* fertilization program. *Obstet. Gynecol.*, **88**, 779–84

21. Zaidi, J., Campbell, S., Pittrof, R., Kyei-Mensah, A., Shaker, A., Jacobs, H. S. and Tan, S. L. (1995). Ovarian stromal blood flow in women with polycystic ovaries – a possible new marker for diagnosis? *Hum. Reprod.*, **10**, 1992–6

22. Tan, S. L., Zaidi, J., Campbell, S., Doyle, P. and Collins, W. (1996). Blood flow changes in the ovarian and uterine arteries during the normal menstrual cycle. *Am. J. Obstet. Gynecol.*, **175**, 625–31

23. Edwards, R. G. (1980). The ovary. In Edwards R. G. (ed.) *Conception in the Human Female*, pp. 343–58. (New York: Academic Press)

24. Simonetti, S., Veeck, L. L. and Jones, H. W. Jr (1985). Correlation of follicular fluid volume with oocyte morphology from follicles stimulated by human menopausal gonadotropin. *Fertil. Steril.*, **44**, 177–80

25. Clark, L., Stanger, J. and Brinsmead, M. (1991). Prolonged follicle stimulation decreases pregnancy rates after *in vitro* fertilization. *Fertil. Steril.*, **55**, 1192–4

26. Wittmaack, F. M., Kreger, D. O., Blasco, L., Tureck, R. W., Mastroianni, L. Jr and Lessey, B. A. (1994). Effect of follicular size on oocyte retrieval, fertilization, cleavage, and embryo quality in *in vitro* fertilization cycles: a 6-year data collection. *Fertil. Steril.*, **62**, 1205–10

27. Tan, S. L., Balen, A., el Hussein, E., Mills, C., Campbell, S., Yovich, J. and Jacobs, H. S. (1992). A prospective randomized study of the optimum timing of human chorionic gonadotropin administration after pituitary desensitization in *in vitro* fertilization. *Fertil. Steril.*, **57**, 1259–64

28. Steiner, H., Staudach, A., Spitzer, D. and Schaffer, H. (1994). Three-dimensional ultrasound in obstetrics and gynecology: technique, possibilities and limitations. *Hum. Reprod.*, **9**, 1773–8

29. Zaidi, J., Jurkovic, D., Campbell, S., Collins, W., McGregor, A. and Tan, S. L. (1995). Luteinized unruptured follicle: morphology, endocrine function and blood flow changes during the menstrual cycle. *Hum. Reprod.*, **10**, 44–9

30. Collins, W., Jurkovic, D., Bourne, T., Kurjak, A. and Campbell, S. (1991). Ovarian morphology, endocrine function and intra-follicular blood

flow during the peri-ovulatory period. *Hum. Reprod.*, **6**, 319–24

31. Kurjak, A., Kupesic-Urek, S., Schulman, H. and Zalud, I. (1991). Transvaginal color flow Doppler in the assessment of ovarian and uterine blood flow in infertile women. *Fertil. Steril.*, **56**, 870–3

32. Kupesic, S. and Kurjak, A. (1997). The assessment of uterine and ovarian perfusion in infertile patients. *Eur. J. Obstet. Gynecol. Reprod. Biol.*, **71**, 151–4

33. Kupesic, S. and Kurjak, A. (1993). Uterine and ovarian perfusion during the periovulatory period assessed by transvaginal color Doppler. *Fertil. Steril.*, **60**, 439–43

34. Scholtes, M. C., Wladimiroff, J. W., van Rijen, H. J. and Hop, W. C. (1989). Uterine and ovarian flow velocity waveforms in the normal menstrual cycle: a transvaginal Doppler study. *Fertil. Steril.*, **52**, 981–5

35. Kupesic, S. and Kurjak, A. (1997). The assessment of normal and abnormal luteal function by transvaginal color Doppler sonography. *Eur. J. Obstet. Gynecol. Reprod. Biol.*, **72**, 83–7

36. Kupesic, S., Kurjak, A., Vujisic, S. and Petrovic, Z. (1997). Luteal phase defect: comparison between Doppler velocimetry, histological and hormonal markers. *Ultrasound Obstet. Gynecol.*, **9**, 105–12

37. Balakier, H. and Stronell, R. D. (1994). Color Doppler assessment of folliculogenesis in *in vitro* fertilization patients. *Fertil. Steril.*, **62**, 1211–16

38. Tekay, A., Martikainen, H. and Jouppila, P. (1995). Blood flow changes in uterine and ovarian vasculature, and predictive value of transvaginal pulsed color Doppler ultrasonography in an *in vitro* fertilization program. *Hum. Reprod.*, **10**, 688–93

39. Oyesanya, O. A., Parsons, J. H., Collins, W. P. and Campbell, S. (1996). Prediction of oocyte recovery rate by transvaginal ultrasonography and color Doppler imaging before human chorionic gonadotropin administration in *in vitro* fertilization cycles. *Fertil. Steril.*, **65**, 806–9

40. Nargund, G., Doyle, P. E., Bourne, T. H., Parsons, J. H., Cheng, W. C., Campbell, S. and Collins, W. P. (1996). Ultrasound-derived indices of follicular blood flow before hCG administration and the prediction of oocyte recovery and preimplantation embryo quality. *Hum. Reprod.*, **11**, 2512–17

41. Nargund, G., Bourne, T., Doyle, P., Parsons, J., Cheng, W., Campbell, S. and Collins, W. (1996). Associations between ultrasound indices of follicular blood flow, oocyte recovery and preimplantation embryo quality. *Hum. Reprod.*, **11**, 109–13

42. Bhal, P. S., Pugh, N., Chui, D., Gregory, L., Walker, S. M. and Shaw, R. W. (1997). Is follicular vascularity an index of pregnancy potential among women undergoing assisted reproduction treatment cycles? [Abstract]. *Hum. Reprod.*, **12**, 72

43. Paulson, R. J., Thornton, M. H., Francis, M. M. and Salvador, H. S. (1997). Successful pregnancy in a 63-year-old woman. *Fertil. Steril.*, **67**, 949–51

44. Walters, D. E., Edwards, R. G. and Meistrich, M. L. (1985). A statistical evaluation of implantation after replacing one or more human embryos. *J. Reprod. Fertil.*, **74**, 557–63

45. Noyes, R. W., Hertig, A. T. and Rock, J. (1997). Dating the endometrial biopsy. *Fertil. Steril.*, **1**, 23

46. Kolb, B. A., Najmabadi, S. and Paulson, R. J. (1997). Ultrastructural characteristics of the luteal phase endometrium in patients undergoing controlled ovarian hyperstimulation. *Fertil. Steril.*, **67**, 625–30

47. Reddy, N., Ryder, T. A., Mobberley, M. A., Nikas, G. and Wiston, R. M. L. (1997). Positive correlation of pregnancy with the presence of endometrial pinopods in oocyte recipients: a preliminary study [Abstract]. *Hum. Reprod.*, **12**, 32

48. Hackeloer, B. J. (1984). Ultrasound scanning of the ovarian cycle. *J. In Vitro Fertil. Embryo Transfer*, **1**, 217–20

49. Fleischer, A. C., Herbert, C. M., Hill, G. A., Kepple, D. M. and Worrell, J. A. (1991). Transvaginal sonography of the endometrium during induced cycles. *J. Ultrasound Med.*, **10**, 93–5

50. Rabinowitz, R., Laufer, N., Lewin, A., Navot, D., Bar, I., Margalioth, E. J. and Schenker, J. J. (1986). The value of ultrasonographic endometrial measurement in the prediction of pregnancy following *in vitro* fertilization. *Fertil. Steril.*, **45**, 824–8

51. Turnbull, L. W., Rice, C. F., Horsman, A., Robinson, J. and Killick, S. R. (1994). Magnetic resonance imaging and transvaginal ultrasound of the uterus prior to embryo transfer. *Hum. Reprod.*, **9**, 2438–43

52. Gonen, Y., Casper, R. F., Jacobson, W. and Blankier, J. (1989). Endometrial thickness and growth during ovarian stimulation: a possible predictor of implantation in *in vitro* fertilization. *Fertil. Steril.*, **52**, 446–50

53. Glissant, A., de Mouzon, J. and Frydman, R. (1985). Ultrasound study of the endometrium during *in vitro* fertilization cycles. *Fertil. Steril.*, **44**, 786–90

54. Fleischer, A. C., Herbert, C. M., Sacks, G. A., Wentz, A. C., Entman, S. S. and James, A. E. Jr (1986). Sonography of the endometrium during conception and nonconception cycles of

in vitro fertilization and embryo transfer. *Fertil. Steril.*, **46**, 442–7

55. Welker, B. G., Gembruch, U., Diedrich, K., al-Hasani, S. and Krebs, D. (1989). Transvaginal sonography of the endometrium during ovum pick-up in stimulated cycles for *in vitro* fertilization. *J. Ultrasound Med.*, **8**, 549–53

56. Li, T. C., Nuttall, L., Klentzeris, L. and Cooke, I. D. (1992). How well does ultrasonographic measurement of endometrial thickness predict the results of histological dating? *Hum. Reprod.*, **7**, 1–5

57. Dickey, R. P., Olar, T. T., Curole, D. N., Taylor, S. N. and Rye, P. H. (1992). Endometrial pattern and thickness associated with pregnancy outcome after assisted reproduction technologies. *Hum. Reprod.*, **7**, 418–21

58. Krampl, E. and Feichtinger, W. (1993). Endometrial thickness and echo patterns [Letter]. *Hum. Reprod.*, **8**, 1339

59. Imoedemhe, D. A., Shaw, R. W., Kirkland, A. and Chan, R. (1987). Ultrasound measurement of endometrial thickness on different ovarian stimulation regimens during *in vitro* fertilization. *Hum. Reprod.*, **2**, 545–7

60. Freidler, S., Schenker, J. G., Herman, A. and Lewin, A. (1996). The role of ultrasonography in the evaluation of endometrial receptivity following assisted reproductive treatments: a critical review. *Hum. Reprod. Update*, **2**, 323–35

61. Gonen, Y., Calderon, M., Direnfeld, M. and Abramovici, H. (1991). The impact of sonographic assessment of the endometrium and meticulous hormonal monitoring during natural cycles in patients with failed donor artificial insemination. *Ultrasound Obstet. Gynecol.*, **1**, 122–6

62. Abdalla, H. I., Brooks, A. A., Johnson, M. R., Kirkland, A., Thomas, A. and Studd, J. W. (1994). Endometrial thickness: a predictor of implantation in ovum recipients? *Hum. Reprod.*, **9**, 363–5

63. Khalifa, E., Brzyski, R. G., Oehninger, S., Acosta, A. A. and Muasher, S. J. (1992). Sonographic appearance of the endometrium: the predictive value for the outcome of *in vitro* fertilization in stimulated cycles. *Hum. Reprod.*, **7**, 677–80

64. Forrest, T. S., Elyaderani, M. K., Muilenburg, M. I., Bewtra, C., Kable, W. T. and Sullivan, P. (1988). Cyclic endometrial changes: ultrasound

assessment with histologic correlation. *Radiology*, **167**, 233–7

65. Smith, B., Porter, R., Ahuja, K. and Craft, I. (1984). Ultrasonic assessment of endometrial changes in stimulated cycles in an *in vitro* fertilization and embryo transfer program. *J. In Vitro Fertil. Embryo Transfer*, **1**, 233–8

66. Sher, G., Herbert, C., Maassarani, G. and Jacobs, M. H. (1991). Assessment of the late proliferative phase endometrium by ultrasonography in patients undergoing *in vitro* fertilization and embryo transfer (IVF/ET). *Hum. Reprod.*, **6**, 232–7

67. Serafini, P., Batzofin, J., Nelson, J. and Olive, D. (1994). Sonographic uterine predictors of pregnancy in women undergoing ovulation induction for assisted reproductive treatments. *Fertil. Steril.*, **62**, 815–22

68. Steer, C. V., Campbell, S., Pampiglione, J. S., Kingsland, C. R., Mason, B. A. and Collins, W. P. (1990). Transvaginal color flow imaging of the uterine arteries during the ovarian and menstrual cycles. *Hum. Reprod.*, **5**, 391–5

69. Steer, C. V., Tan, S. L., Mason, B. A. and Campbell, S. (1994). Midluteal-phase vaginal color Doppler assessment of uterine artery impedance in a subfertile population. *Fertil. Steril.*, **61**, 53–8

70. Sterzik, K., Grab, D., Sasse, V., Hutter, W., Rosenbusch, B. and Terinde, R. (1989). Doppler sonographic findings and their correlation with implantation in an *in vitro* fertilization program. *Fertil. Steril.*, **52**, 825–8

71. Steer, C. V., Campbell, S., Tan, S. L., Crayford, T., Mills, C., Mason, B. A. and Collins, W. P. (1992). The use of transvaginal color flow imaging after *in vitro* fertilization to identify optimum uterine conditions before embryo transfer. *Fertil. Steril.*, **57**, 372–6

72. Zaidi, J., Pittrof, R., Shaker, A., Kyei-Mensah, A., Campbell, S. and Tan, S. L. (1996). Assessment of uterine artery blood flow on the day of human chorionic gonadotropin administration by transvaginal color Doppler ultrasound in an *in vitro* fertilization program. *Fertil. Steril.*, **65**, 377–81

73. Cacciatore, B., Tiitinen, A. and Ylikorkala, O. (1996). Is it possible to improve uterine blood flow in infertile women? [Abstract]. *Ultrasound Obstet. Gynecol.*, **8**(Suppl.1), 204

Uterine and ovarian perfusion changes from reproductive maturity to menopause

15

A. Kurjak and S. Kupesic

INTRODUCTION

In the last few decades, there has been an increasing tendency for women to delay their childbearing into their late 30s and 40s. Many women who defer pregnancy until the mid to late 30s, and especially to the early 40s, will have an infertility problem. The fact that by 45 years of age natural fecundity is minimal presents new challenges for the different specialties involved in the treatment of infertility, especially for experts in ultrasound diagnosis, particularly those involved in transvaginal color and pulsed Doppler. In this chapter we will describe results obtained with this unique non-invasive method for evaluating the normal and abnormal condition of the female pelvis.

THE CAUSES OF DECLINING FERTILITY

The perimenopausal years, extending from the age of 40 years onward, are the transitional years between the reproductive period of life and the postmenopausal period. The decline of fertility among married couples with advancing age has been documented repeatedly. It is believed that the age-related decrease in pregnancy rates is caused by inadequate function of both the ovaries and the endometrium. The decreased ability of the zygote to implant in the uterus and the aging of the oocytes are two major problems. The question of which of these is more important has been resolved by a number of studies.

Some authors have claimed that an age-related decrease in uterine receptivity might be the cause of the decline in fertility. Ezra and Schenker[1] reported an increase in abortions of genetically normal embryos in the older age group, which might be due to uterine dysfunction. The use of sensitive assays for human chorionic gonadotropin suggests that up to 30% of pregnancies are lost between implantation and the 6th week[2]. The frequency of both euploid and aneuploid abortuses increases with maternal age. Experience with young oocytes donated to older women indicates that the major responsibility for the decline in fertility with age can be attributed to aging oocytes rather than to endometrial receptivity. However, some authorities believe that significantly higher pregnancy rates from donated oocytes are due to better oocyte quality. Navot and colleagues[3] investigated 35 infertile women aged 40 years or older who had failed in attempts at conception with their own oocytes. In the analyzed cycles, oocytes were donated by 29 young individuals undergoing *in vitro* fertilization (mean age 33.4 ± 0.7 years). The rate of implantation per embryo transfer was higher (14.7%) with donated oocytes than with the women's own oocytes (3.3%) ($p < 0.01$). To further elucidate the contribution of age to reproductive outcome, pregnancy results were compared between the young donors and the older recipients. Rates for clinical pregnancy and delivery did not differ between the donors (33% and 23%) and the recipients (40% and 30%). These data suggest that the age-related decline in female fertility is attributable to oocyte quality and is correctable by ovum donation.

169

Drews and colleagues[4] reported that similar pregnancy and livebirth rates were obtained when each donor gave oocytes to a woman over 40 years and another under 40 years of age. In a second report, by Serafini and associates[5], uterine receptivity, as reflected by the clinical pregnancy rate, was similar for oocyte recipients over 40 years and young *in vitro* fertilization surrogates when both groups received eggs from young donors. Uterine receptivity declined when surrogate mothers received oocytes from women over the age of 40 years.

In another study, Navot and colleagues[6] evaluated 38 ovum donors donating oocytes throughout 102 ovum donations. Fifty-one cycles were documented in younger recipients (35.8 ± 3.1 years) and 51 in older recipients (44.0 ± 3.1 years). The capacity to conceive and to gestate a conception to term when oocyte quality is controlled appears to be independent of uterine aging through the 5th decade of life. Borini and associates[7] tried to determine the potential of the aging uterus in terms of pregnancy, implantation and abortion rates, and obstetric complications in postmenopausal women aged 50 years and over receiving oocyte donation. They found that women between 50 and 62 years can become pregnant using donated oocytes and adequate hormonal replacement therapy. However, one should be aware of the effect of pregnancy on pre-existing maternal illness, and the increased risk of pre-eclampsia, hypertension and diabetes.

Patients at age 40 years or older who wish to undergo an *in vitro* fertilization (IVF) procedure with their own oocytes require proper counseling from their physician. A realistic view on the following risks should be presented: a 30 to 50% reduced pregnancy potential, and an increased risk of chromosomal abnormalities, abortion and stillbirth[8]. Knowing these risks, additional testing for ovarian reserve may help to identify women with favorable indices in whom IVF, other forms of assisted reproduction, or surgery to restore fertility, are most appropriate.

Toner and associates[9] reported that follicle-stimulating hormone (FSH) is the best predictor of ovarian function after accounting for age, etiology of infertility and semen quality. The combined use of age and basal FSH in counseling patients improves the accuracy of prognosis and may provide an index of functional ovarian reserve ('ovarian age'). Women aged 40 years or more with favorable hormone profiles can do well in assisted reproduction, while women of any age with basal FSH levels greater than 20 IU/l will be poor responders to ovarian stimulation. Furthermore, FSH levels over 25 IU/l are rarely associated with ongoing pregnancy and the best chance for pregnancy exists with an FSH level between 10 and 20 IU/l. Another parameter used in prediction of the 'ovarian age' is basal estradiol (values above 50 pg/ml predict poor ovarian reserve). Therefore, optimal prediction of the ovarian response should involve simultaneous consideration of age, FSH, luteinizing hormone (LH) and estradiol. Provocative tests of ovarian function are probably superior but are not as simple as static tests and are not widely used.

Fitzgerald and colleagues[10] investigated the effect of age on the growth of the follicle and endometrial thickness. Ultrasound scanning was used to confirm ovulation and measurements were taken to assess follicular development and endometrial growth. Older women were reported to have later ovulation, with the mean follicular phase length increasing from 13.9 days (in a group 20–25 years of age) to 15.9 days (in a group 37–45 years of age; $p < 0.05$). The mean maximum follicular diameter prior to rupture was significantly smaller in older women; 16.7 mm in patients 37–45 years of age, compared with 19.6 mm in a group 21–25 years of age, 21.6 mm in a group 26–31 years of age and 21.3 mm in a group 32–36 years of age. The maximum thickness of the endometrium in the luteal phase was greatest for older women: 15.9 mm in the group aged 37–45 years compared with 12.1 mm in the group aged 21–25 years ($p < 0.001$). Serum gonadotropin concentrations during menses were higher with increased age, while mean ovarian steroid concentrations were not different. These data illustrate significant age-related differences in the pituitary–ovarian axis and endometrial thickness, which may have implications for the management of older women in medically assisted reproduction programs.

Meldrum[11] has stressed that reduced implantation with aging may be explained by the high incidence of delayed or absent secretory maturation of the endometrium. A clear decline of implantation with increasing age has been demonstrated in patients using physiological levels of progesterone replacement. When high doses of progesterone have been used, a significant improvement in implantation rate has been demonstrated. Therefore, oocyte donation through the use of oocytes from young donors and an increased level of progesterone replacement for aging recipients corrects these defects.

EFFECT OF ESTRADIOL AND PROGESTERONE ON VASCULAR RESISTANCE

Rhythmic changes in uterine blood flow during the estrous cycle in different species are temporally associated with the daily ratio of estrogen to progesterone in systemic blood[12–14]. The higher the estrogen–progesterone ratio, the greater the blood flow through the uterine vascular bed[15–17]. Progesterone antagonizes the uterine vasodilatory effect of estrogen[18,19], and the magnitude of this inhibition is related to the ratio of the two steroids[18]. The uterine periarterial sympathetic vasoconstrictor nerves have been postulated as being important in regulating uterine blood flow[20]. Exposure to progesterone has been shown to increase, whereas estrogen decreases, the function of uterine periarterial sympathetic vasoconstrictor nerves[21,22]. The results of Ford and colleagues[23] suggest that ovarian steroids alter the function of uterine periarterial sympathetic nerves through changes in α-adrenergic receptor numbers, which may contribute to the marked changes in uterine blood flow observed during the porcine estrous cycle.

To clarify the role played by physiological levels of ovarian hormones in the vascular resistance of uterine arteries, De Ziegler and associates[24] conducted a study in young women deprived of ovarian function who received physiological estradiol and progesterone replacement therapy. Their results showed that in the absence of estrogen production by the ovary, uterine arteries have a high degree of vascular resistance, expressed by narrow systolic Doppler flow waves and high values of the pulsatility index (PI).

According to the hypothesis of Goswamy and Steptoe[25], multiparous women have persistent diastolic flow during the early follicular phase more often than do nulliparous women. A profound modification of the Doppler flow pattern, suggesting a marked decrease in vascular resistance, was detected after the transdermal administration of estradiol (0.1–0.4 mg/day). This observation is in accordance with the hypothesis that the decrease in vascular resistance observed at the time of ovulation is mediated by estradiol[26]. Because estrogen receptors have been identified in the walls of the uterine arteries, it is likely that the effect of estradiol on the uterine waveform is direct. Therefore, it is postulated that the estrogenic effect on the uterine artery vascular resistance is directly related to the plasma level of biologically active estrogens and that a direct dose–effect relationship exists[27]. Other possible mechanisms include modulation by estradiol of the production and/or secretion of certain vasoactive substances, such as prostaglandins[28], calcitonin gene-related peptide[29] and endothelial relaxing factor[30]. Undoubtedly, transvaginal Doppler studies of the uterine arteries are a valuable reflector of the biological efficacy of various estrogenic treatments. This is particularly important for evaluating the effects of postmenopausal hormonal replacement regimens in women who have an increased hepatic metabolism of estrogen and, therefore, lower levels of plasma estradiol.

The influence of progesterone on the PI of the uterine arteries in humans has not yet been determined. In lower mammals, progesterone acts as a vasoconstrictor[31,32]. This raises concern that the progesterone that is added to estrogen replacement therapy, either sequentially or continuously, for endometrial protection[32], may partially or totally reverse the apparent vasodilatory action of estrogen. Hillard and associates[32] used transvaginal color and pulsed Doppler to measure the PI in the uterine arteries before and during the estradiol and estradiol/progesterone treatment. In all patients, the addition of norethindrone acetate (0.7 mg/day) or medroxyprogesterone acetate (10 mg/day) partially antagonized the response to transdermal estradiol. The PI was approximately 34% lower than the pretreatment value during the combined estradiol/ progesterone phase of treatment, but 13% higher when compared with the estradiol-only treatment phase. It remains unclear whether the effects of progesterone on the uterine artery PI are correlated with the clinical reduction in arterial disease protection with estrogen replacement therapy.

RECENT STUDIES

Kurjak and Kupesic analyzed the relationship between ovarian senescence and uterine and ovarian perfusion[33]. The goal of the study was to investigate the influence of age on ovarian and uterine perfusion. A total of 190 patients were analyzed. Of these, 91 were normal cycling patients with documented fertility, 65 were postmenopausal, and 34 were postmenopausal patients receiving hormone replacement therapy (HRT). Signals from the ovarian artery were characterized by low velocity and high impedance. Measurements in the control group were made between the 5th and 10th days of the menstrual calendar and were continued daily until ovulation was documented according to the established clinical criteria. After detectable ovulation, measurements were made at least twice during the luteal phase. The ovary containing the follicle or corpus luteum was considered as 'dominant'. In the postmenopausal group of patients, examinations were performed at random time intervals. The uterine arteries were detected laterally to the cervix at the level of the cervico–corporeal junction. The average value from both uterine arteries was used. Flow velocity waveforms from radial arteries were obtained within the myometrial fibers, while spiral arteries were visualized at the level of the myometrial–endometrial junction. During each procedure the resistance index (RI) was calculated automatically. The resistance index was used as a calculation measurement of the flow velocity waveform: systole minus diastole, divided by systole. The ovarian artery was visualized laterally from the ovary. When the signal was not demonstrated clearly, the sample volume was moved across the ligament until the arterial signal was identified. Longitudinal studies of the ovarian artery in normal cycling patients demonstrated narrow systolic Doppler flow waves with a resistance index of 0.92 ± 0.08 in the early postmenstrual phase. In the periovulatory phase (cycle days 12 to 14), Doppler waveforms obtained from the ovarian artery of the 'dominant' side showed a marked broadening with continuous diastolic flow, indicative of a profound decrease in vascular impedance (RI 0.86 ± 0.04) (Figure 1). Doppler measurements repeated in the luteal phase demonstrated a further rise in end-diastolic flow velocity, which was most obvious at day 21. This finding was reflected by a significant decline in resistance index to 0.83 ± 0.04. The 'nondominant' ovarian artery did not show the cyclic changes described for the side containing the dominant follicle and/or corpus luteum.

There were no significant changes in ovarian artery Doppler measurements in postmenopausal patients whose last menstrual bleeding was 1–5 years ago, when compared with the 'non-dominant' side of healthy fertile controls. When the same cohort was compared with early follicular and luteal phase ovarian flow impedance values for normal controls, significant differences were observed ($p < 0.01$ and $p < 0.001$, respectively). The ovarian artery in the postmenopausal group demonstrated clear interruption of diastolic blood flow signals in 55% of patients. Absent diastolic flow in ovarian arteries was found in

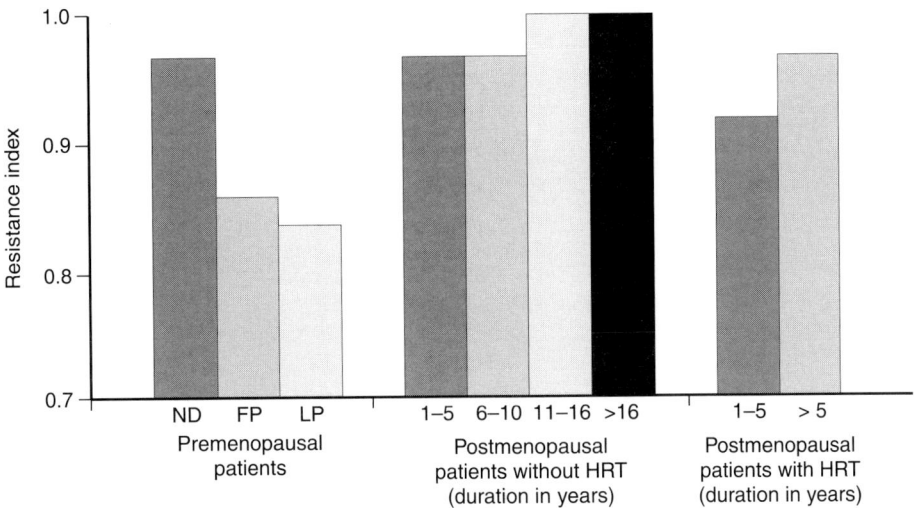

Figure 1 Ovarian artery blood flow in premenopausal patients, and postmenopausal patients with and without hormone replacement therapy (HRT). ND, non-dominant ovarian artery; FP, follicular phase; LP, luteal phase

most patients (84.2%) with menopause of 6–10 years' duration, while interrupted diastolic flow and a resistance index of 1.0 was a constant finding in those with menopause of > 11 years' duration. There was no significant difference when we analyzed the resistance index in the ovarian artery of patients receiving HRT for < 5 years and those receiving it for a longer period of time. No significant difference in terms of ovarian artery impedance was found between patients on HRT and untreated patients. Furthermore, it was not possible to detect velocity waveform signals from the ovarian parenchyma in postmenopausal patients with or without HRT.

The resistance index values of the left and right uterine arteries were correlated highly at each assessment and thus allowed us to use the two values for statistical analysis. The mean resistance index value of the uterine artery during the proliferative phase was 0.88 ± 0.04. Doppler measurements of the uterine artery in the luteal phase demonstrated a decreased resistance index value (0.84 ± 0.04) (Figure 2).

In the group of postmenopausal patients a significant correlation between baseline resistance index and time since menopause was noticed: higher impedance values were obtained in patients with a longer interval since the last menstrual bleeding. Absent diastolic flow in uterine arteries was found in 15% of patients with 1–5 years' duration of menopause (Figure 3). A clear interruption of diastolic blood flow in the uterine artery was demonstrated in 31.6% of patients with menopause duration of between 6 and 10 years, whereas 54.5% of patients with 11–15 years of menopause had this finding. Finally, 79.2% of patients in whom the last menstrual bleeding occurred > 16 years ago demonstrated absent diastolic flow, indicative of a high vascular impedance. In the patients receiving HRT, the uterine artery resistance index was significantly lowered. Increased diastolic flow, and consequently lowered resistance index, were more obvious in patients receiving HRT for more than 6 years. The changes in flow velocity patterns of the radial arteries in premenopausal and postmenopausal patients (with or without HRT) paralleled blood flow dynamics of the uterine arteries. The mean resistance index of the radial artery blood flow declined from 0.74 measured in the proliferative phase to 0.68 in the luteal phase (Figure 4). The values for the resistance index tended to increase during

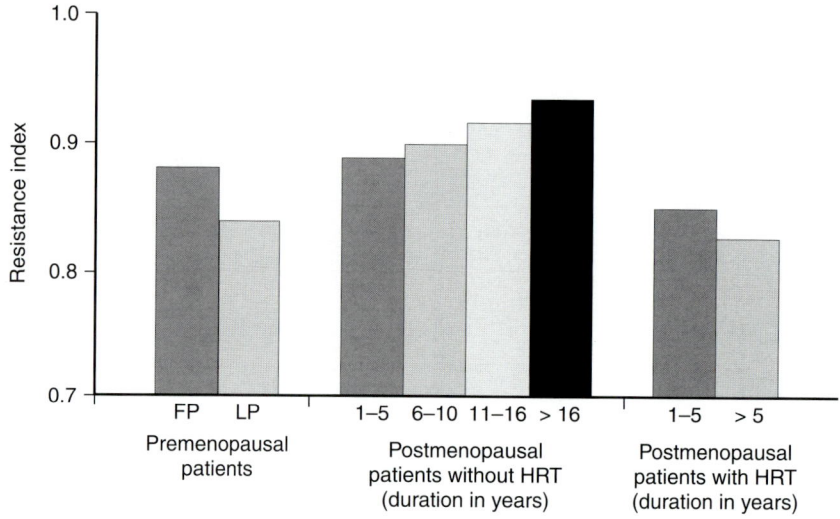

Figure 2 Uterine artery blood flow in premenopausal patients, and postmenopausal patients with and without hormone replacement therapy (HRT). FP, follicular phase; LP, luteal phase

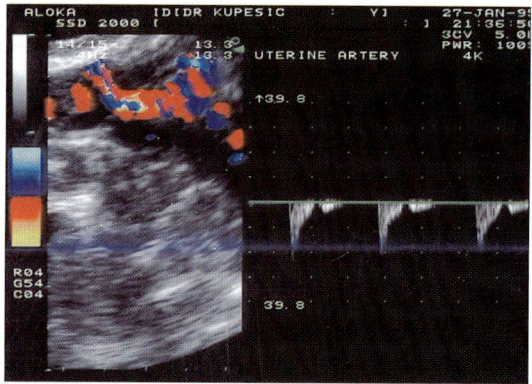

Figure 3 The uterine artery of a postmenopausal patient demonstrates absent diastolic flow

the menopause. Postmenopausal patients receiving HRT showed broadening of systolic flow waves and uninterrupted flow signals during diastole that resulted from decreased radial artery resistance.

A significant difference in the spiral artery resistance occurred between the proliferative (RI 0.64) and luteal (RI 0.50) phases in a group of healthy fertile controls (Figure 5). Visualization of clear Doppler signals from the spiral arteries was possible in only 30% of postmenopausal patients in whom the last menstrual bleeding occurred 1–5 years previously

(Table 1). Furthermore, this group of patients showed significantly increased spiral artery impedance when compared with controls. In patients with menopausal duration of more than 6 years we were unable to obtain any blood flow signals from the periphery of the endometrium. Higher visualization rates ($p < 0.001$) for spiral arteries were demonstrated for patients receiving HRT (Table 2). Spiral artery flow velocity waveforms in these patients were characterized by decreased resistance index values ($p < 0.01$) when compared with postmenopausal patients without HRT.

The results of this Doppler study are concordant with other clinical studies that have demonstrated abrupt changes in ovarian function after the age of 40 years[1,3,34–40]. The addition of color flow imaging has facilitated the measurement of sequential intraovarian blood flow changes. The highest resistance to flow is observed on day 1 of the menstrual cycle, while the lowest occurs on the day of the LH peak. Transvaginal color Doppler reveals areas of vascularity on the follicular rim: the resistance index is around 0.54 when ovulation approaches, declining from 2 days prior to ovulation and reaching its nadir of 0.44 at ovulation. The mature corpus luteum usually measures 1–3 cm in diameter, and shows low

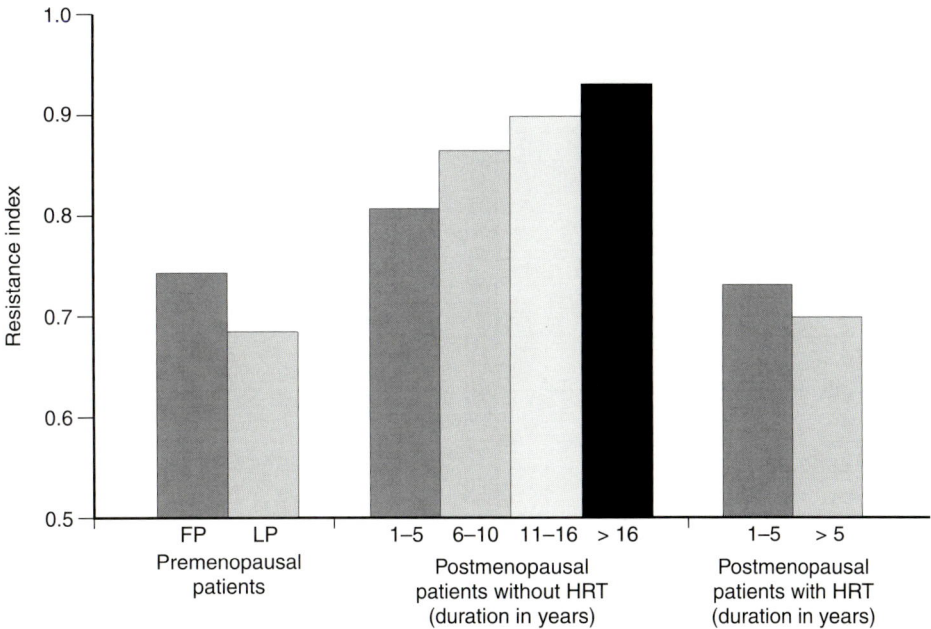

Figure 4 Radial artery blood flow in premenopausal patients, and postmenopausal patients with and without hormone replacement therapy (HRT). FP, follicular phase; LP, luteal phase

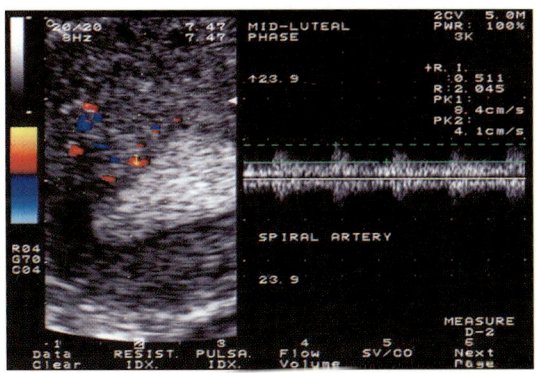

Figure 5 A transvaginal scan demonstrates hyperechogenic layers of the endometrium. The pulsed Doppler waveform analysis obtained from the spiral arteries shows low resistance during the mid-luteal phase of the menstrual cycle (resistance index 0.51)

impedance signals (mean RI 0.43). Regressive changes occur in the corpus luteum as early as the 23rd day after menstruation. Decreased blood velocity and an increased resistance index (mean RI 0.49) are the typical signs of these changes[41-46].

An absence of diastolic flow was common in the early postmenopausal period and was present constantly in patients with > 11 years of menopause. In the postmenopausal group of patients we were not able to detect any intra-ovarian blood flow velocity waveforms. This is probably due to a progressive increase in the amount of fibroblasts and connective tissue and a decrease in the concentration of the circulating estrogens. Therefore, any color flow obtained from the postmenopausal ovary should generate a high index of suspicion for abnormal neovascularization and requires detailed pulsed waveform Doppler analysis.

Our results on uterine arteries clearly demonstrated continuous diastolic flow in all healthy fertile premenopausal controls. In the postmenopausal group, uterine arteries showed an increased degree of vascular impedance expressed by narrow systolic Doppler flow waveforms and high resistance index values. It should be noted that changes in vascular impedance, together with the appearance of absent diastolic flow, were more obvious for the ovarian artery. The fact that

Table 1 Visualization rates of the uterine, radial and spiral arteries in postmenopausal patients

Duration of menopause (years)	No. of patients	Visualization rate (%)		
		Uterine artery	Radial artery	Spiral artery
1–5	15	100	100	30
6–10	14	100	89.5	0
11–15	17	100	76.2	0
> 16	19	100	33.3	0
Total	65	100	76.2	7.6

Table 2 Visualization rates of the uterine, radial and spiral arteries in postmenopausal patients receiving hormone replacement therapy

Duration of menopause (years)	No. of patients	Visualization rate (%)		
		Uterine artery	Radial artery	Spiral artery
1–5	21	100	100	35.7
> 6	13	100	94.1	17.6
Total	34	100	97.7	28.8

the uterine artery resistance index does not change significantly in the first years of menopause supports the thesis that the aging process affects the uterus less than was expected[47]. Changes in the Doppler signal pattern of uterine and radial artery flow observed in response to HRT in our study are indicative of a profound decrease in vascular resistance. Other previous Doppler studies[48–50] showed that physiological amounts of transdermal estradiol markedly decrease uterine artery resistance, suggesting that the uterine environment can be manipulated easily by various hormonal treatments.

Bonilla Musoles and colleagues[51] used transvaginal color Doppler sonography to study the effect of hormone replacement on the uterine arterial blood flow of 203 postmenopausal women. The regimens studied involved estrogen replacement alone, continuous combined estrogen and progestogen, and estrogen followed sequentially by combined estrogen–progestogen. The mean pulsatility index fell to 0.65 ± 0.09 and the mean resistance index fell to 0.87 ± 0.04 during the first month of therapy ($p < 0.0001$). The addition of a progestogen did not alter the effect of

estrogen alone ($p > 0.5$). These findings suggest that the increase in vascular flow occurs even in women who begin therapy long after menopause. Contrary to this study, the same authors used transvaginal color Doppler sonography to study uterine artery blood flow velocity waveforms in 345 normal postmenopausal women who had never been on HRT. Their objective was to establish the standard baseline flow values for normal postmenopausal women. The mean pulsatility index was 3.38 ± 1.04 and the mean resistance index was 0.93 ± 0.09. There was a positive correlation between arterial blood flow impedance and the number of years since menopause. The authors believe that these levels may become important screening parameters for the detection of endometrial carcinoma in postmenopausal women.

Battaglia and colleagues[52] recently published a study aimed at comparing the uterine blood flow variations induced by chemical castration and spontaneous menopause. Thirty infertile patients were studied in the early follicular phase (days 5–7) and then treated with gonadotropin-releasing hormone agonist (GnRH-a). On day 25 from GnRH-a injection, the suppressive effect was checked. The values obtained were compared with those found in 18 postmenopausal women (menopause < 5 years). All the subjects underwent transvaginal ultrasonography, Doppler analysis of uterine arteries, hormonal assay and evaluation of hematological and biochemical parameters. In all infertile patients, the GnRH-a suppressive effect was shown at the 25th day from the injection. Endometrial thickness decreased from 0.6 ± 0.1 mm to 0.3 ± 0.1 mm ($p < 0.05$) and the pulsatility index increased from 2.52 ± 0.31 to 3.02 ± 0.25 ($p < 0.05$). The plasma estradiol level fell from 48.2 ± 4.4 pg/ml to 13.6 ± 7.9 pg/ml ($p < 0.05$). No other hormonal and biochemical parameters were significantly modified by GnRH-a. In postmenopausal women, the values of the studied parameters were similar to those found in the infertile GnRH-a-suppressed patients. These data show that GnRH-a induces vascular modifications similar to those induced soon after menopause and that both are probably exclusively related to hypoestrogenism.

Handa and co-workers[53] wanted to test the hypothesis that a very low-dose regimen of vaginal estrogen would provide effective relief from atrophic vaginitis without endometrial proliferation. Twenty postmenopausal women with symptoms, signs and cytological evidence of atrophic vaginitis were enrolled. Each subject was treated with 0.3 mg of conjugated estrogens, administered vaginally three nights per week for 6 months. They examined the following outcomes: symptoms, vaginal cellular (cytological) maturity, endometrial histology, sonographic evaluation of endometrial thickness, Doppler measures of uterine artery blood flow and serum levels of estrone and estradiol. Pre- and post-treatment data were compared for each subject. Satisfactory relief of symptoms occurred in 19 of 20 cases. Vaginal cellular maturation improved significantly with therapy ($p < 0.01$). There were no significant changes in endometrial thickness, uterine artery blood flow, or serum estrogen levels. Endometrial proliferation was observed in one case. The authors concluded that the relief from atrophic vaginitis can be achieved with 0.3 mg of conjugated estrogens administered vaginally three times per week. Endometrial proliferation may occur rarely at this low dose.

Achiron and colleagues[54] evaluated the endometrial blood flow response to hormone replacement therapy in women with premature ovarian failure who planned to enter an oocyte donation program. Transvaginal color Doppler ultrasound examinations were performed in women with ovarian failure before and during a cycle of standard HRT and in those with normal menstrual cycles. Blood flow response was assessed by visualization of arterial waveforms in the endometrial region. The transvaginal color flow imaging system was used. Resistance indexes were calculated for analysis and correlated with plasma estradiol and progesterone concentrations for 18 women with ovarian failure (study group) and 12 volunteers with normal ovarian cycles (control group). Data for resistance indices were divided into five phases according to the day of the hormonal cycle: 0, pretreatment phase; I, early follicular phase (days 5–7); II, late follicular phase (days 11–13); III, early luteal phase (days 17–21); and IV, late luteal phase (days 23–25). All women with ovarian failure demonstrated continuous forward end-diastolic flow velocities at phase I, whereas none showed this pattern during the pretreatment period (phase 0). Women with ovarian failure had a significantly higher resistance index (0.85 ± 0.10) in the early follicular phase than in the late follicular phase (0.57 ± 0.10), and the resistance index in the early luteal phase (0.67 ± 0.10) was significantly higher than that of the late follicular phase. There was no difference in the resistance index between the early and late luteal phases. A similar pattern of lower resistance index around midcycle was observed in the control group. However, a comparison of the resistance indices between patients with ovarian failure and control patients revealed a significant difference between values in the early follicular phase only (1.0 ± 0.10 vs. 0.68 ± 0.10). In the late follicular phase and during the entire luteal phase, the mean resistance index did not differ between the study and control groups. The authors concluded that standard HRT in women with premature ovarian failure enables restoration of endometrial blood flow to normal. This may imply uterine receptivity for oocyte donation.

These data support the observation that oocytes donated from young women, together with appropriate hormonal support of the endometrium, could overcome problems such as inadequate uterine receptivity and high pregnancy wastage rates[3]. Undoubtedly, transvaginal color and pulsed Doppler is a noninvasive method that can help in better understanding the possible mechanisms involved in the effect of aging on fertility.

References

1. Ezra, Y. and Schenker, J. G. (1993). Appraisal of *in vitro* fertilization. *Eur. J. Obstet. Gynecol. Reprod. Biol.*, **48**, 127–33

2. Wilcox, A. J., Weibereg, C. R., O'Connor, J. F., Baird, D. D., Schlatterer, J. P., Canfield, R. E., Armstrong, E. G. and Nisula, B. C. (1988). Incidence of early loss of pregnancy. *N. Engl. J. Med.*, **319**, 189–94

3. Navot, D., Bergh, P. A., Williams, M. A., Garissi, G. J., Guzman, I., Sandler, B. and Grunfeld, L. (1991). Poor oocyte quality rather than implantation failure as a cause of age-related decline in female fertility. *Lancet*, **337**, 1375–7

4. Drews, M., Bergh, P., Williams, M., Grunfeld, L., Garrisi, G. and Navot, D. (1992). Age-related decline in female infertility is not due to diminished capacity of the uterus to sustain embryo implantation. Presented at the *48th Annual Meeting of the American Fertility Society*, New Orleans, Abstract 0-086, S39

5. Serafini, P., Tran, C., Tan, T., Norbryhn, G. and Batzofin, J. (1992). Oocyte aging is the main factor responsible for the decline in fertility with chronological advancement. Evidence from the IVF surrogacy and egg donation programs. Presented at the *48th Annual Meeting of the American Fertility Society*, New Orleans, Abstract 0-011, S5

6. Navot, D., Drews, M. R., Bergh, P. A., Guzman, I., Karstaedt, A., Scott, R. T. Jr, Garrisi, G. J. and Hofmann, G. E. (1994). Age-related decline in female fertility is not due to diminished capacity of the uterus to sustain embryo implantation. *Fertil. Steril.*, **61**, 97–101

7. Borini, A., Bafaro, G., Violini, F., Bianchi, L., Casadio, V. and Flamigni, C. (1995). Pregnancies in postmenopausal women over 50 years old in an oocyte donation program. *Fertil Steril.*, **63**, 258–61

8. Toner, J. P. and Flood, J. T. (1993). Fertility after the age of 40. *Obstet. Gynecol. Clin. North. Am.*, **20**, 261–72

9. Toner, J. P., Philput, C. B., Jones, G. S. and Muasher, S. J. (1991). Basal follicle-stimulating hormone level is a better predictor of *in vitro* fertilization performance than age. *Fertil. Steril.*, **55**, 784–91

10. Fitzgerald, C. T., Seif, M. W., Killick, S. R. and Elstein, M. (1994). Age-related changes in the female reproductive cycle. *Br. J. Obstet. Gynaecol.*, **101**, 229–33

11. Meldrum, D. R. (1993). Female reproductive aging – ovarian and uterine factors. *Fertil. Steril.*, **59**, 1–5

12. Ford, S. P., Chenault, J. R. and Echterncamp, S. E. (1979). Uterine blood flow of cows during the estrous cycle and early pregnancy: effect of the conceptus on the uterine blood supply. *J. Reprod. Fertil.*, **56**, 53–8

13. Yuthasastrakosol, P., Palmer, W. M. and Howland, B. E. (1975). Luteinizing hormone, oestrogen and progesterone levels in peripheral serum of anoestrous and cyclic ewes as determined by radioimmunoassay. *J. Reprod. Fertil.*, **43**, 57–62

14. Henricks, D. M., Guthlie, H. D. and Handlin, D. L. (1975). Plasma estrogen, progesterone and luteinizing hormone levels during the estrous cycle in pigs. *Biol. Reprod.*, **6**, 210–16

15. Killam, A. P., Rosenfeld, C., Battaglia, F. C., Makowski, E. L. and Meschia, G. (1973). Effect of estrogens on the uterine blood flow in oophorectemized ewes. *Am. J. Obstet. Gynecol.*, **115**, 1045–50

16. Ford, S. P. and Reynolds, L. P. (1983). Role of adrenergic receptors in mediating estradiol-17 beta-stimulated increases in uterine blood flow of cows. *J. Anim. Sci.*, **57**, 665–9

17. Dickson, W. M., Bosc, M. J. and Locatelli, A. (1969). Effect of estrogen and progesterone on uterine blood flow in castrate sows. *Am. J. Physiol.*, **217**, 1431–7

18. Caton, D., Abrams, R. M., Clapp, J. F. and Barron, D. (1974). The effect of exogenous progesterone on the rate of blood flow of the

uterus of ovariectomized sheep. *Q. J. Exp. Physiol.*, **59**, 225–31

19. Resnik, R., Brink, G. W. and Plumer, M. H. (1977). The effect of progesterone on estrogen-induced uterine blood flow. *Am. J. Obstet. Gynecol.*, **128**, 251–5

20. Ford, S. P. (1973). Control of uterine and ovarian blood flow throughout the estrous cycle and pregnancy of the ewe, sow and cow. *J. Anim. Sci.*, **55**(Suppl. 2), 32–4

21. Ford, S. P., Weber, L. J. and Stormshak, F. (1976). *In vitro* response of ovine and bovine uterine arteries to prostaglandin $F_{2\alpha}$ and periarterial sympathetic nerve stimulation. *Biol. Reprod.*, **15**, 58–64

22. Ford, S. P., Weber, L. J. and Stormshak, F. (1977). Role of estradiol-17 beta and progesterone in regulating constriction of ovine arteries. *Biol. Reprod.*, **17**, 480–6

23. Ford, S. P., Reynolds, L. P., Farley, D. B., Bhatnagar, R. K. and van Orden, D. E. (1984). Interaction of ovarian steroids and periarterial alpha-1-adrenergic receptors in altering uterine blood flow during the estrous cycle of gilts. *Am. J. Obstet. Gynecol.*, **5**, 480–4

24. De Ziegler, D., Bessis, R. and Frydman, R. (1991). Vascular resistance of uterine arteries: physiological effects of estradiol and progesterone. *Fertil. Steril.*, **55,** 775–9

25. Goswamy, R. K. and Steptoe, P. C. (1988). Doppler ultrasound studies of the uterine artery in spontaneous ovarian cycles. *Hum. Reprod.*, **3**, 721–5

26. Perrot-Applanat, M., Groyer-Picart, M. T., Garcia, E., Lorenzo, F. and Milgrom, E. (1988). Immunocytochemical demonstration of estrogen and progesterone receptors in muscle cells of uterine arteries in rabbits and humans. *Endocrinology,* **123**, 1511–14

27. Sarrel, P. M. (1990). Ovarian hormones and circulation. *Maturitas*, **590**, 297–8

28. Steinleitner, A., Stancyzk, F. Z., Levin, J. N., d'Ablaing, G., Vijod, M. A. and Shabhagian, V. L. (1989). Decreased *in vitro* production of 6-keto-prostaglandin $F_{1\alpha}$ by uterine arteries from postmenopausal women. *Am. J. Obstet. Gynecol.*, **161**, 1677–81

29. Stevenson, J. C., McDonald, D. W. R., Waren, R. C., Booker, M. W. and Whitehead, M. I. (1986). Increased concentration of circulating calcitonin gene-related peptide during normal human pregnancy. *Br. Med. J.*, **29**, 1329–30

30. Furchgott, R. F. and Zawadzki, J. W. (1980). The obligatory role of endothelial cells in the relaxation of arterial smooth muscle by acetylcholine. *Nature (London)*, **288**, 373–6

31. Resnik, R. (1976). The effect of progesterone on estrogen-induced uterine blood flow. *Gynecol. Invest.*, **128**, 251–4

32. Hillard, T. C., Bourne, T., Whitehead, M. I., Cryford, T. B., Collins, W. P. and Campbell, S. (1992). Differential effects of transdermal estradiol and sequential progestogens on impedance to flow within the uterine arteries of postmenopausal women. *Fertil. Steril.*, **58**, 959–63

33. Kupesic, S., Kurjak, A. and Babic, M. M. (1996). Uterine and ovarian perfusion changes from reproductive maturity to menopause. *ACDS*, **12**, 79–87

34. Wiro, M. S. and Schewchuk, A. B. (1984). Pregnancy outcome in 242 conceptions after artificial insemination with donor sperm and effects of maternal age on the prognosis for successful pregnancy. *Am. J. Obstet. Gynecol.*, **148**, 518–24

35. Van Noord-Zaadstra, B. Y., Looman, C. W. N., Alsbach, H., Rabbena, J. D. F., Te Velde, E. R. and Karbaat, J. (1991). Delaying child bearing: effect of age on fecundity and outcome of pregnancy. *Br. Med. J.*, **302**, 1361–5

36. Menken, J., Trussel, J. and Larsel, U. (1986). Age and infertility. *Science*, **233**, 1389–94

37. Meldrum, D. R. (1993). Female reproductive aging – ovarian and uterine factors. *Fertil. Steril.*, **59**, 1–5

38. Padilla, S. L. and Garcia, J. E. (1989). Effect of maternal age and number of *in vitro* fertilization procedures on pregnancy outcome. *Fertil. Steril.*, **52**, 270–3

39. Check, J. H., Lurie, D., Callan, C., Baker, A. and Benfer, K. (1994). Comparison of the cumulative probability of pregnancy after *in vitro* fertilization–embryo transfer by infertility factor and age. *Fertil. Steril.*, **61**, 257–61

40. Sauer, M. V., Paulson, R. J. and Lobo, R. A. (1993). Pregnancy after 50: application of oocyte donation to women after natural menopause. *Lancet*, **341**, 321–3

41. Bourne, T., Jurkovic, D., Waterstone, J., Campbell, S. and Collins, W. P. (1991). Intrafollicular blood flow during human ovulation. *Ultrasound Obstet. Gynecol.*, **1**, 53–9

42. Collins, W. P., Jurkovic, D., Bourne, T. H., Kurjak, A. and Campbell, S. (1991). Ovarian morphology, endocrine function and intrafollicular blood flow during the peri-ovulatory period. *Hum. Reprod.*, **6**, 319–24

43. Baber, R. J., McSweeney, M. B. and Gill, R. W. (1988). Transvaginal pulsed Doppler ultrasound assessment of blood flow to the corpus luteum in IVF patients following embryo transfer. *Br. J. Obstet. Gynaecol.*, **95**, 1226–30

44. Zalud, I. and Kurjak, A. (1990). The assessment of luteal blood flow in pregnant and nonpregnant women by transvaginal color Doppler. *J. Perinat. Med.*, **18**, 215–21

45. Kurjak, A., Kupesic-Urek, S., Schulman, H. and Zalud, I. (1991). Transvaginal color flow

Doppler in the assessment of ovarian and uterine blood flow in infertile women. *Fertil. Steril.*, **56**, 870–3

46. Kupesic, S. and Kurjak, A. (1993). Uterine and ovarian perfusion during the periovulatory period assessed by transvaginal color Doppler. *Fertil. Steril.*, **60**, 439–43

47. Kurjak, A. and Kupesic, S. (1995). Ovarian senescence and its significance on uterine and ovarian perfusion. *Fertil. Steril.*, **64**, 532–8

48. De Ziegler, D., Bessis, R. and Frydman, R. (1991). Vascular resistance of uterine arteries: physiological effects of estradiol and progesterone. *Fertil. Steril.*, **55**, 775–9

49. Bourne, T. H., Hillard, T. C., Whitehead, M. I., Crook, D. and Campbell, S. (1990). Oestrogens, arterial status, and postmenopausal women. *Lancet*, **335**, 1471–2

50. Hillard, T. C., Bourne, T. H., Whitehead, M. I., Crayford, T. B., Collins, W. P. and Campbell, S. (1992). Differential effects of transdermal estradiol and sequential progestogens on impedance to flow within the uterine arteries of postmenopausal women. *Fertil. Steril.*, **58**, 959–63

51. Bonilla Musoles, F., Marti, M. C. and Ballester, M. J. (1995). Normal uterine arterial blood flow in postmenopausal women assessed by transvaginal color Doppler sonography: the effect of hormone replacement therapy. *J. Ultrasound Med.*, **14**, 497–501

52. Battaglia, C., Artini, P. G., Bencini, S., Bianchi, R., D'Ambrogio, G. and Genazzani, A. R. (1995). Doppler analysis of uterine blood flow changes in spontaneous and medically induced menopause. *Gynecol. Endocrinol.*, **9**, 143–8

53. Handa, V. L., Bachus, K. E., Johnston, W. W., Robboy, S. J. and Hammond, C. B. (1994). Vaginal administration of low-dose conjugated estrogen: systemic absorption and effects on the endometrium. *Obstet. Gynecol.*, **84**, 215–18

54. Achiron, H., Levran, D., Sivan, E., Lipitz, S., Dor, J. and Mashiach, S. (1995). Endometrial blood flow response to hormone replacement therapy in women with premature ovarian failure: a transvaginal Doppler study. *Fertil. Steril.*, **63**, 550–4

The value of color Doppler in oocyte donation programs

16

M. M. Biljan and S. L. Tan

INTRODUCTION

Oocyte donation is a well established method of assisted reproduction and an innovative means of fertility treatment for two groups of patients. The first group includes women without gonadal function because of premature ovarian failure occurring either spontaneously or after surgical castration, as well as women with gonadal dysgenesis with or without chromosomal aberrations. The second group of women are those with functional ovaries who have had repeated failures of fertilization in the course of *in vitro* fertilization (IVF) treatment who are found to be poor responders, and women with no ovulatory problems who are at risk of transmitting genetic disease[1]. Oocyte donation represents a unique physiological configuration, which makes the optimization of ovarian stimulation possible without a negative effect on endometrial receptivity[2]. It is this unique situation which has made oocyte donation more successful than any other assisted conception procedure[3]. In a recent retrospective study, for instance, Remohi and colleagues[4] reported a livebirth rate of 42.6% (95% confidence interval 40.1–45.1%) per treatment cycle and a cumulative livebirth rate of 88.7% (88.1–89.3%) after four treatment cycles.

Oocyte donation, therefore, could offer a solution to a number of otherwise intractable infertility problems. Moreover, the dissociation between ovarian stimulation and preparation of the endometrium provides a unique model to investigate the importance of the effect of different hormones on oocyte and endometrial development. In this review we will address issues related to endometrial preparation, the value of different histological and ultrasonic parameters in predicting implantation following embryo transfer, and differences between different groups of recipients requiring oocyte donation.

ENDOMETRIAL PREPARATION

Unlike the natural ovarian-menstrual cycle, in an oocyte donation program the endometrial preparation is separated from the steroidogenesis related to oocyte development. To achieve a satisfactory endometrial preparation, the internal milieu has to be manipulated by the sequential administration of estrogen and progesterone. Initially, the preparation of the endometrium in recipients was based on close mimicking of the normal menstrual cycle[5]. Estrogen was administered artificially in an incremental fashion, culminating in a late artificial follicular peak, a subsequent postovulatory decrease and a second midluteal rise. Progesterone was started 2 weeks after initiation of the follicular phase. Successful implantation after implementation of this protocol showed that sequential estrogen and progesterone therapy alone, with no other ovarian products, was sufficient for endometrial preparation. A disadvantage of the above protocol is its relative rigidity which results in difficult co-ordination between donor and recipient cycles. To overcome this problem several authors[6–8] have suggested a flexible fixed regimen of endometrial preparation. Such a regimen allows between 2 and 4 weeks of fixed doses of unopposed estrogen administration before the introduction of progesterone and embryo transfer. This fixed regimen produced a similar quality of endometrium and pregnancy rates[6]. It is therefore evident that the human endometrium is not affected adversely when exposed to fixed doses of sequential estrogen and progesterone, and moreover, it maintains its capacity for implantation. It appears that the length of the artificial follicular phase can also be widely manipulated without a detrimental effect on the endometrial histological appearance. Navot and colleagues[7] found no histological difference in endometrial biopsies performed in the mid- and late-luteal phases, in patients exposed to estrogen anywhere between 6 and 18 days prior to progesterone transformation. In a similar study, an unchanged histological picture was reported despite a prolonged follicular phase up to 35 days[8]. However, clinical studies have shown that although histologically similar, the endometrium exposed to a very long or very short artificial follicular phase has lower implantation potential. In a study involving 51 patients, Younis and colleagues[9] reported a 7.7% pregnancy rate in patients exposed for less than 12 or more than 19 days to unopposed estrogen, and a 52% pregnancy rate in patients who had a follicular phase duration ranging between 12 and 19 days. Additionally, Navot and colleagues[10] reported a significantly higher miscarriage rate in the group of patients subjected to short estrogen exposure.

The dose of estrogen required to achieve sufficient endometrial response has not been the subject of sufficient research. Histological studies have shown glandular abnormalities when 6 mg of estradiol was used in the follicular phase. However, a similar pregnancy rate was achieved when this or a lower dose of estrogen was used for endometrial preparation[2]. Moreover, Shapiro and colleagues[11] reported faster growth of ultrasonically similar endometrium when 8 mg estradiol was used. The role of estrogen administration in the luteal phase is less clear. Animal studies have shown reduced pregnancy rates in primates depleted of estrogen during the luteal phase[12]. In humans, however, histological studies performed in the luteal phase show no difference in endometrial appearance, regardless of estrogen exposure in the luteal phase[13]. Before a definite role of estrogen exposure in the luteal phase can be determined, it is essential to prospectively study the differences in pregnancy rate between patients on progesterone only, and those on combined preparations of estrogen and progesterone treatment in the luteal phase.

The mode and dose of progesterone administration varies widely between different programs. Intramuscular injections of progesterone in oil bases[11,14,15], and vaginal micronized progesterone preparations[16,17] appear to be the most popular routes of administration. The intramuscular route is frequently complicated by pain at the injection site. On the other hand, suppositories are associated with discharge that is unacceptable to some patients. The mode of delivery, and the dose of progesterone administered, is not of crucial importance in the majority of patients. Similar pregnancy rates have been reported with serum progesterone levels between 6 and 56 ng/ml[16,18]. Recently, however, it has been reported that older patients may require higher doses of progesterone to achieve the same implantation rates as younger women[19].

ASSESSMENT OF ENDOMETRIAL RECEPTIVITY

While relatively good implantation rates are achieved in oocyte donation programs, still only one out of every five replaced embryos successfully implants. The transfer of more than one embryo increases the pregnancy rate, but carries an increased incidence of multiple gestation[20]. This can be especially dangerous in patients requiring oocyte donation, who are either older or may have additional obstetric risk factors[21-24].

As the probability of pregnancy is related to uterine receptivity, as well as embryo quality, assessment of both these factors is paramount in improving the success of assisted conception. In oocyte donation, embryo quality is relatively constant, as the oocytes come from a uniform cohort of young donors. The assessment of endometrial quality, however, still poses a major obstacle in achieving higher pregnancy rates. Although attempts have been made to assess the functional normality of the endometrium by quantifying the expression of endometrial proteins in response to circulating sex steroids[25], this procedure requires an endometrial biopsy. The potential disadvantage of removing a strip of endometrium to assess uterine receptivity in the same cycle in which embryo transfer is performed is evident. The biopsy may cause trauma and bleeding at the implantation site with a potential reduction in the chance of pregnancy. To avoid this problem, some centers advocate the performance of a mock replacement cycle, with a timed endometrial biopsy which is performed to ascertain the appropriate endometrial response[26]. This, however, requires an additional preparatory cycle, which increases costs and is inconvenient to the patient. The optimal investigation of uterine receptivity should therefore involve a non-invasive procedure which is rapid and easy to perform, and which also provides immediate results. To this end, there has recently been increasing interest in the use of ultrasound in general and color Doppler ultrasound in particular for the assessment of implantation potential.

Ultrasound assessment

Two ultrasound techniques have been proposed for the assessment of endometrial receptivity: the assessment of endometrial appearance, and the assessment of endometrial vascularization by Doppler ultrasound. To be of practical value, the results of any diagnostic test should be available, at the latest, on the day of human chorionic gonadotropin (hCG) administration for the donor, allowing time for hormonal manipulation, delay of embryo transfer, or preparation for embryo cryopreservation.

The value of measuring the endometrial thickness and studying the endometrial reflectivity in the context of assisted conception remains a contentious issue. Gonen and colleagues[27] suggested that endometrial thickness (Figures 1 and 2) on the day before oocyte recovery was significantly greater in the

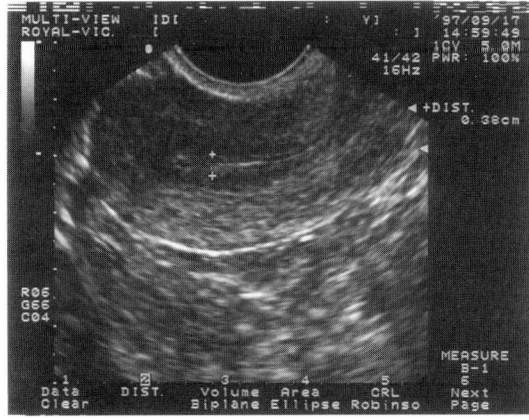

Figure 1 Longitudinal section of the uterus showing a thin endometrium

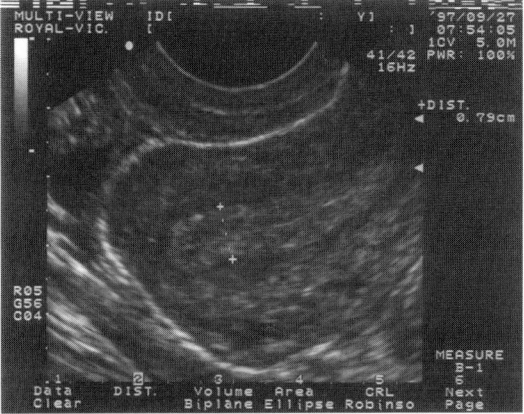

Figure 2 Longitudinal section of the uterus showing a thick endometrium

pregnant than in the non-pregnant woman, and suggested that it may predict the likelihood of implantation. However, Glissant and co-workers[28], Fleischer and colleagues[29], and Welker and co-workers[30] found that measurement of endometrial thickness had no predictive value for pregnancy. Imoedemhe and colleagues[31] compared the endometrial thickness in three groups of patients on three different ovarian stimulation regimens. They found that the endometrial thickness in all three groups of patients was similar and comparable to that observed in a control group of spontaneously ovulating, fertile women, despite significantly higher levels of serum estradiol concentrations in all of the hyper-stimulated cycles. In a group of oocyte recipients, no pregnancies were reported in women who had an endometrial thickness of less than 5 mm, whereas several pregnancies occurred in patients with an endometrium thinner than 7.5 mm[32]. Their findings suggest that there is a maximum endometrial response inducible by estrogen, which is virtually achieved in the normal cycle. With regard to the endometrial appearance, it has been suggested that a multi-layered endometrial pattern (Figures 3 and 4) is associated with a significantly higher pregnancy rate[30,33], and that it may also predict the likelihood of fertilization[33,34].

Doppler studies of uterine arteries

Uterine blood flow

In general, blood flow studies have been confined to arteries, as Doppler studies of the venous circulation provide no information on flow impedance and it is assumed that changes in venous circulation are a poor predictor of functional changes in organ perfusion.

Initial studies of Doppler ultrasound in assisted conception cycles were performed using the transabdominal approach. However, the transabdominal approach requires the presence of a distended bladder which increases the distance between the Doppler probe and the vessels under investigation so that low pulse repetition frequencies, which are relatively inaccurate, have to be used. Another disadvantage of the abdominal approach is that the distended bladder may alter blood flow in the smaller arteries[35]. Finally, patients can rarely tolerate an uncomfortably full bladder long enough for the Doppler study to be completed. In contrast, vaginal sonography obviates the need for a full bladder and the ultrasound probe can be placed close to the vessel under investigation, so that the optimal pulse repetition frequency can be chosen. Recently, Steer and colleagues have investigated the accuracy of transvaginal and transabdominal Doppler assessment of the uterine artery in the subfertile population. They found

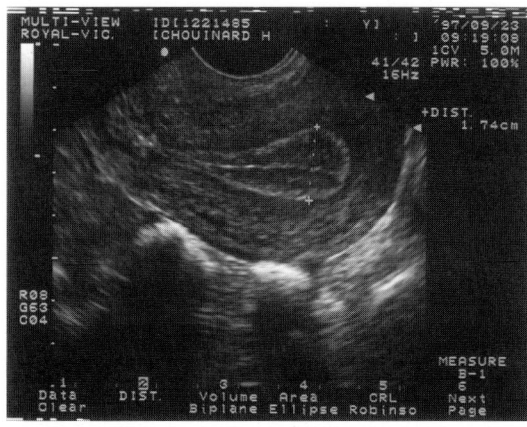

Figure 3 A multilayered endometrium with the so-called triple line appearance

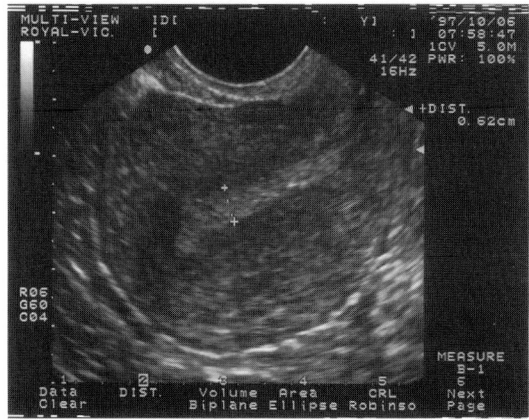

Figure 4 Hyperechogenic non-multilayered endometrium

transvaginal assessment to be easier to perform and significantly more reproducible[35]. With regard to the size of blood vessels, it is unlikely that blood flow in large vessels such as the external or internal iliac arteries would significantly affect physiological changes during the implantation period and there have been, therefore, no attempts to investigate these vessels. So far, the most commonly studied blood vessel in relation to implantation has been the uterine artery (Figure 5). However, with the development of power Doppler, some attention has also been drawn to the importance of smaller uterine blood

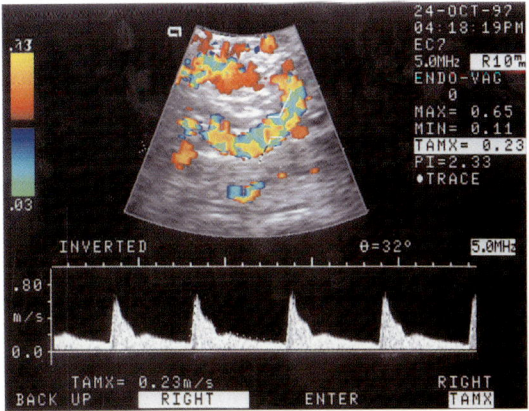

Figure 5 Transvaginal color Doppler ultrasound showing the right uterine artery

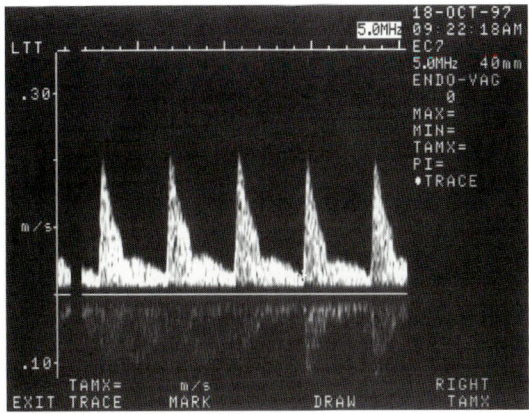

Figure 7 Flow velocity waveform of the uterine artery

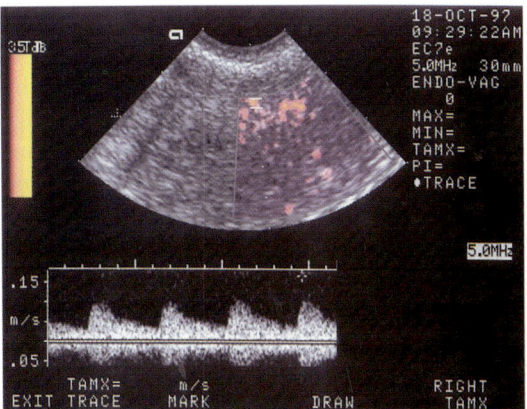

Figure 6 Power Doppler ultrasound of subendometrial blood flow

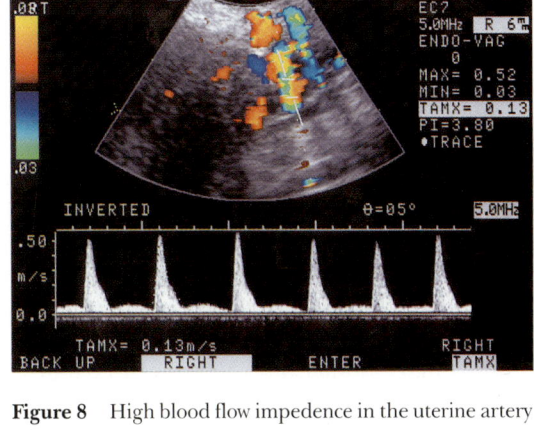

Figure 8 High blood flow impedence in the uterine artery

vessels, such as the subendometrial and arcuate arteries (Figure 6)[36]. When measuring the flow within uterine arteries, signals are measured at the uterine arteries and their ascending branches located in the outer third of the myometrium. The graphic display of the temporal changes in Doppler frequency, which shifts across the full cross-section of the vessel throughout each cardiac cycle, is called the flow velocity waveform (Figure 7). The maximum outline of the flow velocity waveform indicates the degree of resistance to flow in the artery under investigation. Absence of Doppler frequency shifts during the diastolic phase of the cycle is typically found in large arteries, such as the external iliac artery, supplying high-resistance vascular beds. In contrast, high end-diastolic velocities are usually present in smaller arteries supplying organs such as the uterus and ovaries. The flow velocity waveform is most easily quantified by calculating an index of resistance or impedance to blood flow. The indices most commonly used clinically are the resistance index (RI) and the pulsatility index (PI). Both indices are based on the ratio between the peak systolic and end-diastolic velocities, and they are both independent of the angle of insonation. This is important since flow velocity waveform analysis can, therefore, be used for blood flow studies even in small arteries which are not clearly visualized, and which have an undefined angle of insonation. Of the various indices, we favor use of the PI because it has been demonstrated to correlate most closely with changes in blood flow volume[37] and can be used even when there is absence of diastolic velocities or reverse flow in the diastolic phase.

Clinical application

Taylor and colleagues[38] were the first to point out the possibility of investigating normal ovarian and uterine blood flow by means of Doppler ultrasound. Soon after, Feichtinger and colleagues[39] described an increase of systolic blood flow velocity with time in the internal iliac artery and the ovarian artery during ovarian stimulation. The use of Doppler ultrasound to investigate implantation potential was then suggested by Goswamy and Steptoe[40]. Using the transabdominal route, these authors examined, in the late luteal phase, 153 patients who had a history of three previous unsuccessful IVF attempts in spite of the transfer of good quality embryos. They reported a 55% incidence of poor perfusion, defined as an absence of end-diastolic flow, in this group of patients and postulated that perhaps suboptimal flow could be an independent cause of infertility. Sterzik an colleagues[41] performed transvaginal Doppler ultrasound on 45 patients undergoing IVF treatment on the day of follicular aspiration. While no difference was observed between the pregnant (12 patients) and the non-pregnant patients in either the number of follicles developed or embryos transferred, a significantly higher PI was seen in the non-pregnant group. Similarly to previous studies, they observed no pregnancies in the group of patients who had no end-diastolic flow (Figure 8). Steer and colleagues[42] were the first to use transvaginal color Doppler to study the uterine arteries in infertility. Daily measurements of the PI of both uterine arteries were made in 23 normally cycling women. They noted that the lowest uterine artery PI was found 9 days after the luteinizing hormone (LH) peak, which is consistent with a maximum uterine perfusion at the time of peak luteal function and expected implantation.

Steer and colleagues also showed that the uterine artery impedance was different in the midluteal phase in women with subfertility compared with those with normal fertility[43]. They used transvaginal color Doppler to study the uterine arterial blood flow in 82 women undergoing IVF treatment on the day of embryo transfer[44]. The PI was calculated and the patients were grouped according to whether the PI was low (1–1.99), medium (2–2.99) or high (3.0+) (Figure 8). There were no pregnancies in the high PI group and the PI was significantly lower in the women who became pregnant, as compared with those who did not. Moreover, the authors found a significant correlation between uterine blood flow indices and biochemical markers of uterine receptivity, including 24-kDa protein, uterine estradiol receptor and endometrial histology dating[45]. Similar findings have since been reported by others. Coulam and colleagues found that significantly more non-conceptional than conceptional cycles ($p < 0.001$) had a high uterine artery PI (> 3.3)[46]. Interestingly, Tekay and colleagues[47] were not able to confirm data reported by other groups. In their study, which included only 30 non-selected patients, the authors found no difference in uterine perfusion between pregnant and non-pregnant patients. This difference could be attributed to an inconsistency in patient preparation and timing of Doppler investigations. In an interesting study, Dickey and colleagues[48] examined the influence of patient position on Doppler readings. In their study, the patients were first examined in the recumbent and subsequently in the upright position. After standing for 9–14 min, the uterine artery blood flow decreased by an average of 34% and the PI increased by 70%. In addition, the number of cycles with absent end-diastolic flow increased. We have recently shown that the time of the day when Doppler measurements are made could also have a major impact on results. We found that blood flow in the uterine arteries follows a circadian rhythm, with the PI values being lowest during the early morning hours and increasing towards the evening[49]. To obtain consistent and comparable data it is, therefore, important to allow patients to remain in a recumbent position and to perform investigations on all patients at approximately the same time of the day.

Although blood flow impedance on the day of embryo transfer may be able to predict pregnancy, it would be more useful to detect flow abnormalities earlier in the cycle. To investigate this we recently measured uterine artery PI in 135 women undergoing IVF on the day of hCG injection[50]. We found significantly diminished implantation rates in women with uterine artery PI > 3.0. The ability to predict implantation before the administration of hCG allows the clinician the option to delay giving hCG until uterine artery PI improves. An alternative approach would be to try to improve uterine perfusion by the administration of glyceryl trinitrate (GTN). In a preliminary study Cacciatore and colleagues reported, in a group of patients with increased uterine artery PI, a 20% increase in uterine blood flow following the administration of GTN throughout the normal menstrual cycle[51]. It has been suggested that the administration of GTN may increase pregnancy rates in women with poor uterine perfusion. However, no randomized studies have been performed to address this issue.

In a study investigating intrauterine circulation, Achiron and colleagues[36] defined subendometrial flow as a pulsatile flow detected within 10 mm of the endometrial surface (Figure 6). In their study, these authors investigated subendometrial flow in 18 patients with premature ovarian failure (POF) and 12 healthy women. They observed decreased vascular impedance in the late follicular phase with a gradual increase during the early and late luteal phases in both groups of patients. In the patients with POF, they observed a significantly higher vascular resistance in the early follicular phase. This difference disappeared after administration of hormone replacement therapy. These authors concluded that hormone replacement therapy enables normalization of subendometrial blood flow, and creates a vascular status that is compatible with

pregnancy. Moreover, increased subendometrial blood flow resistance could be a sign of diminished implantation potential.

SPECIFIC CHARACTERISTICS OF DIFFERENT PATIENT GROUPS REQUIRING OOCYTE DONATION

Initially intended for young women with premature ovarian failure[1,5,52] or heritable genetic defects[1,53], this technique has more recently been applied to menopausal women[54–56], women who have a history of unsuccessful IVF treatments[1,56,57], and women with a history of recurrent miscarriages[58]. Here we will examine the differences between these groups of patients, and offer some suggestions regarding their preparation for oocyte donation treatment cycles.

Older patients (> 40 years)

Oocyte donation provides a unique model in which the contribution of uterine and embryo factors can be separated. In animal studies it has been shown that the decline in fecundity is at least partly due to age-related morphological and physiological changes of the uterus[59,60]. In humans the role of uterine aging is less clear. To investigate the effect of aging on the uterus, Sauer and colleagues[61] studied 122 functionally agonadal women, aged 25 to 60 years, during a hormone replacement cycle leading to oocyte donation. Ultrasound scans and endometrial biopsies performed on day 21 of the cycle in this group of patients showed no age-related difference in either ultrasonic appearance, endometrial histology or the presence of estrogen or progesterone receptors. In a separate study, Guanes and colleagues[62] investigated the age-related difference in uterine response to early pregnancy. They longitudinally followed 21 patients who achieved a singleton pregnancy following oocyte donation and found no difference in either hormonal levels or uterine blood vessel resistance between younger and older patients. These data suggest that the increase in miscarriage rate seen in older patients is not due to decreased uterine perfusion. The best model to assess the effect of age on uterine receptivity is to share oocytes from the same donor between recipients of different ages. This study model was used in two prospective[63,64] and two retrospective[65,66] analyses. In a prospective study, Navot and colleagues[63] found no difference in either the pregnancy rate or the pregnancy loss rate between younger and older patients. In a similar study, however, Cano and colleagues[64] observed significantly higher pregnancy loss rates in a group of older patients. They concluded that the mechanisms for placental formation are age-related. In a retrospective study, Borini and colleagues[65] found reduced pregnancy rates in patients over the age of 40 years. In another retrospective study, Abdalla and colleagues[66] compared pairs of patients separated by at least 5 years of age receiving oocytes from the same donors. Cycles where similar fertilization rates and similar numbers and quality of embryos were replaced were included in the analysis. The findings suggested no difference in implantation, pregnancy, miscarriage or livebirth rates between younger and older patients. Finally, Meldrum[19] recently reported a marked decrease in the livebirth rate in women above age 40 years. However, when the luteal progesterone dosage was increased from 50 to 100 mg/day, recipients older than 40 years of age had a marked increase in pregnancy rate when compared to younger patients.

From the above, it appears to be clear that unlike the quality of oocytes which declines with age, endometrial receptivity remains constant, perhaps compromised only marginally by retardation of steroid synthesis. In practice, oocyte donation using oocytes from young donors, and possibly using hormonal preparations with an increased dosage of progesterone, is likely to result in high pregnancy rates in older patients.

Patients with chromosomal abnormalities

Turner's syndrome

Another group of patients requiring oocyte donation are women with Turner's syndrome.

This syndrome is characterized by the complete or partial absence of one of the X chromosomes that results in multiple somatic abnormalities and ovarian dysgenesis[67]. The majority of women with this condition have streak ovaries with the absence of any follicular structure. Therefore, for most Turner's syndrome patients, the only possibility of achieving pregnancy is through oocyte donation. In the literature there are many sporadic reports of pregnancy in Turner's syndrome patients following oocyte donation[1,68]. From these reports it is unclear whether differences exist in achieving pregnancy in Turner's syndrome patients when compared with other patients requiring oocyte donation. It is also unclear whether these women require a different hormonal preparation to achieve satisfactory endometrial preparation. Li and colleagues[69] suggested that the endometria of women with Turner's syndrome respond suboptimally to steroid hormonal preparation. They hypothesized that this may be related to a reduced concentration of steroid hormone receptors. Rogers and colleagues[70] reported a series of six patients with Turner's syndrome who received hormone replacement therapy. Eleven endometrial biopsies were obtained from these patients prior to oocyte donation treatment, and were assessed by electron microscopy using a freeze-fracture technique. Nine of the 11 biopsies had no discernible tight junctions; the other two biopsies had reduced and disorganized junctional structures. Recently Biljan and associates have investigated the effect of a standard hormone regimen on endometrial preparation and levels of serum hormonal markers of implantation[71]. In this study the authors compared five Turner's syndrome patients with two comparable groups of patients, women with idiopathic premature ovarian failure (POF) and women who had surgical castration. The Turner's syndrome patients, when exposed to the same doses of estrogen and progesterone, had significantly higher uterine artery resistance, thinner endometrium and lower levels of placental protein 14 in the serum. In a separate study[72] the same authors investigated the

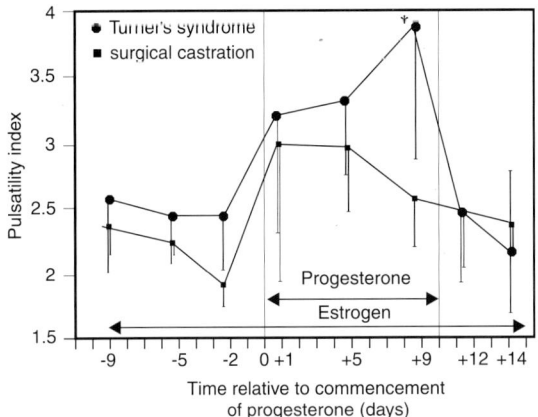

Figure 9 Increased impedence in uterine arteries of Turner's syndrome patients when compared with other patients with premature ovarian failure due to surgical removal of ovaries. [*]$p < 0.05$. From reference 71 with permission

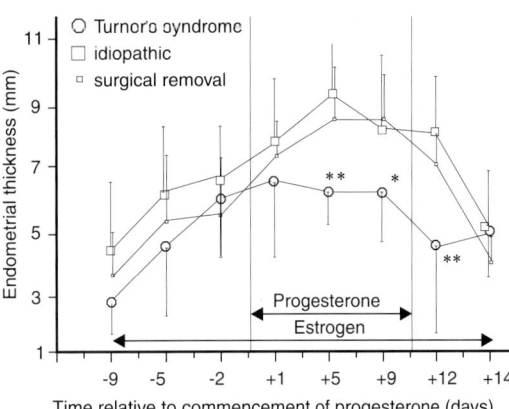

Figure 10 Thinner endometrium in Turner's syndrome patients when compared with other patients with premature ovarian failure. [*]$p < 0.05$; [**]$p < 0.01$. From reference 72, with permission

difference in uterine impedance between Turner's syndrome patients and other patients with POF exposed to the same hormonal replacement therapy regimen and found significantly increased resistance and thinner endometrium in Turner's syndrome patients (Figures 9 and 10). On the basis of these results the authors concluded that Turner's syndrome patients might need a different hormonal preparation in order to achieve the same pregnancy rates. Following this study, Press and colleagues[73] compared 11 Turner's syndrome patients and 38 patients with normal karyotype undergoing 91 cycles of oocyte donation. Although the pregnancy rates in the two groups were comparable, the Turner's syndrome patients required higher doses of estrogen to achieve the same endometrial thickness. Moreover, the Turner's syndrome patients had higher miscarriage rates. Subsequently, Yaron and colleagues[74] investigated seven Turner's syndrome patients and 15 controls in an oocyte donation program, and found significantly lower pregnancy and higher miscarriage rates in the Turner's syndrome patients. Finally, Khastgir and colleagues[75] retrospectively analyzed a group of 29 Turner's syndrome patients who had 68 cycles of oocyte donation. They also found that Turner's syndrome patients required

higher doses of estrogen to achieve the same endometrial thickness. Moreover, significantly lower pregnancy rates were recorded in patients who were exposed to standard rather than higher levels of estrogen prior to embryo transfer. Interestingly, although the pregnancy rate in this series was 41.2%, the birth rate was only 19.1%. High miscarriage rates reported in all of the above studies could be explained by previously reported hormonal and endometrial deficiencies.

Turner's syndrome patients have an altered response to estrogen and require higher doses of estrogen to achieve the levels of vascular and endometrial preparation required to achieve and maintain pregnancy. In Turner's syndrome patients we always perform a mock cycle, where patients are given increasing doses of estrogen until satisfactory endometrial thickness and vascularization are achieved. Thereafter, this dose is given in the oocyte donation treatment cycle.

Other chromosomal abnormalities

Endometrial response in other genetic diseases is not clear. Although successful pregnancies have been achieved in pure gonadal dysgenesis with 46,XY patients (Swyer's syndrome)[76], XXX syndrome[1], Blackfan–Diamond syndrome[77] and Noonan syndrome[1], there is insufficient evidence regarding the specific response in any of these conditions to hormonal stimulation with estrogen. However, in all these cases, prior to the actual treatment cycle, as in Turner's syndrome patients, we perform a mock cycle to assess the individual response to medication.

Patients developing premature ovarian failure following chemotherapy or radiotherapy

The disease-free period following aggressive cancer chemotherapy or radiotherapy has increased dramatically in the last few years. Unfortunately, this type of treatment frequently leads to permanent damage to ovarian function. Although several reports of the spontaneous return of ovarian function[78,79] or the re-initiation of ovarian function by the administration of high doses of human gonadotropins[80] have been published, the only realistic hope for this group of patients to achieve a pregnancy is through oocyte donation. To date, however, there exist no data on either endometrial responsiveness to hormone replacement treatment or vascular resistance in this group of patients. Sporadic clinical data pertaining to these patients undergoing oocyte donation, however, suggests severe endometrial incompetence[1,53]. In a retrospective study, Pados and colleagues[1] reported no clinical pregnancies in 25 patients with a history of POF due to either chemo- or radiotherapy. The authors concluded that antineoplastic treatment has a detrimental and destructive effect on the fine structure of the endometrium, resulting in a low likelihood of implantation. These conclusions, however, have not been confirmed in any histological or ultrasound studies. It would, therefore, be of considerable interest to investigate the features of endometrial response in these patients, as well as to explore the types of hormone replacement treatment which might improve implantation potential.

SUMMARY

Pregnancy and delivery rates for oocyte donation are higher than for any other assisted conception technique. A simplified, fixed endometrial preparation appears to yield similar endometrial quality and pregnancy rates when compared to more elaborate regimens where the dose of estrogen is gradually increased. Older patients, patients with premature ovarian failure following chemotherapy, and Turner's syndrome patients, however, may require different endometrial preparation to achieve the same pregnancy rate. Implantation rates following oocyte donation are still relatively low. Measurements of the minimal endometrial thickness and endometrial appearance, as well as the assessment of uterine artery and subendometrial blood flow impedance can successfully identify patients with low implantation potential. More research is required to find methods of improving the implantation rates in these patients.

References

1. Pados, G., Camus, M., van Waesberghe, L., Liebaers, I., van Steirteghem, A. and Devroey, P. (1992). Oocyte and embryo donation: evaluation of 412 consecutive trials. *Hum. Reprod.*, **7**, 1111–17
2. Younis, J. S., Simon, A. and Laufer, N. (1996). Endometrial preparation: lessons from oocyte donation [Review]. *Fertil. Steril.*, **66**, 873–84
3. Medical Research International and the Society for Assisted Reproductive Technology (1997). *In vitro* fertilization and embryo transfer (IVF–ET) in the United States; 1990 results from the IVF–ET registry. *Fertil. Steril.*, **57**, 15–24
4. Remohi, J., Gartner, B., Gallardo, E., Yalil, S., Simon, C. and Pellicer, A. (1997). Pregnancy and birth rates after oocyte donation. *Fertil. Steril.*, **67**, 717–23
5. Lutjen, P., Trounson, A., Leeton, J., Findlay, J., Wood, C. and Renou, P. (1984). The establishment and maintenance of pregnancy using

in vitro fertilization and embryo donation in a patient with primary ovarian failure. *Nature (London)*, **307**, 174–5

6. Serhal, P. F. and Craft, I. L. (1987). Ovum donation – a simplified approach. *Fertil. Steril.*, **48**, 265–9

7. Navot, D., Anderson, T. L., Droesch, K., Scott, R. T., Kreiner, D. and Rosenwaks, Z. (1989). Hormonal manipulation of endometrial maturation. *J. Clin. Endocrinol. Metab.*, **68**, 801–7

8. Younis, J. S., Mordel, N., Ligovetzky, G., Lewin, A., Schenker, J. G. and Laufer, N. (1991). The effect of a prolonged artificial follicular phase on endometrial development in an oocyte donation program. *J. In Vitro Fertil. Embryo Transfer*, **8**, 84–8

9. Younis, J. S., Mordel, N., Lewin, A., Simon, A., Schenker, J. G. and Laufer, N. (1992). Artificial endometrial preparation for oocyte donation: the effect of estrogen stimulation on clinical outcome. *J. Assisted Reprod. Genet.*, **9**, 222–7

10. Navot, D., Bergh, P. A., Williams, M., Garrisi, G. J., Guzman, I., Sandler, B., Fox, J., Schreiner-Engel, P., Hofmann, G. E. and Grunfeld, L. (1991). An insight into early reproductive processes through the *in vivo* model of ovum donation. *J. Clin. Endocrinol. Metab.*, **72**, 408–14

11. Shapiro, H., Cowell, C. and Casper, R. F. (1993). The use of vaginal ultrasound for monitoring endometrial preparation in a donor oocyte program. *Fertil. Steril.*, **59**, 1055–8

12. Finn, C. A. (1977). The implantation reaction. In Wynn, R. M. (ed.) *Biology of the Uterus*, pp. 245–308 (New York: Plenum Press)

13. de Ziegler, D., Bergeron, C., Cornel, C., Medalie, D. A., Massai, M. R. and Milgrom, E. (1992). Effects of luteal estradiol on the secretory transformation of human endometrium and plasma gonadotropins. *J. Clin. Endocrinol. Metab.*, **74**, 522–31

14. Navot, D., Laufer, N., Kopolovic, J., Rabinowitz, R., Birkenfeld, A., Lewin, A., Granat, M., Margalioth, E. J. and Schenker, J. G. (1986). Artificially induced endometrial cycles and establishment of pregnancies in the absence of ovaries. *N. Engl. J. Med.*, **314**, 806–11

15. Paulson, R. J., Hatch, I. E., Lobo, R. A. and Sauer, M. V. (1997). Cumulative conception and livebirth rates after oocyte donation: implications regarding endometrial receptivity. *Hum. Reprod.*, **12**, 835–9

16. Lutjen, P. J., Findlay, J. K., Trounson, A. O., Leeton, J. F. and Chan, L. K. (1986). Effect on plasma gonadotropins of cyclic steroid replacement in women with premature ovarian failure. *J. Clin. Endocrinol. Metab.*, **62**, 419–23

17. Brooks, A. A., Johnson, M. R., Pawson, M. E., Thomas, A., Phelan, L. K. and Abdalla, H. I.

(1996). Endometrial thickness: individual and mean growth profiles for different hormone replacement regimens. *Hum. Reprod.*, **11**, 2724–31

18. Kogosowski, A., Yovel, I., Lessing, J. B., Amit, A., Barak, Y., David, M. P. and Peyser, R. (1990). The establishment of an ovum donation program using a simple fixed-dose estrogen-progesterone replacement regimen. *J. In Vitro Fertil. Embryo Transfer*, **7**, 244–8

19. Meldrum, D. R. (1993). Female reproductive aging – ovarian and uterine factors [Review]. *Fertil. Steril.*, **59**, 1–5

20. Yaron, Y., Amit, A., Kogosowski, A., Peyser, M. R., David, M. P. and Lessing, J. B. (1997). The optimal number of embryos to be transferred in shared oocyte donation: walking the thin line between low pregnancy rates and multiple pregnancies. *Hum. Reprod.*, **12**, 699–702

21. Wolff, K. M., McMahon, M. J., Kuller, J. A., Walmer, D. K. and Meyer, W. R. (1997). Advanced maternal age and perinatal outcome: oocyte recipiency versus natural conception. *Obstet. Gynecol.*, **89**, 519–23

22. Sauer, M. V., Paulson, R. J. and Lobo, R. A. (1996). Oocyte donation to women of advanced reproductive age: pregnancy results and obstetrical outcomes in patients 45 years and older. *Hum. Reprod.*, **11**, 2540–3

23. Michalas, S., Loutradis, D., Drakakis, P., Milingos, S., Papageorgiou, J., Kallianidis, K., Koumantakis, E. and Aravantinos, D. (1996). Oocyte donation to women over 40 years of age: pregnancy complications. *Eur. J. Obstet. Gynecol. Reprod. Biol.*, **64**, 175–8

24. Antinori, S., Versaci, C., Panci, C., Caffa, B. and Gholami, G. H. (1995). Fetal and maternal morbidity and mortality in menopausal women aged 45–63 years. *Hum. Reprod.*, **10**, 464–9

25. Huhtala, M., Seppala, M., Julkenen, M. and Kolstein, R. (1992). Characteristics, biological action and clinical studies of endometrial proteins. In Grudzinkas, G. and Chard, T. (eds.) *Implantation*. (London: Springer-Verlag)

26. Sauer, M. V., Paulson, R. J. and Moyer, D. L. (1997). Assessing the importance of endometrial biopsy prior to oocyte donation. *J. Assisted Reprod. Genet.*, **14**, 125–7

27. Gonen, Y., Casper, R. F., Jacobson, W. and Blankier, J. (1989). Endometrial thickness and growth during ovarian stimulation: a possible predictor of implantation in *in vitro* fertilization. *Fertil. Steril.*, **52**, 446–50

28. Glissant, A., de Mouzon, J. and Frydman, R. (1985). Ultrasound study of the endometrium during *in vitro* fertilization cycles. *Fertil. Steril.*, **44**, 786–90

29. Fleischer, A. C., Herbert, C. M., Hill, G. A., Kepple, D. M. and Worrell, J. A. (1991).

Transvaginal sonography of the endometrium during induced cycles. *Ultrasound Med.*, **10**, 93–5

30. Welker, B. G., Gembruch, U., Diedrich, K., al-Hasani, S. and Krebs, D. (1989). Transvaginal sonography of the endometrium during ovum pick-up in stimulated cycles for *in vitro* fertilization. *J. Ultrasound Med.*, **8**, 549–53

31. Imoedemhe, D. A., Shaw, R. W., Kirkland, A. and Chan, R. (1987). Ultrasound measurement of endometrial thickness on different ovarian stimulation regimens during *in vitro* fertilization. *Hum. Reprod.*, **2**, 545–7

32. Abdalla, H. I., Brooks, A. A., Johnson, M. R., Kirkland, A., Thomas, A. and Studd, J. W. (1994). Endometrial thickness: a predictor of implantation in ovum recipients? *Hum. Reprod.*, **9**, 363–5

33. Gonen, Y. and Casper, R. F. (1990). Prediction of implantation by the sonographic appearance of the endometrium during controlled ovarian stimulation for *in vitro* fertilization (IVF). *J. In Vitro Fertil. Embryo Transfer*, **7**, 146–52

34. Smith, B., Porter, R., Ahuja, K. and Craft, I. (1984). Ultrasonic assessment of endometrial changes in stimulated cycles in an *in vitro* fertilization and embryo transfer program. *J. In Vitro Fertil. Embryo Transfer*, **1**, 233–8

35. Steer, C. V., Williams, J., Zaidi, J., Campbell, S. and Tan, S. L. (1995). Intra-observer, inter-observer, inter-ultrasound transducer and intercycle variation in color Doppler assessment of uterine artery impedance. *Hum. Reprod.*, **10**, 479–81

36. Achiron, R., Levran, D., Sivan, E., Lipitz, S., Dor, J. and Mashiach, S. (1995). Endometrial blood flow response to hormone replacement therapy in women with premature ovarian failure: a transvaginal Doppler study. *Fertil. Steril.*, **63**, 550–4

37. Tan, S. L., Zaidi, J., Campbell, S., Doyle, P. and Collins, W. (1996). Blood flow changes in the ovarian and uterine arteries during the normal menstrual cycle. *Am. J. Obstet. Gynecol.*, **175**, 625–31

38. Taylor, K. J., Burns, P. N., Wells, P. N., Conway, D. I. and Hull, M. G. (1985). Ultrasound Doppler flow studies of the ovarian and uterine arteries. *Br. J. Obstet. Gynaecol.*, **92**, 240–6

39. Feichtinger, W., Putz, M. and Kemeter, P. (1988). Transvaginale Doppler-sonographie zur Blutflussmessung in kleinen becken. *Ultraschall Med.*, **9**, 30–4

40. Goswamy, R. K. and Steptoe, P. C. (1988). Doppler ultrasound studies of the uterine artery in spontaneous ovarian cycles. *Hum. Reprod.*, **3**, 721–6

41. Sterzik, K., Grab, D., Sasse, V., Hutter, W., Rosenbusch, B. and Terinde, R. (1989).

Doppler sonographic findings and their correlation with implantation in an *in vitro* fertilization program. *Fertil. Steril.*, **52**, 825–8

42. Steer, C. V., Campbell, S., Pampiglione, J. S., Kingsland, C. R., Mason, B. A. and Collins, W. P. (1990). Transvaginal color flow imaging of the uterine arteries during the ovarian and menstrual cycles. *Hum. Reprod.*, **5**, 391–5

43. Steer, C. V., Tan, S.L., Mason, B. A. and Campbell, S. (1994). Midluteal-phase vaginal color Doppler assessment of uterine artery impedance in a subfertile population. *Fertil. Steril.*, **61**, 53–8

44. Steer, C. V., Campbell, S., Tan, S. L., Crayford, T., Mills, C., Mason, B. A. and Collins, W. P. (1992). The use of transvaginal color flow imaging after *in vitro* fertilization to identify optimum uterine conditions before embryo transfer. *Fertil. Steril.*, **57**, 372–6

45. Steer, C. V., Tan, S. L., Dillon, D., Mason, B. A. and Campbell, S. (1995). Vaginal color Doppler assessment of uterine artery impedance correlates with immunohistochemical markers of endometrial receptivity required for the implantation of an embryo. *Fertil. Steril.*, **63**, 101–8

46. Coulam, C. B., Bustillo, M., Soenksen, D. M. and Britten, S. (1994). Ultrasonographic predictors of implantation after assisted reproduction. *Fertil. Steril.*, **62**, 1004–10

47. Tekay, A., Martikainen, H. and Jouppila, P. (1995). Blood flow changes in uterine and ovarian vasculature, and predictive value of transvaginal pulsed color Doppler ultrasonography in an *in vitro* fertilization program. *Hum. Reprod.*, **10**, 688–93

48. Dickey, R. P., Hower, J. F., Matulich, E. M. and Brown, G. T. (1994). Effect of standing on nonpregnant uterine flow. *Ultrasound Obstet. Gynecol.*, **4**, 480–7

49. Zaidi, J., Jurkovic, D., Campbell, S., Pittrof, R., McGregor, A. and Tan, S. L. (1995). Description of circadian rhythm in uterine artery blood flow during the peri-ovulatory period. *Hum. Reprod.*, **10**, 1642–6

50. Zaidi, J., Pittrof, R., Shaker, A., Kyei-Mensah, A., Campbell, S. and Tan, S. L. (1996). Assessment of uterine artery blood flow on the day of human chorionic gonadotropin administration by transvaginal color Doppler ultrasound in an *in vitro* fertilization program. *Fertil. Steril.*, **65**, 377–81

51. Cacciatore, B., Tiitinen, A. and Ylikorkala, O. (1996). Is it possible to improve uterine blood flow in infertile women? [Abstract]. *Ultrasound Obstet. Gynecol.*, **8**(Suppl. 1), 204

52. Barri, P. N., Coroleu, B., Martinez, F., Parera, N., Veiga, A., Calderon, G., Boada, M. and Belil, I. (1992). Indications for oocyte donation. *Hum. Reprod.*, **7**(Suppl. 1), 85–8

53. Sauer, M. V., Paulson, R. J., Ary, B. A. and Lobo, R. A. (1994). Three-hundred cycles of oocyte donation at the University of Southern California: assessing the effect of age and infertility diagnosis on pregnancy and implantation rates. *J. Assisted Reprod. Genet.*, **11**, 92–6

54. Sauer, M. V., Paulson, R. J. and Lobo, R. A. (1990). A preliminary report on oocyte donation extending reproductive potential to women over 40. *N. Engl. J. Med.*, **323**, 1157–60

55. Serhal, P. F. and Craft, I. L. (1989). Oocyte donation in 61 patients. *Lancet*, **1**, 1185–7

56. Sauer, M. V., Paulson, R. J. and Lobo, R. A. (1992). Reversing the natural decline in human fertility. An extended clinical trial of oocyte donation to women of advanced reproductive age. *J. Am. Med. Assoc.*, **268**, 1275–9 [erratum appears in *J. Am. Med. Assoc.*, **269**, 476]

57. Burton, G., Abdalla, H. I., Kirkland, A. and Studd, J. W. (1992). The role of oocyte donation in women who are unsuccessful with *in vitro* fertilization treatment. *Hum. Reprod.*, **7**, 1103–5

58. Remohi, J., Gallardo, E., Levy, M., Valbuena, D., de los Santos, M. J., Simon, C. and Pellicer, A. (1996). Oocyte donation in women with recurrent pregnancy loss. *Hum. Reprod.*, **11**, 2048–51

59. Harman, S. M. and Talbert, G. B. (1974). Effect of maternal age on synchronization of ovulation and mating and on tubal transport of ova in mice. *J. Gerontol.*, **29**, 493–8

60. Adams, C. E. (1975). Effects of maternal age on ovulation, fertilization and embryonic development. In Blandau, R. J. (ed.) *Aging Gametes*, pp. 231–48. (Basel: Kerger)

61. Sauer, M. V., Miles, R. A., Dahmoush, L., Paulson, R. J., Press, M. and Moyer, D. (1993). Evaluating the effect of age on endometrial responsiveness to hormone replacement therapy: a histologic, ultrasonographic and tissue receptor analysis. *J. Assisted Reprod. Genet.*, **10**, 47–52

62. Guanes, P. P., Remohi, J., Gallardo, E., Valbuena, D., Simon, C. and Pellicer, A. (1996). Age does not affect uterine resistance to vascular flow in patients undergoing oocyte donation. *Fertil. Steril.*, **66**, 265–70

63. Navot, D., Drews, M. R., Bergh, P. A., Guzman, I., Karstaedt, A., Scott, R. T. Jr, Garrisi, G. J. and Hofmann, G. E. (1994). Age-related decline in female fertility is not due to diminished capacity of the uterus to sustain embryo implantation. *Fertil. Steril.*, **61**, 97–101

64. Cano, F., Simon, C., Remohi, J. and Pellicer, A. (1995). Effect of aging on the female reproductive system: evidence for a role of uterine senescence in the decline in female fecundity. *Fertil. Steril.*, **64**, 584–9

65. Borini, A., Bianchi, L., Violini, F., Maccolini, A., Cattoli, M. and Flamigni, C. (1996). Oocyte donation program: pregnancy and implantation rates in women of different ages sharing oocytes from a single donor. *Fertil. Steril.*, **65**, 94–7

66. Abdalla, H. I., Wren, M. E., Thomas, A. and Korea, L. (1997). Age of the uterus does not affect pregnancy or implantation rates; a study of egg donation in women of different ages sharing oocytes from the same donor. *Hum. Reprod.*, **12**, 827–9

67. Turner, H. H. (1938). A syndrome of infantilism, congenital webbed neck, and cubitus valgus. *Endocrinology*, **23**, 566–74

68. Abdalla, H. I., Baber, R., Kirkland, A., Leonard, T., Power, M. and Studd, J. W. (1990). A report on 100 cycles of oocyte donation; factors affecting the outcome. *Hum. Reprod.*, **5**, 1018–22

69. Li, T. C., Dockery, P., Ramsewak, S. S., Klentzeris, L., Lenton, E. A. and Cooke, I. D. (1991). The variation of endometrial response to a standard hormone replacement therapy in women with premature ovarian failure. An ultrasonographic and histological study. *Br. J. Obstet. Gynaecol.*, **98**, 656–61

70. Rogers, P. A., Murphy, C. R., Leeton, J., Hoise, M. J. and Beaton, L. (1992). Turner's syndrome patients lack tight junctions between uterine epithelial cells. *Hum. Reprod.*, **7**, 883–5

71. Biljan, M. M., Taylor, C. T., Matijevic, R., Jones, S. V., Fraser, W. D., Diver, M. J. and Kingsland, C. R. (1995). The differences in endometrial and vascular response to standard hormone replacement treatment between Turner's syndrome patients who had surgical castration and patients with primary ovarian failure [Abstract]. *Hum. Reprod.*, **10**, FC16

72. Biljan, M. M., Taylor, C. T., Matijevic, R., Jones, S. V., Garden, A. S., Fraser, W. D., Diver, M. J. and Kingsland, C. R. (1995). Exaggerated effects of progestogen on uterine artery pulsatility index in Turner's syndrome patients receiving hormone replacement therapy. *Fertil. Steril.*, **64**, 1104–8

73. Press, F., Shapiro, H. M., Cowell, C. A. and Oliver, G. D. (1995). Outcome of ovum donation in Turner's syndrome patients. *Fertil. Steril.*, **64**, 995–8

74. Yaron, Y., Ochshorn, Y., Amit, A., Yovel, I., Kogosowki, A. and Lessing, J. B. (1996). Patients with Turner's syndrome may have an inherent endometrial abnormality affecting receptivity in oocyte donation. *Fertil. Steril.*, **65**, 1249–52

75. Khastgir, G., Abdalla, H., Thomas, A., Korea, L., Latarche, L. and Studd, J. (1997). Oocyte donation in Turner's syndrome: an analysis of the factors affecting the outcome. *Hum. Reprod.*, **12**, 279–85

76. Bianco, S., Agrifoglio, V., Mannino, F., Cefalu, E. and Cittadini, E. (1992). Successful

pregnancy in a pure gonadal dysgenesis with karyotype 46,XY patient (Swyer's syndrome) following oocyte donation and hormonal treatment. *Acta Eur. Fertil.*, **23**, 37–8

77. Aird, I. A., Biljan, M. M., Stevenson, P. and Kingsland, C. R. (1996). Successful pregnancy following oocyte donation in a patient with Diamond–Blackfan syndrome and premature ovarian failure. *Hum. Reprod.*, **11**, 1123–5

78. Hague, W. M., Tan, S. L., Adams, J. and Jacobs, H. S. (1987). Hypergonadotropic amenorrhea – etiology and outcome in 93 young women. *Int. J. Gynaecol. Obstet.*, **25**, 121–5

79. Nasir, J., Walton, C., Lindow, S. W. and Masson, E. A. (1997). Spontaneous recovery of chemotherapy-induced primary ovarian failure: implications for management. *Clin. Endocrinol.*, **46**, 217–19

80. Chatterjee, R., Mills, W., Katz, M., McGarrigle, H. H. and Goldstone, A. H. (1993). Induction of ovarian function by using short-term human menopausal gonadotrophin in patients with ovarian failure following cytotoxic chemotherapy for haematological malignancy. *Leuk. Lymphoma*, **10**, 383–6

Combined Doppler and hormonal studies of uterine receptivity

17

D. de Ziegler, N. de Quay and R. Fanchin

INTRODUCTION

The functional assessment of the uterine vasculature with transvaginal pulsed and color Doppler has offered the prospect of determining the quality of endometrial receptivity. Because of their non-invasive nature, pulsed and color Doppler can be performed during the actual *in vitro* fertilization (IVF) cycle, and particularly before deciding whether to transfer the embryos. Some paradoxes exist, however, between Doppler data published in different fields of gynecology. In women whose ovaries are inactive, the effects of estrogen have been universally recognized as vasodilative. It can therefore be seen as paradoxical that a sizeable fraction of women who undergo IVF and whose estradiol levels are very high have nonetheless high uterine artery resistance values. Hence, it is important to study the physiopathology of the vascular effects induced by controlled ovarian hyperstimulation (COH) in order to understand and take full benefit of the results obtained.

EFFECTS OF ESTRADIOL

In the egg donation model, Navot and colleagues[1] established that the duration of the estradiol priming phase normally occurring during the follicular phase of the menstrual cycle could be as short as 5 days without impacting on endometrial receptivity. In the model, 5 days of exposure to estradiol only sufficed for priming an adequate endometrial proliferation and induction of progesterone receptors. More importantly, these authors also showed that such a short follicular phase nonetheless permitted the establishment of pregnancy. However, they also noticed that in the subgroup of women whose donor egg cycle included a 'short' estradiol-only phase of 5–10 days, an unexpectedly high miscarriage rate was observed, although no causal relationship could be established. It appears, therefore, that a consensus now exists to support the concept that estradiol exerts a 'permissive' rather than a 'controlling' role for the priming of endometrial receptivity[2–4]. In a recent study in the egg donation model, Remohí and associates[5] observed a positive correlation ($p < 0.004$) between endometrial thickness on the day of oocyte retrieval and implantation rates, although it only explained 5% of the variance ($r^2 = 0.05$). There were, however, no correlations between serum estradiol levels and implantation rates. The impact of estradiol on endometrial thickness is a complex one which involves exogenous factors in which are combined both the amount of estradiol and the duration of exposure, as well as an array of as yet unclarified endogenous factors (growth factors, weight, etc.). Moreover, as alluded to later in this chapter, other ovarian factors such as androgens are likely to be instrumental in the endometrial effects described in COH.

In the absence of estrogen, Doppler studies of uterine arteries have shown elevated resistance scores as expressed by high pulsatility index (PI) data. In women deprived of ovarian function, whether during reproductive age as a result of premature ovarian failure (POF)[6] or after having reached the normal age of menopause[7], there is now a consensus that PI is uniformly high in the absence of other local factors such as hyperplasia and/or cancer. Indeed, despite numerous controversies over the vascular status of uterine arteries in various other physiological conditions, all recent Doppler data have linked the estrogen-deprived state with high uterine artery resistance, making this a finding that has never been challenged (Figure 1). Similarly, it has been clearly established, and also not challenged, that in women whose ovaries are absent or inactive, minimal amounts of exogenous estradiol, such as are administered for bone-sparing objectives in menopausal women, suffice to induce a prompt, profound and persistent drop in uterine artery PI values[6,7] (Figure 2). From this early work, it had been concluded that the doses of estradiol that induce a complete correction of the post-menopausal increase in bone loss also exert maximal vasodilation properties on uterine arteries as expressed by PI values < 2.5. Optimistic conclusions have been drawn from this early work, suggesting that even minimal amounts of estradiol, clearly less than the quantities produced by the ovaries during COH for IVF or even during the menstrual cycle, have nearly maximal vasodilative effects on the uterine arterial system.

In a distinct trial, we looked at the effects of endogenous estradiol and compared our results to historical data obtained with exogenous estradiol. We studied over 100 women undergoing menopausal changes at a physiological age. Participants were women of 42 to 58 years of age who attended a private menopause clinic. All underwent a pelvic ultrasound scan with uterine artery Doppler assessment on cycle days 2 to 4 when still cycling, or randomly otherwise. None of these women had received hormonal treatments in the past 6 months. Uterine artery Doppler evaluations showed an inverse correlation between estradiol levels and PI data when estradiol levels were ⩽ 60 pg/ml (Figure 3). Conversely, when estradiol levels were > 60 pg/ml, PI values were low but no correlation was found between estradiol levels and PI results. This again was taken as reflecting that maximal vasodilation of the uterine arterial system is achieved with early follicular phase levels of estradiol. Therefore, similar results are found when estrogen is of endogenous or

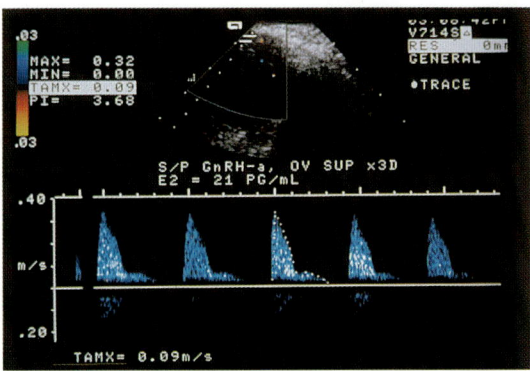

Figure 1 Uterine artery Doppler investigation of estrogen deprivation. In the estrogen-deprived state, uterine artery Doppler shows high resistance flow waves characterized by minimal to no diastolic flow. Computation of the pulsatility index shows a high value, typically > 3

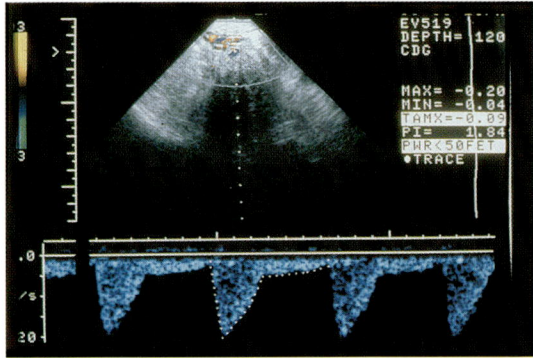

Figure 2 Uterine artery Doppler investigation of the effects of exogenous estradiol. In women whose ovaries are absent or inactive, exogenous estradiol induces a prompt, profound and persistent decrease in uterine artery resistance characterized by a widening of the flow wave and the presence of uninterrupted diastolic flow

exogenous source. Conversely, higher estradiol levels (such as encountered in the preovulatory phase or in COH for IVF) are of no apparent consequence for uterine artery PI.

The permanence of the vasodilative effects of estradiol after menopause has been questioned. Studying uterine artery flow in untreated menopausal women, Bourne and colleagues observed an inverse correlation between baseline uterine artery PI values and the time since menopause[7]. In our study in prematurely menopausal women[6] we observed very high baseline uterine artery PI values.

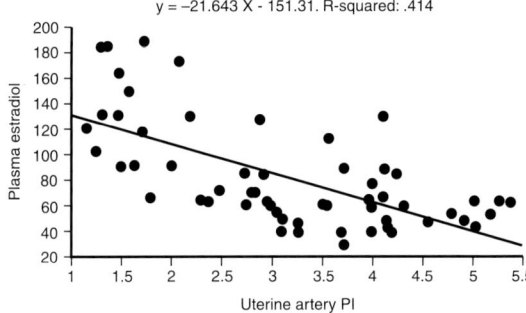

$y = -21.643 X - 151.31.$ R-squared: .414

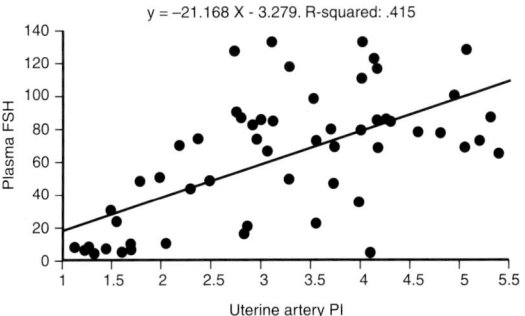

$y = -21.168 X - 3.279.$ R-squared: .415

Figure 3 Uterine artery Doppler investigation of the effects of endogenous estradiol. In women undergoing menopausal changes, an inverse correlation was found between the plasma estradiol level and the uterine artery pulsatility index (PI) when estradiol levels are < 200 pmol/l

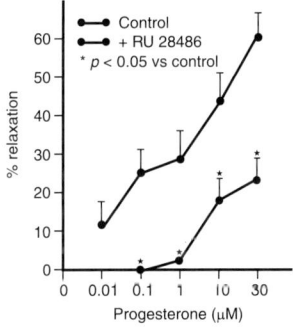

Figure 4 The vascular effects of progesterone. Progesterone induces relaxation of human placental arteries and veins, a phenomenon partially antagonized by the antiprogestin RU-486. From reference 9, with permission

This was in agreement with the observations of Bourne and colleagues, as all our patients had a long interval since menopause. However, our patients were remarkable in that they all had been off estradiol therapy for only a short time (6 weeks). Hence, a paradox exists between the persistence of some vasodilation after menopause but not after exogenous estradiol treatment. This was taken as indicating that the moderately increased PI values observed in newly menopausal women reflect some degree of persistent estrogen production during the first years after menopause rather than a remnant effect of estradiol on vessels.

EFFECTS OF PROGESTERONE AND SYNTHETIC PROGESTINS

Because progesterone antagonizes the proliferative effects exerted by estradiol on endometrial glands and stroma, it has been feared that similar dualistic relationships governed all estradiol–progesterone interactions[8]. Along these lines, it has been postulated that progesterone, or its often used surrogates in hormone replacement therapy, the synthetic progestins, may antagonize the vasodilative properties of estradiol. An original paper by Omar and colleagues[9], however, showed that in an *in vitro* model progesterone induces a vasodilation of human placental arteries and veins (Figure 4). This phenomenon has been linked to relaxing effects exerted by progesterone on smooth muscles, including in organs other than the uterus such as the colon[10] and ductus deferens[11], and in vessel walls. Interestingly, these relaxing properties of progesterone and/or some of its metabolites in smooth muscle including vascular smooth muscle[12-15] have been found to potentiate the isuprenaline-induced relaxation seen in the vascular system.

Vasodilative properties of progesterone in the uterine vascular system had been already suspected from morphological studies on endometrial capillaries conducted throughout the menstrual cycle. Using morphometric techniques, Peek and associates[16] observed that the largest diameter for endometrial capillaries was reached during the luteal phase. In agreement with the lack of anti-vasodilative effects of progesterone, we did not observe that vaginal administration of progesterone altered the low uterine artery PI found in menopausal women receiving exogenous estradiol[6]. Divergent findings were found, however, when uterine artery Doppler was studied after administration of synthetic progestins. Bourne and colleagues[7] observed that synthetic progestins such as medroxyprogesterone acetate (MPA) reversed the vasodilative effects of estradiol by approximately 50%, a finding later confirmed by Hillard and associates[17].

The mechanisms underlying the differences between progesterone and synthetic progestins have not been elucidated[18]. One can speculate that the difference resides in divergent non-genomic effects of the two types of products. Aside from its genomic effects mediated after binding to the progesterone receptor (PR), progesterone also exerts membrane-mediated effects not requiring genomic activation, mostly mediated by locally produced metabolites of progesterone. For example, 3α-OH, $5\alpha/\beta$-reduced metabolites of progesterone increase the resting potential of cells by activation of the γ-aminobutyric acid (GABA)-controlled Cl^- pumping system, which in turn decreases cellular excitability. Conversely, the symmetric metabolites of the synthetic progestin MPA fail to cause the allosteric activation of the $GABA_A$ system that underlies the progesterone-mediated decrease in cellular excitability[19]. That the difference between the effects of progestrone and synthetic progestins is of clinical relevance is shown by a study by Adams and colleagues[20]. Studying the impact of hormone replacement therapy on coronary deposition of plaque in a monkey model, these authors observed that MPA but not progesterone antagonizes the beneficial effects of estradiol on plaque deposition[20]. In keeping with this data, Miyagawa and associates observed that MPA interferes with the protection exerted by estradiol against coronary vasospasm[21].

UTERINE DOPPLER IN IVF

In an original study, Steer and colleagues[22] assessed uterine artery resistance with trans-vaginal pulsed Doppler in 82 women of 22 to 42 years of age who were undergoing IVF. Nineteen women (23.2%) who had a PI > 3.0 did not become pregnant. Conversely, an above-average pregnancy rate of 44% was found in women with a PI < 3.0. There were, however, no differences in the number of embryos transferred in the two groups. This led the investigators to conclude that uterine artery resistance (PI) assessed by Doppler measurement is a clinically usable reflector of endometrial receptivity. In a further trial, the same investigators used transvaginal Doppler for studying uterine artery resistance in women receiving exogenous estradiol and progesterone after suppression of their ovarian function[23]. This was prescribed for priming the endometrium before transferring cryopreserved embryos. Eighty-six women received a long acting gonadotropin-releasing hormone agonist (GnRH-a) preparation to suppress their pituitary gland and ovaries before receiving exogenous estradiol (2–6 mg/day) and progesterone (100 mg/day, intramuscularly). After a preparation, or 'mock', cycle during which an endometrial biopsy was performed (day 21), the treatment was repeated for an actual transfer cycle. Embryos were transferred on the 3rd or 4th day of progesterone administration, depending on their stage of maturation when cryopreserved, as commonly done in donor egg IVF. Here again, the authors observed a higher PI value in women who did not become pregnant as compared to those who did. These latter data are puzzling, however, in that the results contradict the observation of a vasodilative response to estradiol administration reported by many[6,7]. Considering the body of data published on uterine artery Doppler, we are tempted to propose the following explanation for this data paradox. It is possible that some of the patients in the study by Steer and colleagues (those with high PI values in estradiol and progesterone cycles) may have displayed an effect of their past IVF cycle during which an ovarian factor ('third factor') exerted a vasopressive effect. No information is available, however, on the time lapse between the IVF and embryo transfer cycle.

The high predictability of Doppler data for implantation outcome in IVF reported by Steer and colleagues[22] (Figure 5) has not been reproduced by others, or at least not in such

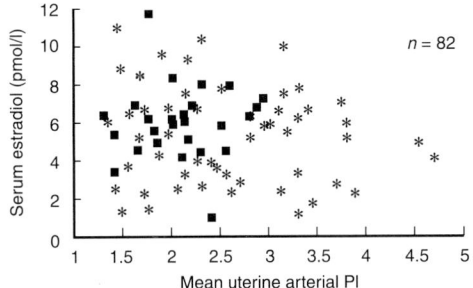

Figure 5 The uterine artery pulsatility index (PI) in *in vitro* fertilization (IVF). Uterine artery resistance evaluated by pulsed Doppler and PI computation reflects endometrial receptivity. Women with a PI > 3 did not become pregnant. Because estradiol levels are elevated in IVF, these results indicate that in IVF a factor likely to result from the ovarian hyperstimulation antagonizes the vasodilative properties of estradiol. From reference 22, with permission

absolute or extreme terms. We did not observe that the differences between women becoming pregnant and those who did not were discriminative enough. In particular, our data did not allow postponing embryo transfer in women who did not score on the uterine Doppler measurements above a given limit. More pessimistic are the results of Favre and colleagues[24]. Studying a population of 198 women undergoing IVF, these authors observed no difference in uterine artery PI values between women who became pregnant and those who did not[24]. Uterine artery resistance was lower, however, in women who received a combination of GnRH-a and human menopausal gonadotropin (hMG) as compared to hMG alone. Similarly, Tekay and associates[25] showed no difference in uterine Doppler data between conception and non-conception IVF cycles. Despite the limited difference in uterine artery Doppler indices observed by these latter authors, it remains unquestionable that a sizeable fraction of women undergoing IVF have high uterine PI values despite high estradiol levels. Tekay and associates[25] reported individual PI values between 2.13 and 6.72 in the non-conception IVF cycles despite the high estradiol levels characteristic of hMG treatments. Kupesic and Kurjak measured uterine flow in radial and spiral arteries in spontaneous cycles and COH cycles[26]. In spontaneous

cycles, the mean PI reached 2.2 at the time of ovulation, while a higher value (3.1) was observed in COH cycles[26]. In cycling women, Kurjak and colleagues observed the lowest impedance to flow in the uterine vasculature during the mid-luteal phase[27]. Despite the negative characteristics of the data reported by Favre and colleagues[24], they indicate that women whose PI values are markedly increased fail to become pregnant. These authors found that the cut-off value of 3 taken by Steer and colleagues[22] for PI values predicting an unreceptive endometrium was too low for practical use in their own population of IVF women. They concluded, however, that when the PI value exceeded 2 SD above the mean ($\geqslant 3.55$), no pregnancy was obtained.

From these Doppler data it can safely be concluded that some IVF women have high uterine artery PI values on the day of oocyte retrieval and/or embryo transfer and that this is of poor prognosis for the prospect of embryo implantation and pregnancy. We will discuss in a later section of this chapter the possible mechanism(s) underlying this finding and the practical lesson to be learned for improving the management and outcome of IVF cycles. We must unfortunately conclude that to this date a consensus has not been established as to whether a universal cut-off value can be safely established upon which the decision of transferring embryos immediately or later (after cryopreservation) can be taken. However, new technical improvements in uterine Doppler measurements will permit assessment of the impedance to flow further down the vascular tree of uterine vascularization (Figure 6), and will improve the predictability of uterine Doppler results in IVF.

DOPPLER DATA NOT EXPLAINED BY THE VASODILATIVE EFFECTS OF ESTRADIOL: THE THIRD FACTOR HYPOTHESIS

To our knowledge there has been no report of resistance to the vasodilative effects of estradiol in women whose ovaries are absent or inactive. Hence, it is puzzling to observe, as

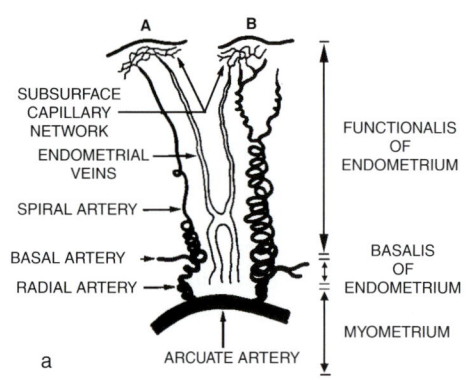

a

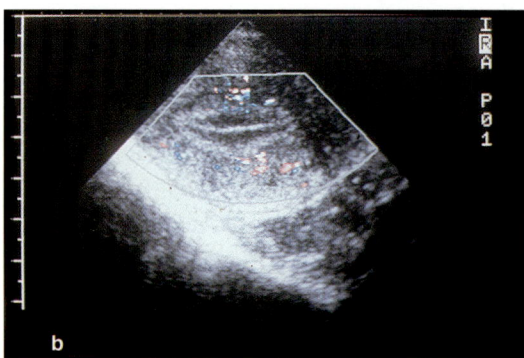

b

Figure 6 Assessment of vascular resistance. (a) The uterine artery and its functional branches. (b) New high-resolution ultrasound probes have permitted the extension of color and pulsed Doppler evaluation further down the uterine vascular tree. This offers new prospects for assessing endometrial receptivity with transvaginal Doppler

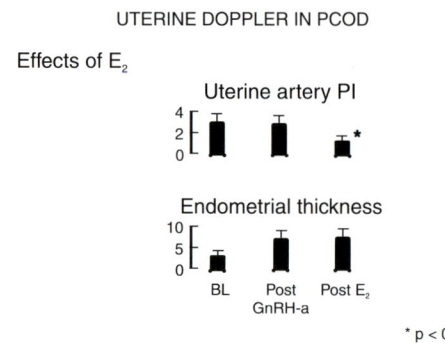

UTERINE DOPPLER IN PCOD

Effects of E_2

Figure 7 The uterine artery Doppler pulsatility index (PI) and endometrial thickness, at baseline (BL), after gonadotropin-releasing hormone agonist (GnRH-a) and estradiol (E_2) add-back therapy, in polycystic ovarian disease (PCOD). Baseline uterine artery PI values are elevated in PCOD despite plasma estradiol levels in the early follicular phase range. Suppression of ovarian function, including the ovarian production of androgens, did not modify PI values. Add-back of bone-sparing quantities of estradiol, however, induced a prompt decrease in uterine artery PI, indicating that in PCOD a gonadotropin-dependent (suppressible by a gonadotropin-releasing hormone agonist) factor antagonizes the vasodilative effects of estradiol. From reference 28 with permission

first reported by Steer and colleagues[22], that in IVF a fraction of women have elevated PI values at the time of embryo transfer, despite the markedly elevated estradiol levels.

In women with polycystic ovaries, we observed[28] that uterine artery resistance exceeds the findings normally expected from plasma estradiol levels. As illustrated in Figure 7, the baseline uterine artery PI was approximately 3 in women suffering from polycystic ovarian disease (PCOD). A subgroup of these patients who were markedly hirsute underwent a 3-month treatment with a GnRH-a in order to suppress their ovarian function, including the production of androgens. This did not impact on uterine artery resistance, which remained elevated while estradiol levels dropped to reach the menopause range.

Subsequently, all these women received estradiol as part of a hormonal add-back strategy. Within 2 weeks of receiving minimal amounts of estradiol, as commonly prescribed for bone-sparing purposes in menopausal women, uterine artery PI decreased, reaching values less than 2, as commonly expected in estrogenized women[29]. We interpreted these results as indicating that no alterations exist in PCOD in the uterine artery response to estradiol. Rather, the results led us to postulate that a gonadotropin-dependent ovarian factor (suppressible by GnRH-a), other than estradiol and progesterone (the 'third factor'), is responsible for increasing the uterine artery resistance through specific vasoactive properties or by interfering with the vasodilative properties of estradiol. Findings made in PCOD led us to suspect that analogies exist with the situation prevailing in COH. Because COH is characterized by the hyperstimulation of the ovary by gonadotropins, we were led to postulate that here again the elevated PI values observed in some women might result from a direct effect of an ovarian factor produced in excessive amounts as a result of COH. Stated differently, we hypothesized that the ovarian hyperstimulation in COH may induce a polycystic-like phenomenon, resulting in increased uterine artery resistance in some individuals. We named this concept the 'third factor hypothesis'.

Because PCOD is characterized by an increase in the production of ovarian androgens, we postulated that the ovarian factor other than estradiol and progesterone suspected to interfere with the vasodilative properties of estradiol, the 'third factor', may be the androgens. To challenge this hypothesis we conducted an extensive survey of the hormonal profile observed in response to hMG in normal IVF candidates. For this, we studied the hormonal profile observed during the 24 h that follow the last injection of hMG in an IVF cycle[30]. Nine IVF cycles were studied. All patients were ovulating regularly and all had shown adequate response to COH in prior IVF embryo transfer cycles. Body mass index, expressed as weight/height^2 x 100, did not exceed 25. Indications for IVF were tubal ($n = 4$), male factor ($n = 3$) and idiopathic ($n = 2$) infertility. COH was initiated after endogenous gonadotropins were suppressed by intramuscular injection of a long-acting preparation of GnRH-a. Ovarian stimulation was initiated 18 days later, provided that pituitary desensitization was confirmed. The initial dose of hMG was set at 300 IU/day for 6 days. Further hMG doses and the timing of human chorionic gonadotropin (hCG) administration were determined on the basis of estradiol levels and ultrasound findings. On the last day of COH, the dose of hMG was set arbitrarily at 225 IU. Women whose clinical conditions dictated either lower or higher doses of hMG were not permitted to participate in the study. Just before the last hMG administration of 225 IU, study participants were hospitalized for 24 h and serial blood sampling was started. Samples were obtained every 30 min for 1 h, hourly for 4 h and every 3 h for the remaining part of the 24-h post-hMG observation period. As illustrated in Figure 8, plasma progesterone, testosterone and androstenedione increased progressively after

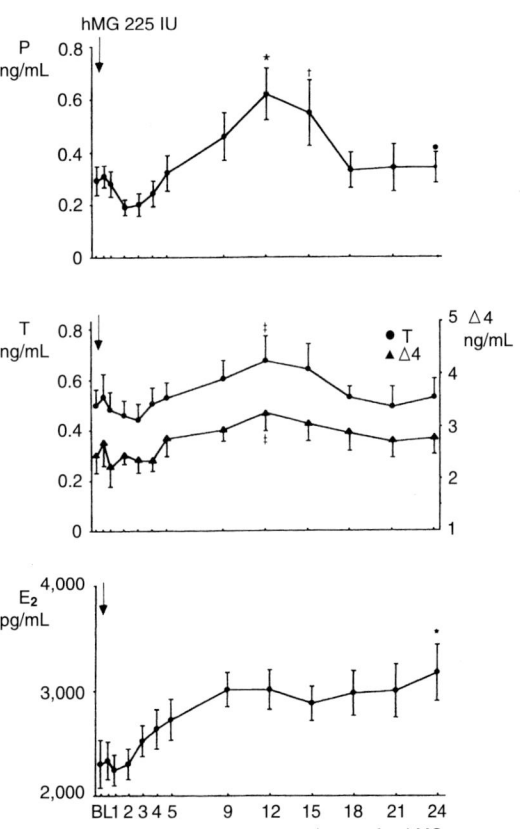

Figure 8 Plasma progesterone and testosterone levels after human menopausal gonadotropin (hMG) administration in *in vitro* fertilization. In controlled ovarian hyperstimulation (COH) for IVF, hMG administration (225 IU) induces an elevation in plasma progesterone, testosterone and androstenedione which culminates approximately 12 h after hMG administration. The hMG-induced increase in ovarian production of androgens may alter endometrial receptivity in IVF and increase the uterine artery pulsatility index. From reference 30, with permission

hMG administration, peaking 12 h later ($p < 0.05$). Thereafter, plasma progesterone, testosterone and androstenedione decreased progressively throughout the observation period, ultimately reaching values not different from baseline. The mean number of oocytes retrieved was 9.1 ± 1.5, not an unexpected finding.

Because the observed increase in androgens 12 h after an evening injection of hMG coincided with the circadian increase in adrenal activity, we repeated the study after suppression of the adrenal function with daily administration of dexamethasone[31]. In this latter study, we observed that daily administration of dexamethasone (1 mg) decreased baseline androgen levels and the levels at the end of hMG administration. From these data, we realized that COH does more than just increase the ovarian production of estradiol and progesterone. Particularly, we noted that hMG (and follicle-stimulating hormone (FSH), unpublished data) also increase the ovarian production of androgens (testosterone and androstenedione), a phenomenon likely to have clinical significance, at least in some women. Indeed, we believe that in sensitive individuals, ovarian androgens and/or other (peptidic) factors may alter uterine artery resistance and ultimately endometrial receptivity to embryo implantation. It is probably advisable in these cases to limit the magnitude of the ovarian stimulation and/or suppress baseline production by suppressing the adrenal component of androgen production. However, contradicting our fears, hCG administration was not associated with an increase in plasma androgen levels. Hence, it is the hMG/ FSH component of COH (and not hCG) that needs to be minimized when sub-receptivity of the endometrium is feared. Conversely, it is likely that an as yet unidentified factor protects from the deleterious impact of androgens on the endometrium by rendering the ovarian production of androgens insensitive to hCG toward the end of COH.

CONCLUSION

Pulsed and color Doppler studies of uterine artery impedance to flow offer a novel non-invasive approach for assessing endometrial receptivity. In particular, they offer the advantage over other approaches, and especially those involving endometrial sampling, of being usable in the actual cycle during which conception is sought. The results of Doppler studies should be compared to the rest of the information provided by ultrasound evaluations, including the assessment of endometrial echogenicity and uterine contractility. Doppler studies are to be seen as one of the new refinements of ultrasound analyses, and their findings integrated in the overall ultrasound assessment of uterine receptivity. We much favor this integrated concept over the one-parameter-does-all approach which claims that a single measurement of uterine artery PI can safely and reliably predict the reproductive outcome. Other ultrasound refinements, such as the assessment of uterine contractility, have made findings in COH (increased contractility at the time of embryo transfer) that differ from findings in the menstrual cycle (uterorelaxing effects of progesterone). Future work will determine if both of these changes, increased PI values and uterine contractility in COH, are possibly linked (third factor?) or result from distinct physiopathological phenomena.

References

1. Navot, D., Bergh, P. A., Williams, M., Garrisi, G. J., Guzman, I. and Sandler, B., (1991). An insight into the early reproductive process through the *in vivo* model of ovum donation. *J. Clin. Endocrinol. Metab.*, **72**, 408–14
2. de Ziegler, D. (1995). Hormonal control of endometrial receptivity. *Hum. Reprod.*, **10**, 4–7
3. Edgar, D. H. (1995). Oestrogen and human implantation. *Hum. Reprod.*, **10**, 2–3
4. Ghosh, D. and Sengupta, J. (1995). Another look at the issue of peri-implantation oestrogen. *Hum. Reprod.*, **10**, 1–2
5. Remohí, J., Ardiles, G., García-Velasco, J. A., Gaitán, P., Simón, C. and Pellicer, A. (1997). Endometrial thickness and serum oestradiol concentrations as predictors of outcome in oocyte donation. *Hum. Reprod.*, **12**, 2271–6
6. de Ziegler, D., Bessis, R. and Frydman, R. (1991). Vascular resistance of uterine arteries: physiological effects of estradiol and progesterone. *Fertil. Steril.*, **55**, 775–9
7. Bourne, T., Hillard, T. C., Whitehead, M. I., Crook, D. and Campbell, S. (1990). Oestrogens,

arterial status, and postmenopausal women. *Lancet*, **335**, 1471–2

8. Sarrel, P. M. (1995). How progestins compromise the cardioprotective effects of estrogens. *Menopause: J. N. Am. Menopause Soc.*, **2**, 187–90

9. Omar, H. A., Ramirez, R. and Gibson, M. (1995). Properties of a progesterone-induced relaxation in human placental arteries and veins. *J. Clin. Endocrinol. Metab.*, **80**, 370–3

10. Gill, R. C., Bowes, K. L. and Kingma, Y. J. (1985). Effects of progesterone on canine colonic smooth muscle. *Gastroenterology*, **88**, 1941–7

11. Morshita, S. (1986). Prompt effect of progesterone on the adrenergic response of smooth muscle. *Jpn. J. Pharmacol.*, **42**, 289–96

12. Foster, P. S., Goldie, R. G. and Paterson, J. W. (1983). Effects of steroids on β-adrenoreceptor-mediated relaxation of pig bronchus. *Br. J. Pharmacol.*, **78**, 441–5

13. Miller, V. M. and Vanhoutte, P. M. (1991). Progesterone and modulation of endothelium-dependent responses in canine coronary arteries. *Am. J. Physiol.*, **261**, R1022–7

14. Kubli-Garfias, C. (1987). Modulatory action of 5-reduced androgens and progestins on the excitability of CNS and smooth muscle. *J. Steroid Biochem.*, **27**, 631–4

15. Jiang, C. W., Sarrel, P. M., Lindsay, D. C., Poole-Wilson, P. A. and Collins, P. (1992). Progesterone induces endothelium-independent relaxation of rabbit coronary artery *in vitro*. *Eur. J. Pharmacol.*, **211**, 163–7

16. Peek, M., Landgren, B.-M. and Johannisson, E. (1992). The endometrial capillaries during the menstrual cycle: a morphometric study. *Hum. Reprod.*, **7**, 906–11

17. Hillard, T. C., Bourne, T. H., Whitehead, M. I., Crayford, T. B., Collins, W. P. and Campbell, S. (1992). Differential effects of transdermal estradiol and sequential progestogens on impedance to flow within the uterine arteries of postmenopausal women. *Fertil. Steril.*, **58**, 959–63

18. Whitehead, M. I., Hillard, T. C. and Crook, D. (1990). The role and use of progestogens. *Obstet. Gynecol.*, **75**, 59S–76S

19. McAuley, J. W., Kroboth, P. D., Stiff, D. D. and Reynolds, I. J. (1993). Modulation of (3H) flunitrazepam binding by natural and synthetic progestational agents. *Pharmacol. Biochem. Behav.*, **45**, 77–83

20. Adams, M. R., Register, T. C., Golden, D. L., Wagner, J. D. and Williams, J. K. (1997). Medroxyprogesterone acetate antagonizes inhibitory effects of conjugated equine estrogens on

coronary artery atherosclerosis. *Arterioscler. Thromb. Vasc. Biol.*, **17**, 217–21

21. Miyagawa, K., Rösch, J., Stanczyk, F. and Hermsmeyer, K. (1997). Medroxyprogesterone interferes with ovarian steroid protection against coronary vasospasm. *Nature Med.*, **3**, 324–7

22. Steer, C. V., Campbell, S., Tan, S. L., Crayford, T., Mills, C., Mason, B. A. and Collins, W. P. (1992). The use of transvaginal color flow imaging after *in vitro* fertilization to identify optimum uterine conditions before embryo transfer. *Fertil. Steril.*, **57**, 372–6

23. Steer, C. V., Tan, S. L., Dillon, D., Mason, B. A. and Campbell, S. (1995). Vaginal color Doppler assessment of uterine artery impedance correlates with immunohistochemical markers of endometrial receptivity required for the implantation of an embryo. *Fertil. Steril.*, **63**, 101–8

24. Favre, R., Bettahar, K., Grange, G., Ohl, J., Arbogast, E., Moreau, L. and Dellenbach, P. (1993). Predictive value of transvaginal uterine Doppler assessment in an *in vitro* fertilization program. *Ultrasound Obstet. Gynecol.*, 350–3

25. Tekay, A., Martikainen, H. and Jouppila, P. (1996). Comparison of uterine blood characteristics between spontaneous and stimulated cycles before embryo transfer. *Hum. Reprod.*, **11**, 364–8

26. Kupesic, S. and Kurjak, A. (1993). Uterine and ovarian perfusion during the periovulatory period assessed by transvaginal color Doppler. *Fertil. Steril.*, **60**, 439–43

27. Kurjak, A., Kupesic-Urek, S., Shulman, H. and Zalvd, I. (1991). Transvaginal color Doppler in the assessment of ovarian and uterine perfusion in infertile women. *Hum. Reprod.*, **6**, 870–4

28. de Ziegler, D. and Cedars, M. I. (1992). Doppler: a refinement to standard transvaginal ultrasonography for the gynecologist. *Semin. Reprod. Endocrinol.*, **10**, 34–44

29. de Ziegler, D. and Bouchard, P. (1993). Understanding endometrial physiology and menstrual disorders in the 1990s. *Obstet. Gynecol.*, **5**, 378–88

30. Fanchin, R., de Ziegler, D., Castracane, V. D., Taieb, J., Olivennes, F. and Frydman, R. (1995). Physiopathology of premature progesterone elevation. *Fertil. Steril.*, **64**, 796–801

31. Fanchin, R., Righini, C., Olivennes, F., Taieb, J., de Ziegler, D. and Frydman, R. (1997). Premature plasma progesterone and androgen elevation are not prevented by adrenal suppression in *in vitro* fertilization. *Fertil. Steril.*, **67**, 115–19

Infection as a cause of infertility

18

M. Toth and F. Chervenak

INTRODUCTION

Infection of the upper genital tract frequently leads to infertility. It is estimated that in about one-third of cases, infertility is caused by tubal obstruction. Permanent damage to the Fallopian tube can be the result of pelvic inflammatory disease[1,2].

Pelvic inflammatory disease (PID) is common, having an estimated annual incidence in Western society of 1% among women aged 16–34 years. PID is the infection of the tubes, ovaries and the uterus (the upper genital tract) that can result in permanent obstruction of the tubes, chronic pelvic pain, an ectopic pregnancy and other pregnancy complications. Recent data show a strong correlation between miscarriage and a history of PID[3]. A variety of aerobic and anaerobic bacteria have been implicated in the etiology of PID, but only *Neisseria gonorrhea* and *Chlamydia trachomatis* are considered really serious pathogens. Because both bacteria are sexually transmitted, sexual behavior is a major risk factor in contracting PID. Consistent with this finding is the pattern of risk factors related to sexual behavior: young age at first intercourse, high frequency of intercourse, and a large number of life-time sexual partners all increase the risk of PID. Barrier methods of contraception appear to reduce the risk of PID, as does oral contraception. The increased risk of PID in users of the intrauterine device (IUD) appears to be confined to new users and women at high risk for sexually transmitted diseases. Douching and cigarette smoking may also be associated with the development of PID, but the evidence is weak. Effective preventive measures are based on modifying sexual behavior[4].

The mechanism leading to tubal damage seems to be different in gonococcal and chlamydial salpyngitis. *In vitro* experiments showed that *N. gonorrhea* elicited more serious damage to tubal tissue than did *C. trachomatis*. The reverse is true *in vivo*[5]. Because of the clinical symptoms and readily available accurate bacterial testing, the diagnosis of gonococcal PID is relatively easy. The treatment, unless a rare, resistant bacterial strain is isolated from the patient, is effective and simple. The opposite is true for chlamydial infection. Present in 60–70% of cases, this bacterium has evolved as the most important and most common pathogen in PID.

CHLAMYDIAL INFECTIONS

There are few branches of medicine on which chlamydial infections and their sequelae do not impinge. *Chlamydia trachomatis* is responsible for many millions of cases of blindness, urethritis, epididymitis, infertility and ectopic pregnancy annually. It is also the most common cause of female upper genital tract infection (PID), which affects more than a million women every year in the USA alone[6].

Recent evidence suggests that pregnancy loss or pregnancy complications are also more common after chlamydial infection. *Chlamydia* may also have a role in the etiology of coronary heart disease. In the majority of cases the infection is subclinical, but even a mild-appearing initial disease may lead to serious long-term sequelae[3].

Bacterial identification was greatly aided by the invention of polymerase and ligand chain reaction technologies, which are capable of amplifying bacterial DNA. In a small study of women with high-risk sexual behavior, we found polymerase chain reaction (PCR) to be ten times more sensitive than regular

Chlamydia culture. Tumor necrosis factor (TNF), a cytokine, produced by macrophages, is usually elevated in the infected tubal tissue of women with PID. Its measurement may help to confirm or to rule out upper genital tract infection[7].

A complicated immunological process is thought to be responsible for scar tissue formation in women infected with *Chlamydia*. This process may be mediated by heat shock proteins. The 57-kDa membrane protein of the bacterium belongs to the family of the 60-kDa heat shock proteins. These highly antigenic substances are present in many bacteria and also in man[8]. Chlamydial heat shock proteins are capable of sensitizing human T lymphocytes. Because of the 50% homology between the human and the chlamydial heat shock proteins, lymphocytes that were sensitized by *Chlamydia* can also respond to human heat shock protein that is released by the host cells under environmental stress. The result is a delayed hypersensitivity reaction which continues to cause progressive tissue damage. Another possibility is the continued presence of undetectable *Chlamydia* in host tissue. This low-grade, so-called 'persistent' chlamydial infection can have a continuous stimulating effect on the host immune system[5].

Silent *Chlamydia* infection

Chlamydial infection is asymptomatic in about two-thirds of cases. Often, the diagnosis is made after irreversible injury to the upper genital tract has already developed. Thus, tubal damage and infertility may occur in asymptomatic women without any clinical evidence of a current or prior episode of pelvic infection. Many women are first told of having a pelvic infection at the time of their infertility work-up. In a much disputed publication, Wolner-Hanssen recently referred to this disease as 'overstated'[9]. According to his opinion, careful, very detailed questioning of an infertility patient frequently reveals past symptoms of an unrecognized, low-grade pelvic infection. Others, like Beatty and colleagues[10], believe that *Chlamydia* can exist in a non-infectious but immunologically active

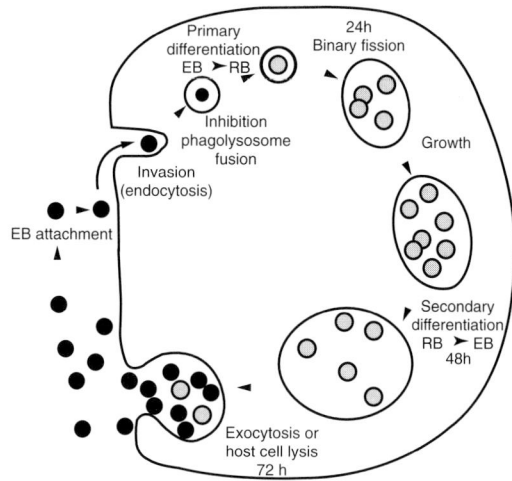

Figure 1 Schematic diagram of the developmental cycle of *Chlamydia trachomatis*. Small, dark structures represent elementary bodies (EB). Larger, stippled structures represent reticulate bodies (RB)

form in which it evades detection by conventional methods like culture or even PCR. In this persistent state the organism is seldom detected but continues to stimulate the immune system of the host. The host response will then lead to progressive tissue damage of the reproductive system.

Chlamydia is an obligate, intracellular parasite because it is unable to make ATP on its own. It exists as two cell types with distinct morphological properties: the elementary body is the infectious particle, which is metabolically inert, and the reticulate body is non-infectious and metabolically active. During the growth cycle of the bacterium, a reticulate body will differentiate into a large number of elementary bodies that will infect more host cells (Figure 1).

The primary host response to *Chlamydia* infection is the release of interferon[10]. *In vitro* exposure of *Chlamydia* to this cytokine results in the formation of atypical (aberrant) reticulate bodies that fail to differentiate into infectious progeny. In this reversible, persistent state the highly antigenic 60-kDa heat shock protein production by the bacterium continues, while the synthesis of bacterial wall or major outer membrane proteins (MOMP) comes to a halt[10].

Because most of the conventional tests for *Chlamydia* (PCR, ligand chain reaction, cultures, enzyme-linked immunosorbent assay, etc.) are based on MOMP detection, persistent infection is undetectable by these methods. Direct antigen identification by methods such as immunoperoxidase staining (IPS) or *in situ* hybridization (ISH) have to be used to localize *Chlamydia* in the persistent state (Figure 2).

Detection of chlamydial antigenic material in culture-negative subjects

In collaboration with the Departments of Obstetrics and Gynecology and Pathobiology of the University of Washington, Seattle, we have developed antigen detection methods (ISH, IPS) to identify persistent *Chlamydia* infection in PCR-negative men and women. In a pilot study, ovarian biopsy specimens from 19 PCR-negative women with tubal factor infertility were analyzed by both methods. Samples of prostates from 10 culture-negative men undergoing prostatectomy for benign hypertrophy, semen samples from PCR-negative sexual partners of 14 women with tubal infertility, and 10 endometrium–tube sample-pairs from ectopic pregnancies were examined by IPS only. We found seven positive results among the 19 ovarian specimens tested for *Chlamydia* antigen or DNA (36%). Of the 10 hypertrophic prostates examined, four (40%) tested positive. Of the 14 semen samples examined, three (21%) tested positive. Tissue samples of three cases of ectopic pregnancy were positive by IPS. All patients with positive findings were also seropositive for *Chlamydia*, which indicates a past infection.

These data led to four very important conclusions: (1) *Chlamydia trachomatis* antigen and nucleic acid can be frequently demonstrated in asymptomatic, PCR- or culture-negative men and women with chronic infection; (2) *Chlamydia* antigens may have an etiologic role in benign prostate hypertrophy and ectopic pregnancy; (3) antigenic material may be sexually transmissible; and (4) IPS and ISH identify temporarily inactive bacteria that may continue to act as immunostimulants and

Events mediated by IFN-γ	Characteristics of persistent Chlamydia
Induction of IDO by IFN-γ	Morphologically large aberrant chlamydial forms
Reduced level of intracellular tryptophan	Non-infectious but viable
Isufficient tryptophan for normal chlamydial growth	Continued heat shock protein 60 production
Development of chlamydial persistence	Dramatic decrease in levels of MOMP, 60-kDa OMP and LPS

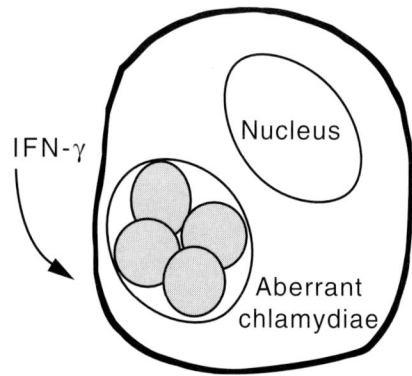

Figure 2 The mechanism for persistent *Chlamydia* infection is interferon-γ (IFN-γ)-mediated. Enzymes induced by this cytokine will reduce intracellular tryptophan levels. In the absence of this amino acid, chlamydial growth is slowed down. IDO, indoleamine 2,3-dioxygenase; LPS, lipopolysaccharide; OMP, outer membrane protein; MOMP, major outer membrane proteins

potentially reactivate as *Chlamydia* infection (Figures 3 and 4). These findings put a new perspective on our view of chlamydial infections. It now seems plausible that very small amounts of the bacteria or its fragments can stimulate an immune response in the host strong enough to cause permanent tubal damage. This could explain why, in some cases, Patton and colleagues were unable to clear neglected chlamydial infections even with 3 months of antibiotic treatment[11]. The sexual transmissibility of the antigenic material raises the possibility of a pathogenic role for these substances in currently unexplained conditions like bacterial vaginosis, recurrent miscarriage and idiopathic preterm birth. Finally, an

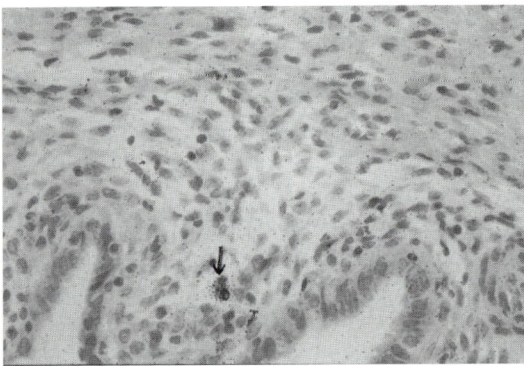

Figure 3 Chlamydial antigenic material in the ovary of a culture- and polymerase chain reaction (PCR)-negative woman by *in situ* hybridization (arrow). The deep penetration of the bacterium into the parenchyma indicates that the infection occurred at the time of ovulation

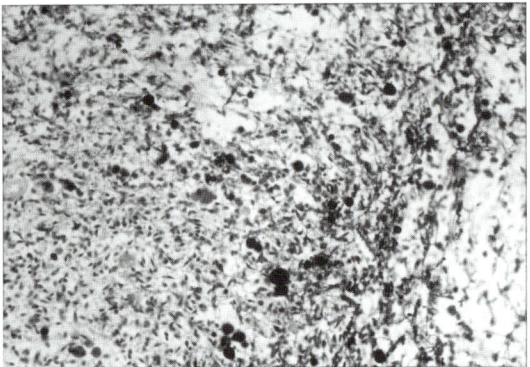

Figure 4 The dark areas represent chlamydial antigenic material (CAM) in culture- and polymerase chain reaction (PCR)-negative semen by an immunoperoxidase antigen detection method. This positive finding raises the possibility for sexual transmission of CAM

asymptomatic, low-grade persistent infection can reactivate in the immune-compromised host. This can happen at the time of a concurrent viral or other bacterial infection or in pregnancy which is a natural state of immune compromise. The reactivated infection will then lead to pregnancy loss, as we have previously shown[12].

Color Doppler ultrasound in the detection of silent chlamydial infection of the ovary

Silent *Chlamydia* infection of the upper genital tract may result in irreversible scarring of the tubes, ovaries and the pelvic side walls. This is

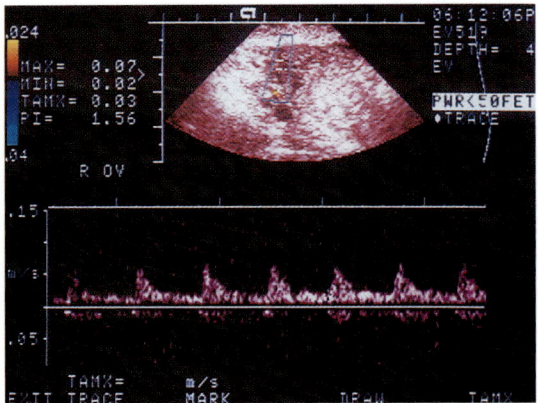

Figure 5 Increased resistance (pulsatility index = 1.56) in the ovarian parenchyma of an infertile, anovulatory woman. The area of decreased blood flow was biopsied and tested positive for chlamydial antigenic material by immunoperoxidase staining

more likely to occur in repeat or prolonged, neglected infection. Extension of the scarring to the ovaries may result in endocrine functional problems like anovulation and premature ovarian failure. Because of the irreversible nature of tissue damage, early diagnosis is mandatory.

Silent ovarian infection is best diagnosed by identifying chlamydial antigenic material (CAM) in the biopsy specimen obtained at the time of a diagnostic laparoscopy. Earlier we found color Doppler ultrasound useful to identify infertility patients with chronic silent PID by measuring ovarian blood flow indices. An elevated resistance index in the ovarian parenchyma correlated well with chronic PID[13] (Figure 5). More recently we used color Doppler-assisted office mini-laparoscopy to localize scar tissue in the ovary. Mini-laparoscopy and ovarian biopsy were performed in 39 patients with suspected tubal factor infertility. Intra-operative color Doppler was used in 19 patients to identify the area of highest resistance within the ovaries. Targeted biopsies of these sites were performed (Figure 6). The remaining 20 patients had random ovarian sampling. The tests were done in the follicular phase. The ovarian biopsy specimens were analyzed for CAM by *in situ* hybridization and immunoperoxidase staining. The results showed that the

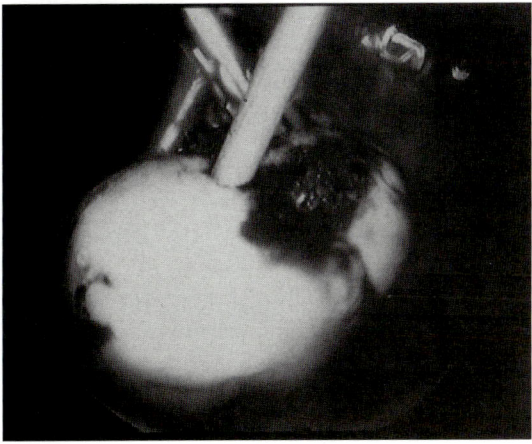

Figure 6 Needle biopsy of an area of increased resistance in the ovary as indicated by color Doppler ultrasound. The Doppler results are shown in Figure 5

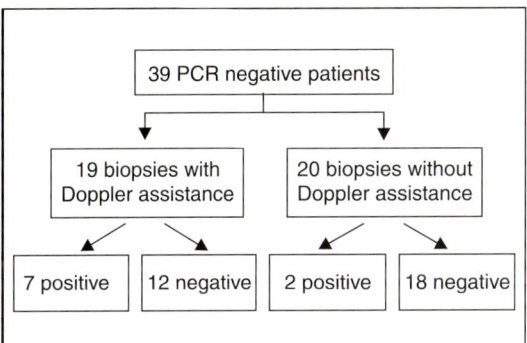

Figure 7 The use of color Doppler increased the yield on ovarian chlamydial antigenic material (CAM) detection ($p < 0.01$). Ovaries which were biopsied after identifying areas with the highest resistance indices were more likely to be positive for *Chlamydia* antigens. PCR, polymerase chain reaction

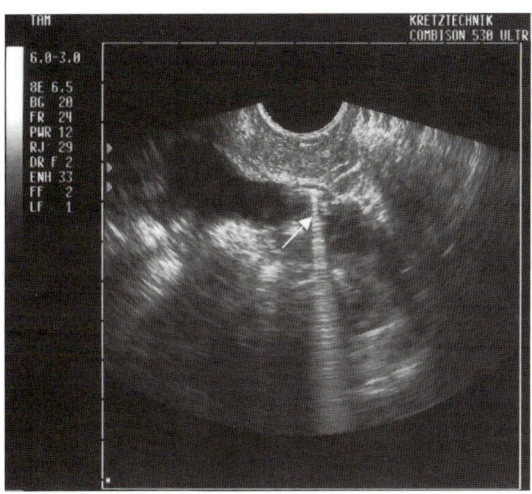

Figure 8 Antibiotic hysterosalpyngo-sonography of the left tube. A mixture of clindomycin and gentamycin solution is injected into the uterine cavity and the tubal patency is confirmed by visualizing the 'fimbrial jet' (arrow). The procedure can be used to open up early tubal blockage

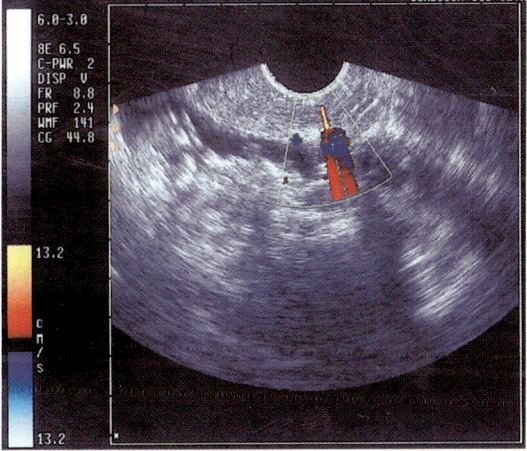

Figure 9 Tubal patency is easily confirmed by color Doppler. The free passage of fluid through the fimbria is better visualized in color

Doppler-assisted group had a significantly higher yield of positive findings than the random group (36% vs. 10%) (Figure 7). We concluded that color Doppler greatly enhanced the detection of *Chlamydia*-infected cases. As the scarring progresses, perfusion of the ovarian stroma diminishes. The higher the resistance, the less likely that ovulation will occur. As the disease further progresses, larger and larger areas of the ovary become under-perfused. This is recognized through the absence of capillary flow. Any large, entirely avascular area in the ovarian parenchyma of an asymptomatic infertility patient should be biopsied and tested for the presence of *Chlamydia* antigenic material. Our preliminary data suggest that in the presence of peri-ovarian or peritubal adhesions these sites are usually positive for *Chlamydia* antigens.

HYSTEROSALPYNGO-CONTRAST-SONOGRAPHY (HyCoSy) IN THE DIAGNOSIS AND MANAGEMENT OF TUBAL DISEASE

The use of different contrast materials in the evaluation of tubal patency is well established. Echovist® and Albunex® are the two most widely used contrast materials for the procedure. HyCoSy is a reliable and simple test for tubal patency, which, when properly done, has a diagnostic yield equal to that of the hysterosalpyngogram (HSG)[14].

During these procedures, which are now included in the routine work-up of our infertility patients, we observed that a healthy tube completely cleared the contrast material from its lumen within 5 min after the injection was stopped. This phenomenon is probably due to the intact function of the endosalpynx and ciliae. Infected tubes with damaged endosalpynx, however, retained Echovist for hours or even days.

We always use antibiotic lavage before and after the HSG procedure. The purpose of local antibiotic treatment is two-fold: first, it mechanically clears removable obstructions like a mucus plug from the tubal lumen, and second, it can break open fresh peritubal or fimbrial adhesions (Figure 8). In addition, the assessment of the pelvis and tubes by three-dimensional ultrasound, which is the next step in the work-up, is easier when there is some fluid in the cul-de-sac.

ASSESSMENT OF THE FALLOPIAN TUBE BY THREE-DIMENSIONAL ULTRASOUND

First, under sterile circumstances, a ballooned HSG catheter is placed into the uterine cavity and routine transvaginal assessment of the pelvis is performed. We use the Voluson 350D machine (Kretz-technik, ZipF, Austria). The tubes are usually found around the ovaries or between the ovary and the iliac vessels. If the tube is not visualized, antibiotic solution is injected into the uterus and the 'fimbrial jet' identified on the screen (Figure 8). It is then confirmed by color Doppler (Figure 9). Absence of the 'fimbrial jet' suggests a blocked tube that is further investigated with a contrast-enhanced study. Once the position of the fimbriated end is established by visualizing the jet, the volume mode is turned on and volume-acquisition of the area commences. Three-dimensional rendering is aimed at visualization of the fimbriae. The finger-like projections are usually visible in normal cases. Loss of most of the fine, velvety structures suggests blunted fimbria that may be adherent to surrounding tissue (Figures 10 and 11). In many cases it is possible to visualize the distended tubal lumen with septae or papillary projections in it (Figure 12).

THE ROLE OF INFECTION IN MALE INFERTILITY

This is a controversial issue. The ambiguity is due to the currently conflicting literature, coupled with present limitations in evaluating the significance of diagnostic tests such as semen cultures and pyospermia. Certain ejaculate infections can be traced back to sexually transmitted bacteria such as *Chlamydia* or *Neisseria*. While the adverse effect of these bacteria on the male reproductive tract is well understood, their relevance for male infertility is a matter of debate.

A recent British study suggests that routine bacterial culture of the semen followed by antibiotic treatment does not improve *in vitro* fertilization (IVF) outcome[15]. The study also warns that antibiotic treatment of the male could alter the urethral and seminal flora in favor of resistant anaerobic bacteria. Thus, giving antibiotics to the male partner may increase the likelihood of inoculation of pathogenic, antibiotic-resistant bacteria from the vagina into the embryo-culture system during oocyte collection. This can lead to adverse IVF outcome[15]. Others have found infection of the endometrium in infertile women correlated with positive semen cultures[16].

Much attention has been paid to the role of different sperm antibodies. These IgG- and IgM-type immunoglobulins are thought to be

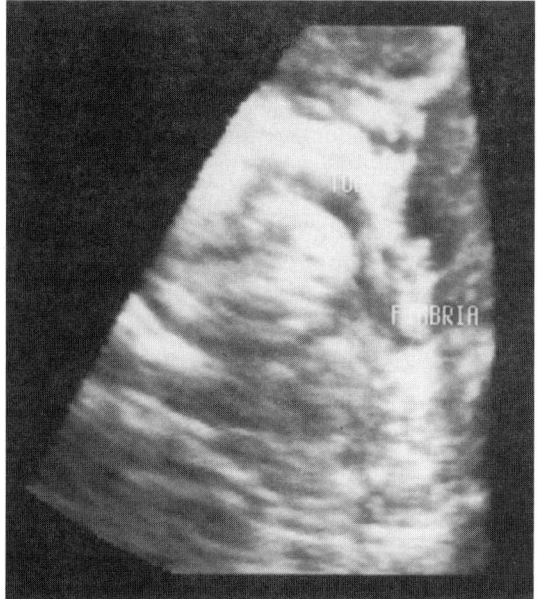

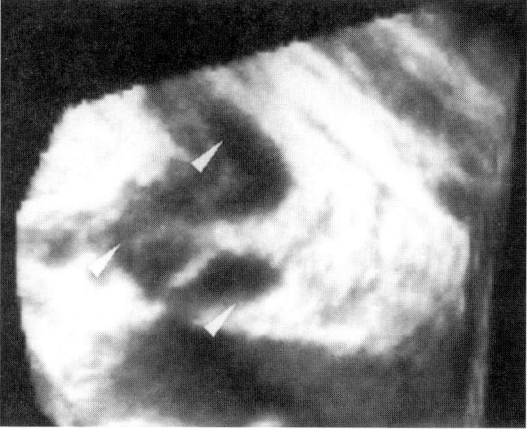

Figure 12 Three-dimensional ultrasound of the Fallopian tube in an asymptomatic infertility patient with very early hydrosalpynx. The fluid accumulation is noticeable along the entire course of this tube (arrows), as it runs towards the iliac vein (bottom of the picture). The intraluminal septations are suggestive of chronic tubal damage

Figure 10 Three-dimensional ultrasound of an infected Fallopian tube. The fimbria is extensively damaged. Only three to four normal projections are visible at the top portion of the fimbriated end

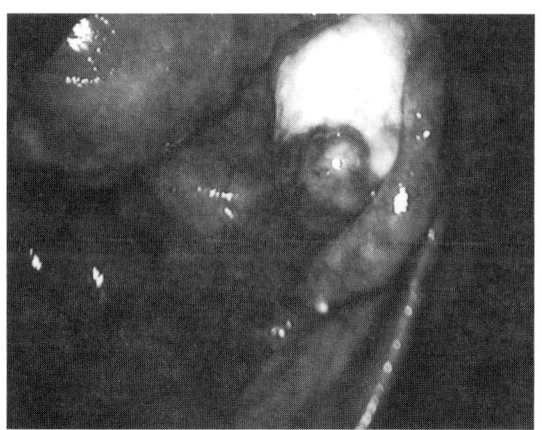

Figure 11 The same case as in Figure 10. Laparoscopy confirms the extensive tubal damage in this asymptomatic, culture- and polymerase chain reaction (PCR)-negative infertile woman. There is an almost complete loss of fimbrial structure and the tubal wall is thickened and scarred. Note the ovary with the corpus luteum cyst

associated with tubal infertility. It is known that the production of these antibodies can be upregulated by bacteria, but in PCR semen

studies Dieterle and colleagues could not find any correlation between *Chlamydia* infection in the semen and sperm antibodies[17].

We found decreased motility in PCR-negative sperm that was positive for chlamydial antigenic material by *in situ* hybridization or immunoperoxidase staining. In a larger study, we are now looking for a possible association between seminal CAM, heat shock protein and sperm antibodies in infertile couples.

In our opinion, an infertile couple should be treated for sexually transmitted bacteria in the semen (*Chlamydia*, *Neisseria*, *Mycoplasma* and *Trichonomas*). Treatment for non-sexually transmitted seminal bacteria should be decided on an individual basis, monitoring semen quality.

CONCLUSIONS

Infection frequently causes infertility. The disease may be silent or may produce vague symptoms only. An infection-oriented work-up is mandatory to identify any damage to the reproductive tract and the patient at risk. Only early intervention can be successful. Permanent damage to the tubes can occur after repeated or neglected infection. This is due to the immunological process that is put into motion at the initial exposure to the bacteria.

Heat shock proteins and their antibodies have become the focus of research. The immune response triggered by these molecules is thought to be causing the tissue damage in the Fallopian tubes. It is interesting that the latest research has found that the immune response protective of a subsequent pregnancy may be through 'blocking' antibody production[18]. This twist in the behavior of the human immune system is fascinating. In addition, Lichtenwalner and associates recently showed that the HLA type has an effect on the immune response to bacteria[19]. This test may help identify women who are at increased risk for tubal damage. In a further development, Dean and colleagues found that only certain genetic variants of *Chlamydia trachomatis* were associated with severe PID. The majority of the bacteria caused mild disease only[20].

Persistent chlamydial infection plays a very important role in silent pelvic infections. In our opinion these latent bacteria or antigenic particles can boost a full immune response that progressively maintains scar tissue formation.

These antigens have the potential to become full bacterial infection at any time.

Ultrasound has become an invaluable tool in the diagnosis and management of pelvic infection. Ultrasound readily identifies advanced tissue damage in the pelvis, such as hydrosalpynx or tubo-ovarian abscesses. Color Doppler is useful to select areas in the infected ovary that are replaced by scar tissue. Biopsy of these areas will frequently yield *Chlamydia* antigens. Hysterosalpyngo-sonography with an antibiotic solution is used to assess tubal damage. It can break open early tubal occlusions and peritubal adhesions. Finally, with three-dimensional ultrasound it is now possible to visualize early damage to the fimbriated end of the tube and recognize early intraluminal changes like septation and fluid accumulation.

In summary, there has been a lot of progress made in the field of infectious disease research, but none of the results mentioned here will supercede a carefully planned prevention program. Only regular bacterial screening of the young, sexually active male and female population with the most sensitive tests available will be effective in preventing infertility that is caused by infection.

References

1. Expert Committee on Pelvic Inflammatory Disease (1991). Research directions for the 1990s. *Sex. Trans. Dis.*, **18**, 46–64
2. Gales, W. and Wasserheit, J. N. (1991). Genital chlamydial infections. *Am. J. Obstet. Gynecol.*, **161**, 1771–81
3. Toth, M., Chaundray, A. and Witkin, S. S. (1993). Pregnancy outcome following pelvic infection. *Infect. Dis. Obstet. Gynecol.*, **1**, 12–15
4. Jossens, O. R., Schachter, J. and Sweet, R. (1994). Risk factors associated with pelvic inflammatory disease. *Obstet. Gynecol.*, **83**, 989–96
5. Beatty, W. L., Byrne, G. I. and Morrison, R. P. (1994). Repeated and persistent infection with *Chlamydia. Trends Microbiol. (England)*, **2**, 94–8
6. Patton, D. L., Halbert, S. A., Kuo, C. C., Wang, S.-P. and Holmes, K. K. (1993). Host response to primary *Chlamydia trachomatis* infection. *Fertil. Steril.*, **6**, 829–39
7. Toth, M., Jeremias, J., Ledger, W. and Witkin, S. (1992). *In vivo* tumor necrosis factor production in women with acute salpyngitis. *Surg. Gynecol. Obstet.*, **174**, 359–62
8. Eckert, L. O., Hawes, S. E., Wolner-Hanssen, P. *et al.* (1997). Prevalence and correlates of antibody to *Chlamydia* heat shock protein. *Infect. Dis.*, **175**, 1453–8
9. Wolner-Hanssen, P. (1995). Silent pelvic inflammatory disease. Is it overstated? *Obstet. Gynecol.*, **86**, 321–5
10. Beatty, W. L., Byrne, G. I. and Morrison, R. P. (1993). Morphologic and antigenic characterization of interferon-mediated persistent *Chlamydia trachomatis* infection *in vitro*. *Proc. Natl. Acad. Sci. USA*, **90**, 3998–4002
11. Patton, D. L., Askienazy-Elbhar, M., Henry-Suchet, J., Campbell, L. A. and Cappuccio A. (1994). Detection of *Chlamydia trachomatis* in Fallopian tube tissue in women with

postinfectious tubal infertility. *Am. J. Obstet. Gynecol.*, **171**, 95–101

12. Toth, M., Witkin, S. S., Ledger, W. J. and Thaler, H. (1998). The role of infection in the etiology of preterm birth. *Obstet. Gynecol.*, **71**, 723–6

13. Toth, M., Chervenak, F. A., Witkin, S. S. and Ledger, W. J. (1992). Color Doppler ultrasound in the diagnosis of pelvic inflammatory disease. Presented at the *Annual Meeting of the Infectious Disease Society for Obstetrics and Gynecology*, San Diego, California, August. Abstr. 7

14. Deichert, U., van de Sant, M., Lauth, G., *et al.* (1988). Dietransvaginale Hysterokontrastsonographie. *Geburt. Freuenh.*, **48**, 835–44

15. Liversedge, N. H., Jenkins, J. M. and Kea, S. D. (1996). Antibiotic treatment based on seminal cultures from asymptomatic male partners in *in vitro* fertilization is unnecessary. *Hum. Reprod.*, **11**, 1227–31

16. Taylor, S. and Frydman, R. (1996). Hysteroscopy and sperm infection. *Contracept. Fertil. Sexuality*, **24**, 549–51

17. Dieterle, S., Mahoney, J. B. and Luinstra, K. E. (1995). Chlamydial immunoglobulin IgG and IgA antibodies in serum and semen are not associated with the presence of *Chlamydia* DNA or rRNA in semen from male partners of infertile couples. *Hum. Reprod.*, **10**, 315–19

18. Nip, M. M., Miller, D., Taylor, P., Gannon, M. J. and Hancock, K. W. (1994). Expression of heat shock protein 70kDa in human endometrium of normal and infertile women. *Hum. Reprod.*, **9**, 1253–6

19. Lichtenwalner, A. B., Patton, D. L., Cosgrove Sweeney, Y. T. and Gaur, L. K. (1997). Evidence of genetic susceptibility to *Chlamydia trachomatis*-induced pelvic inflammatory disease in the pig-tailed macaque. *Infect. Immun.*, **65**, 2250–3

20. Dean, D., Oudens, E., Bolan, G., Padian, N. and Schachter, J. (1995). Major outer membrane variants of *Chlamydia trachomatis* are associated with severe upper genital tract infections. *J. Infect. Dis.*, **172**, 1013–22

Ectopic pregnancy

19

I. E. Timor-Tritsch and A. Monteagudo

INTRODUCTION

Ectopic pregnancy is defined as a gestation implanted outside the uterine cavity. Its incidence and risk factors are discussed below, but first there is a short explanation of why it is dealt with here, in a book that devotes its efforts towards solving the problems of infertility.

The first reason is that an inordinately high number of ectopic pregnancies are the result of infertility treatments. They occur in the very patients who, throughout the weeks, months or even years of treatment have become attached to and in many ways 'dependent' on their doctors, whom they respect and upon whom they rely. It is this doctor who should detect the first signs (biochemical or sonographic) of the woman's pregnancy. Sometimes, this pregnancy resides outside the uterus. It is therefore the task of the very same infertility specialist to be able to handle the transvaginal ultrasound probe skilfully, and swiftly to recognize this life-threatening medical emergency.

The second reason is that early and appropriate treatment or management for an ectopic pregnancy can be provided by the same infertility specialist, by the proper and intensive use of ultrasonography. Thus, transvaginal sonography (TVS) becomes the leading tool in treating as well as following up the clinical course of the disease if alternative treatments (other than surgical) are considered.

ETIOLOGY

Multiple etiologies of this disease unique to humans are entertained. The most logical of the reasons for ectopic pregnancy is the interference with the transport of the fertilized eggs. This may result from peritubal adhesions, previous surgery of the tubes (incomplete tubal ligation, previous surgery for infertility or ectopic gestation in the tube), previous infection of the tubes, tubal diverticula[1-9] or other, more rare causes. It seems important to mention that tubal sterilization is an important risk factor for ectopic pregnancy. If pregnancy occurs after a surgical sterilization procedure, 12.3% have been found in those having the procedure performed through laparotomy and 51% in those women who underwent the surgery through laparoscopy[9].

Although embryos implanted outside the uterine cavity have the same rate of *chromosomal abnormalities* as those correctly implanted *in utero*[10], it seems that ectopic pregnancies have more cases of faulty embryogenesis[11], although this has not been confirmed.

Hormonal imbalance during the menstrual cycle is also implicated in the possible etiology of this disease. If one gives credit to the ciliary and myoelectrical activity of the Fallopian tubes, it is easy to understand that estrogens increase this activity and progestins decrease it[12]. Extremely large amounts of estrogens may bring about a powerful contraction of the isthmus, preventing the transport of the fertilized eggs into the uterine cavity. If this theory is correct, one has to recognize the contribution of Pulkkinen and Talo[13], who researched this activity as a possible causative factor in tubal ectopic pregnancy. This may also support the observation that large doses of estrogens given as a 'morning after' contraceptive treatment[14] or as ovarian hormonal hyperstimulation[15] result in a larger than usual percentage of ectopic pregnancies.

Other factors may include transabdominal transfer of the eggs from an ovary to the contralateral tube. According to Berry and associates[16] and Walters and colleagues[17], about one-third to one-half of tubal gestations demonstrated a contralateral corpus luteum. This concept was suggested years before by Iffy[18,19], and corroborates the fact that a delay in fertilization due to the distance travelled by the eggs causes late and ectopic implantation. The fertilized egg may even be too large to fit through the narrow isthmus.

As far as the risk factors for ectopic pregnancies are concerned, they fall into the following categories: previous tubal pregnancy, pelvic inflammatory disease, currently used intrauterine contraceptive device and previous surgery for infertility. An exhaustive analysis and critical evaluation of the various risk factors involved was compiled by Stoval and Ling[20].

DIAGNOSIS

Clinical presentation

The classic presentation of a patient with shoulder pain and fainting spells leading to the diagnosis of ruptured ectopic pregnancy is rarely seen. Today's typical picture is that of a patient with some degree of uterine bleeding, who has missed a period and used the readily available pregnancy tests, which indicate the presence of an early pregnancy.

Physical examination will reveal abdominal tenderness or peritoneal irritation in the presence (or sometimes the absence) of a palpable adnexal mass. Dizziness and nausea may help in confirming the suspicion of an ectopic gestation. Patients may be encountered in the office, emergency room or even through the telephone.

Astute clinicians should consider all the presenting signs and symptoms as the 'rule-out-ectopic' case until an intrauterine pregnancy is diagnosed or the ectopic pregnancy is found. This is true regardless of how atypical the presentation may be. It is of primary importance to know whether the patient is indeed pregnant. If a pregnancy test has been performed and the pregnancy ascertained, one can proceed to the next step, which is sonographic imaging.

If the office or the emergency room is equipped with an ultrasound machine with a transvaginal probe and the clinician is familiar with its use (I wholeheartedly recommend this to all practicing obstetricians and gynecologists), one can proceed immediately to this imaging modality even before the results of the pregnancy test are available. Most of the time a decision can be reached right there and then, in the physician's office or the emergency room, sometimes without receiving the results of other tests, saving valuable time and effort for both the patient and her health care provider[21].

At times, the sonographic evaluation may become more complex and an imaging specialist has to be involved. However, a patient suspected of an ectopic pregnancy should never be permitted to leave the office or the emergency room without the diagnosis properly ruled out. If the diagnosis of ectopic pregnancy is confirmed, appropriate measures should be provided. Both can be arrived at with the knowledge and handling of the ultrasound machine or, if such a test cannot be administered by the physicians on the spot, at least there should be an understanding of the importance to obtain sonographic evaluation immediately.

The role biochemical markers of ectopic pregnancy

The most important development in the detection, correct diagnosis and management of ectopic pregnancy has been the introduction of qualitative and quantitative human chorionic gonadotropin (hCG) assessment, which continues to be not only more and more sensitive and easily available, but also less and less expensive. These tests can be performed on urine or blood. The qualitative or semi-qualitative quick tests can be carried out in the physician's office. There are various standards for reporting the levels of hCG. Usually, the β subunits of hCG are tested. The International Reference Preparation (IRP) and the Second International Standard are the most used. It must be understood that the

Second International Standard values are about half of the IRP values. It is also important to use the same laboratory if serial values are to be compared. Most qualitative tests are considered to be positive with an hCG level of 30 mIU/ml (IRP). The sensitivity of the currently used monoclonal antibody tests achieves levels of detection as low as 50 IU/ml (IRP), therefore these are useful adjuncts to transvaginal sonography in establishing a correct diagnosis.

The most important use of the quantitative hCG determination in conjunction with ultrasonography is that of understanding the value of the 'discriminatory zone' of hCG. The discriminatory zone represents the level of hCG above which all normal intrauterine chorionic sacs will be detected by ultrasound. This concept was introduced by Kadar and co-workers[22], using transabdominal ultrasound. Its value was 6000–6500 mIU/ml (IRP). Nyberg and associates[23] used the Second International Standard and a different transducer and were able to see the intrauterine pregnancy (IUP) at levels of 1800 mIU/ml. There is now almost a consensus in considering the discriminatory zone to be about 1000 mIU/ml with the use of a transvaginal transducer of at least 5 MHz[24–27]. This level at which the normal IUP is detected varies with different authors and the use of different equipment as well as the operator's experience. The discriminatory zone may also be different in a multimyomatous uterus.

Progesterone levels are also used to monitor the pregnancy and some think that this has a role in the differential diagnosis of early pregnancy failure. Low levels of serum progesterone were suggested to be indicative of ectopic gestation[28–35]. Cut-off levels of 15–20 mg/ml are used, below which ectopic pregnancy is likely to be diagnosed. A single measurement of 0.5 mg/ml or less indicates a non-viable pregnancy, regardless of its location. From the literature, it appears that levels of progesterone, as a screening test, can help in diagnosing ectopic pregnancy. However, if quick hCG determination and transvaginal sonography are readily available the use of serum progesterone levels is not practical and may waste time and money.

For the sake of completeness, we must mention the attempts to use other biochemical markers in the diagnosis of ectopic pregnancy. Some of these are α-fetoprotein, C-reactive protein, CA-125, pregnancy-associated plasma protein-A (PAPP-A), renin, relaxin and Schwangerschafts protein-1 in alphabetical order, rather than order of their relative importance[20]. Their role in the quick diagnosis of ectopic pregnancy may be only historical, since the advent of quick hCG determination and of ultrasound scans.

Culdocentesis will also be mentioned here in a historical sense. Once it was of prime importance to obtain blood from the peritoneal cavity and observe whether it coagulated or not. Non-coagulating blood supported the diagnosis of ectopic pregnancy. Since the availability of TVS, even the smallest amount of peritoneal fluid can easily be diagnosed. If this sonographic evaluation of pelvic fluid is available and it is properly placed in the diagnostic process, the role of culdocentesis as a diagnostic means must justifiably be excluded. The article of Vermesh and co-workers[36] clearly states that, if hCG determination and TVS are available, culdocentesis has limited or no value in the diagnostic algorithm.

Curettage and subsequent 'floating' of the obtained tissue in water, after its thorough washing to get rid of blood, is a simple and valid procedure to prove the existence of placental tissue. It can be used in a bleeding patient who is amenable to the fact that this is performed at a time when no viable IUP or an obvious ectopic pregnancy is detected by TVS and if villi are seen (villi are easily identified with the naked eye with some experience). If persons performing chorionic villus sampling are able to detect as little as 20–30 μg of villi in a Petri dish (sufficient sample to perform chromosomal analysis) with the naked eye, one can do the same thing with tissue obtained by curettage. If villi are found, this will practically rule out the presence of an ectopic pregnancy.

Laparoscopy has been, and still is, considered the ultimate diagnostic test for ectopic pregnancy. The procedure requires an experienced operator, complex equipment, an operating room, an anesthesiologist and experienced nursing staff. These may not be readily available at night. The advantage of the procedure is that, once an ectopic pregnancy is diagnosed, it can be treated at the same time. At times, however, false-negative cases have been described. We know that, when a tubal ectopic pregnancy is about 5–10 mm in size, the hCG should be about 1000–1500 mIU/ml. This chorionic ectopic sac should be seen on TVS. However, if the hCG level is below 1000 mIU/ml or if the tubal ectopic pregnancy is not developing normally, owing to its small size, it will often be missed, even by experienced laparoscopists, provided it is not bleeding through the fimbriae. Such cases can, however, be treated expectantly or by parenteral methotrexate administration. The medical treatment under sonographic control is discussed later.

The role of ultrasound in the diagnosis of ectopic pregnancy

Ultrasonography, but more precisely transvaginal sonography, has become the 'gold standard' laboratory modality for the effective and fast diagnosis of ectopic pregnancy. Even more importantly, and understandably more frequently, it will effectively rule out an ectopic pregnancy, by detecting a normal or pathological IUP. As a first-line modality, it should be said that transabdominal sonography (TAS) has some value in successfully detecting a very small number of oddly located ectopic gestations, mainly high up in the pelvis – outside the effective 'reach' of a 5-MHz vaginal probe (usually about 12–14 cm). In general, TAS has low sensitivity, specificity and positive predictive value for this task. It is therefore natural that TVS has become the test of choice in the clinical work-up of the patient suspected of ectopic pregnancy (Figure 1). The clinical value of TVS in achieving this goal is well documented[37–44].

By now, the technique of transvaginal scanning is almost common knowledge and is sufficiently described in different textbooks. If,

at her first visit for the problem, the patient presents with a full bladder, TAS can or should be performed first. After the bladder is emptied, a thorough bimanual palpatory examination should precede the transvaginal ultrasound examination. If, however, for any reason, the bladder of a patient suspected of ectopic pregnancy has to be filled, this should be done by drinking water, in the view of a possible surgical procedure under general anesthesia.

Using TVS, a rather rigid scanning routine should be followed. The scanning should obviously start by looking at the cervix and the area of the internal os. It is frustrating if, after a prolonged scanning period looking at the uterus and the adnexa, one misses a cervical pregnancy. Because of its rarity, it is unlikely that a second chance would be presented to the examiner.

The strict routine, as said before, should start with the uterus, examining its various areas – the cervix, the cavity and the cornual area. Then the adnexa and the cul-de-sac should follow. These sites and the possible findings are described, but before the description of the specific sites and their sonographic findings, several important statements should be made. These observations are the results of personal experience and reviewing the literature time and again.

(1) If the diagnosis of ectopic pregnancy is a possibility, then a transvaginal probe is a necessity.

(2) An inconclusive TAS scan is not an acceptable end-point.

(3) An ectopic pregnancy should be recognized not by its appearance but by its location.

(4) In a patient with significant cul-de-sac fluid without hormonal ovulation induction and a positive pregnancy test, the bleeding ectopic pregnancy must be found.

The uterus

For practical purposes an intrauterine pregnancy in patients who are not at risk for ectopic

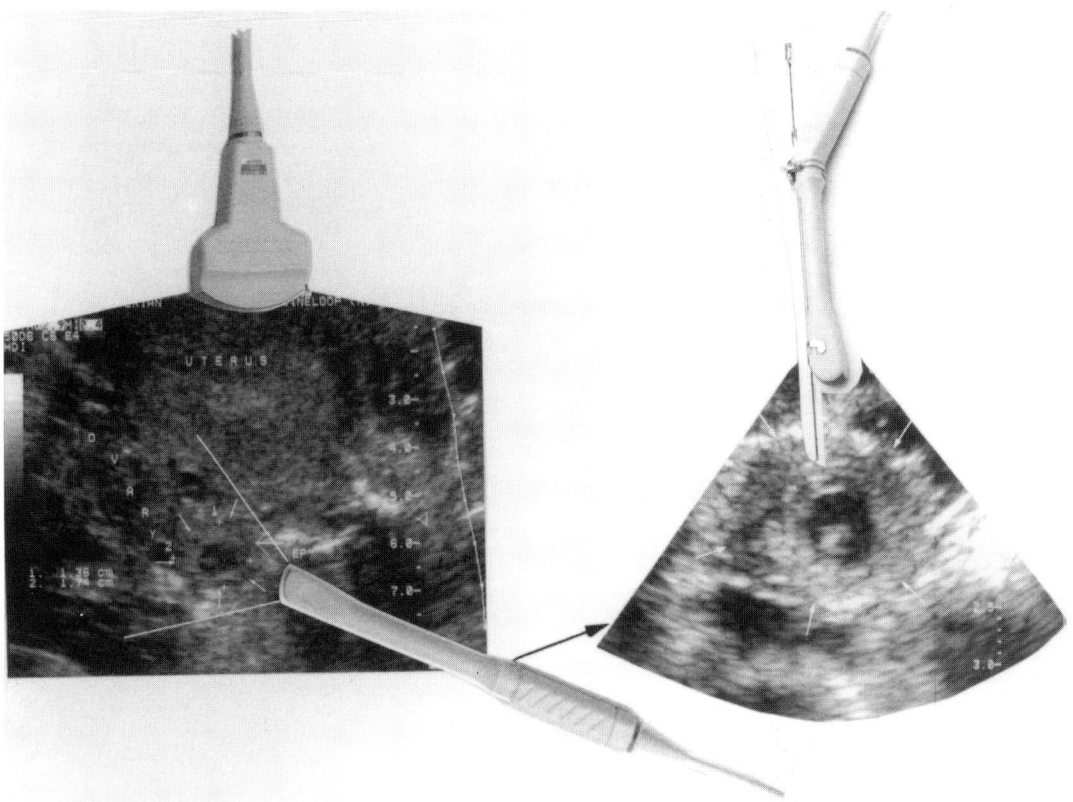

Figure 1 Picture illustrating that an image generated by the transabdominal probe (left) has two disadvantages in diagnosing a tubal ectopic pregnancy: the relatively large distance of about 6 cm from the transducer and the low resolution. Compare the high-resolution picture generated by the vaginal transducer on the right, placed about 1.5–2 cm from the clear tubal ring containing the ectopic pregnancy outlined by small arrows

pregnancy excludes an ectopic pregnancy. The rare risk of heterotopic, intra- and extrauterine pregnancy is duly acknowledged in the literature. The first effort, therefore, is directed towards carefully scrutinizing the cervix (for that rare, but possible, cervical gestation) and the endometrial cavity. There are three diagnostic and two non-diagnostic sonographic intracavitary findings. The first diagnostic sign is the finding of *normal early intrauterine gestation*. The problem usually is the detection of a very early pregnancy at 4–5 postmenstrual weeks. The true early intrauterine chorionic sac, measuring several millimeters, is implanted and should be visible on one side of the cavity line – at the depth of the hyperechoic endometrium (Figure 2).

The second sign is that of an *abnormal, non-developing, non-living intrauterine pregnancy* with some embryonic or extraembryonic structures (e.g. fetal pole, yolk sac).

The third diagnostic sign is a *thick* (usually more than 1–1.5 cm) *hyperechoic endometrium* in a patient with a positive pregnancy test (Figure 3b).

Non-diagnostic sonographic signs of ectopic pregnancy are: *shifting fluid in the cavity*, termed 'pseudogestational sac' of ectopic pregnancy (this definition was coined using TAS) and heterogeneous undefined uterine content, i.e. the remnants of a failed IUP intermixed with blood. If a dilatation and curettage (D & C) is performed in these cases, the villi of the placenta should be identified if the tissue is floated in water. These last two sonographic pictures of the uterus are only partially helpful; therefore they can be considered as non-diagnostic. These findings present the greatest

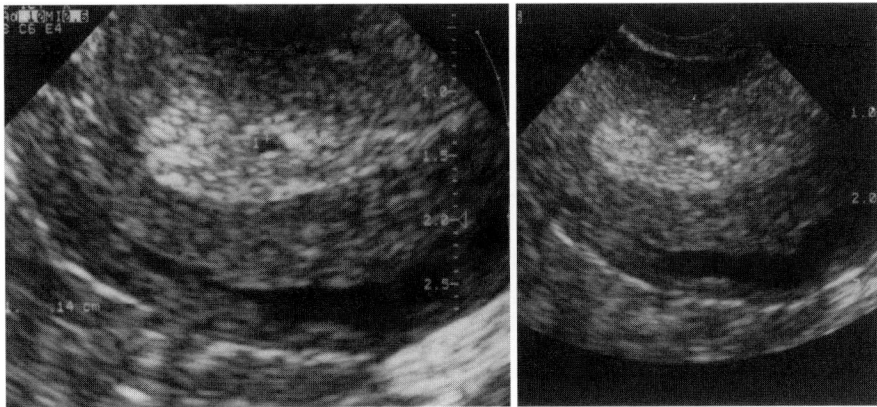

Figure 2 Transvaginal sonographic picture of a normal early intrauterine pregnancy at 4 postmenstrual weeks and 3 days. Note the thin but clearly recognizable hyperechoic chorionic ring and the sac, located somewhat off-center, which will not shift

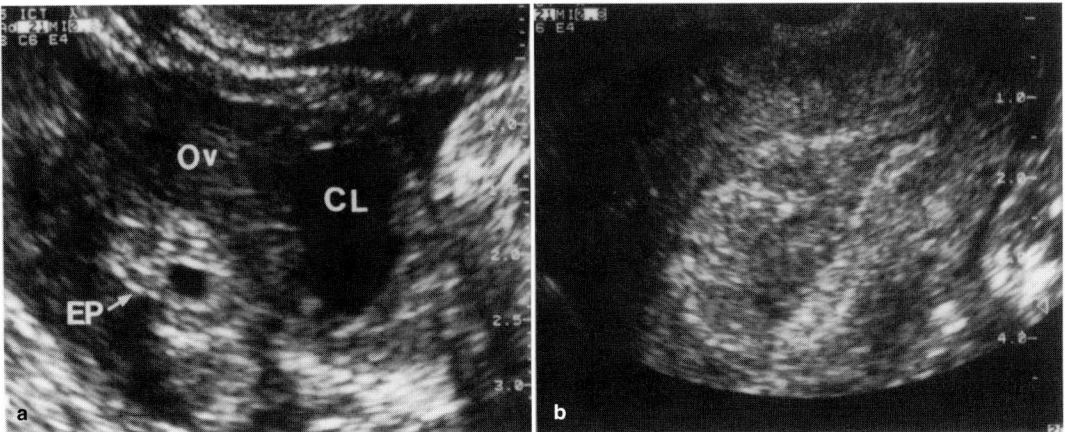

Figure 3 A 4-week and 5-day (from the last menstrual period) tubal gestation. (a) The ovary (Ov) and corpus luteum (CL) are on the same side of the ectopic pregnancy (EP). Note the difference in their echogenicity, since this is pathognomonic. (b) The 'robust', echogenic decidual reaction measuring about 2.8 cm in thickness on the sagittal section of the uterus corroborates the sonographic diagnosis

challenge to the examiner. Once these findings are encountered in the presence of a positive hCG test, they should be interpreted as a decidual reaction or an early pregnancy failure. If no adnexal findings are detected and no cul-de-sac fluid is present, such non-diagnostic endocavitary findings enable continuous TVS follow-up with occasional hCG testing. An even better approach is to perform curettage and examine the products visually (in the way already described) and/or histologically.

The *pseudogestational sac* is a special case of a decidual reaction. It will always be found in the middle of the uterine cavity, flanked by symmetrically thick hyperechoic endometrium. Its shape changes owing to the shifting fluid, as a result of the slow myometrial contractions around it. A short (1- or 2-min) observational period focused upon this structure without changing the scanning plane will be useful to detect the unstable shape and shifting of the intracavitary fluid. A true intrauterine

Table 1 Comparison of transvaginal sonographic features of intrauterine pregnancies and the pseudogestational sac of ectopic pregnancies

	Pseudogestational sac	*Intrauterine pregnancy*
Location	along the cavity line, between the endometrial lining	'buried' in the endometrium, on either side of the cavity line
Borders	no 'double ring', may be irregular	'double ring' with echoic inner ring (trophoblast)
Shape and size	may change during the same or close subsequent examination	steady shape and location
Content	no embryonic or extraembryonic structures; sometimes amorphous material	after 5 menstrual weeks; extraembryonic and embryonic structures
Color flow pattern	flow is seen within the decidua only at a more advanced gestational age	trophoblastic, low-resistance flow present; 'hot flow' pattern

chorionic sac will stay fixed and, as said before, will be seen on one side or the other of the usually hyperechoic cavity live. Color Doppler studies may be helpful in differentiating between an early IUP and intracavitary fluid.

With TVS it is less likely that a small intracavitary fluid collection in the case of an ectopic pregnancy will be confused with a small chorionic sac of 4–5 postmenstrual weeks[45]. Table 1 lists the comparative features of an early IUP and a central intracavitary fluid collection referred to as the 'pseudogestational sac of ectopic pregnancy'.

Lately, Ackerman and co-workers[46] reported that the subendometrial or subdecidual layer of the uterus in a small (14%) but significant number of patients revealed a cystic structure no larger than 2–3 mm in size. They called this structure a 'decidual cyst'.

The adnexa

Evaluating the adnexa is extremely important, since most ectopic gestations are found in this region of the pelvis. The examiner should be familiar with the rarely seen sonographic appearance of the normal tube with its fimbrial end (Figure 4). This can be seen only if fluid, of any kind, surrounds it. An unequivocal adnexal finding providing the convincing diagnosis of an ectopic pregnancy would be that of a clear 'tubal ring' containing embryonic fetal pole with or without heart beats and

extraembryonic (yolk sac) structures. This may occur as frequently as 15–25% of the time, depending upon the mix of the patient population examined[47–49].

At the very early period, such as 4.5–5 postmenstrual weeks, only a hyperechoic tubal ring surrounding the sonolucent chorionic sac will be evident (Figure 3a).

On the basis of the sequential appearance of extraembryonic and embryonic structures in a normal intrauterine pregnancy[50] and assuming that about 15–20% of ectopic pregnancies will have a normally growing embryo, one can assess the expected sonographic picture in such ectopic gestations. At 5 postmenstrual weeks, in addition to a 2–4-mm sonolucent chorionic sac surrounded by an echogenic trophoblastic ring within the tubal ring (i.e. tubal wall), a yolk sac should appear. At 6 postmenstrual weeks, the heart beats within an embryonic pole of several millimeters will be detectable. Figure 5 demonstrates a tubal ectopic pregnancy of 6 postmenstrual weeks and 1 day, with a live embryo. At 7 postmenstrual weeks an embryo of approximately 10–13 mm with a small cranial sonolucency appears. Figure 6 shows an ectopic pregnancy of 7 postmenstrual weeks and 2 days with a yolk sac. At 8 postmenstrual weeks, the monolocular sonolucency in the embryonic head (the head reaching the approximate size of the yolk sac, i.e. 4–5 mm) can be seen. At 9 postmenstrual weeks, the falx will appear in

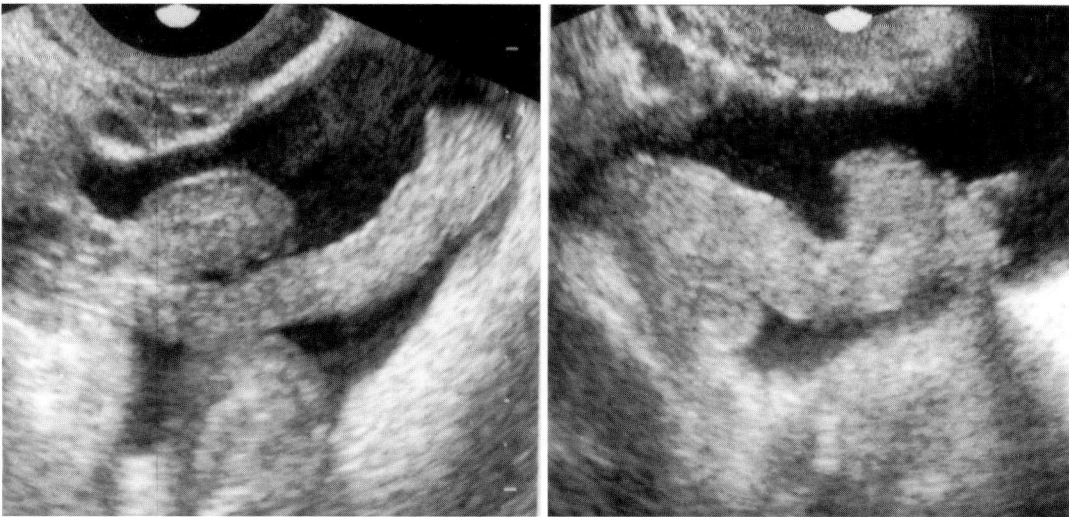

Figure 4 The normal left ovary and Fallopian tube are surrounded by fluid which enables their clear imaging. Fluid around the tube acts as a contrast medium. This is probably the only way the normal tube can be imaged

the head, and the physiological midgut herniation (starting to be evident about 1 week earlier) becomes easily located at the abdominal insertion of the tiny umbilical cord[51]. Figure 7 shows a live tubal ectopic pregnancy of 9 postmenstrual weeks with the yolk sac as well as the appropriate sized embryo.

It is important to emphasize here that normal-appearing structures of a live or non-live embryo/fetus should not be misdiagnosed as an IUP. The difference between an IUP and an ectopic pregnancy is the surrounding myometrium, the presence of which is necessary to reassure the patient of an IUP. Further clarification of this statement is necessary: in the case of an isthmic or cornual pregnancy the myometrial 'envelope' will appear extremely thin (about 2–4 mm). In the case of a cervical pregnancy, there is obviously a somewhat thicker myometrial layer; however, the recognition of these two ectopic rare pregnancies should be relatively easy, owing to their location.

Pellerito and co-workers[52] claim that about 85% of ectopic pregnancies are formed on the same side of the corpus luteum. This raises an important differential diagnostic issue, namely to be able reliably to differentiate the tubal ectopic pregnancy from the ipsilateral corpus

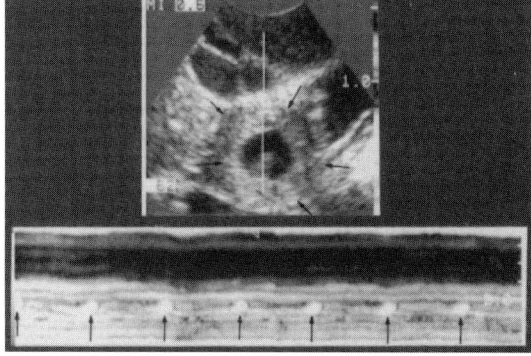

Figure 5 An intact tubal ectopic pregnancy (arrows) of 6 postmenstrual weeks and 1 day, with heart beats displayed on the gray scale and on the M-mode sweep

luteum (Figures 3 and 6). To the rescue comes the fact that the corpus luteum and the unruptured tubal ectopic pregnancy are of different sonographic properties. The corpus luteum is found in the ovary and its echogenicity is slightly (or at times even more prominently) lower than that of the trophoblastic tissue of the tubal ring. The problem in comparing echogenicity arises when (in about 15%) these two structures are on opposing sides. Our advice is that, in these cases, the operator should take advantage of the split-screen feature offered by most ultrasound machines.

One of the suspected structures should be 'frozen' on the left side of the screen, the other (without changing the controls of the panel) on the right side of the screen. Thus, it is easy to compare the relative echogenicities of the two. Almost invariably, the tubal ring will be of a more prominent echogenicity. Of course, color Doppler or power Doppler imaging is even

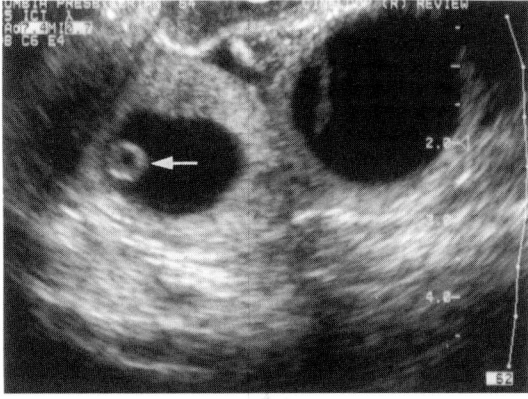

Figure 6 The side-by-side location of the hyperechoic tubal ring on the left side of the picture, containing the yolk sac (arrow) and the less echogenic thin-walled corpus luteum on the right. This was a live, tubal ectopic pregnancy of 7 postmenstrual weeks and 2 days

more helpful and will demonstrate conspicuously the more 'color-rich' corpus luteum. Needless to say, this is a gestalt approach and relies on the experience of the more sophisticated ultrasound users.

Another problem in finding an ectopic pregnancy in the adnexa arises in patients undergoing artificial reproductive technologies or simple hormonal superovulation. Besides the increased risk of ectopic pregnancy in these patients, dictating a much more labor-intensive sonographic work-up, there will be a large number of 'artificial' corpora lutea resembling the tubal ring of an ectopic pregnancy (Figure 8). To examine each of these structures presents a challenge to even the most experienced sonologist/sonographer.

Brown and Doubilet[53] analyzed the sonographic criteria available for the correct diagnosis of ectopic pregnancy. They proposed that, as the sonographic criteria for the diagnosis of ectopic pregnancy become less stringent, the sensitivity of making the diagnosis increases and the specificity decreases; the positive predictive value decreases and the negative predictive value increases. Table 2 demonstrates this.

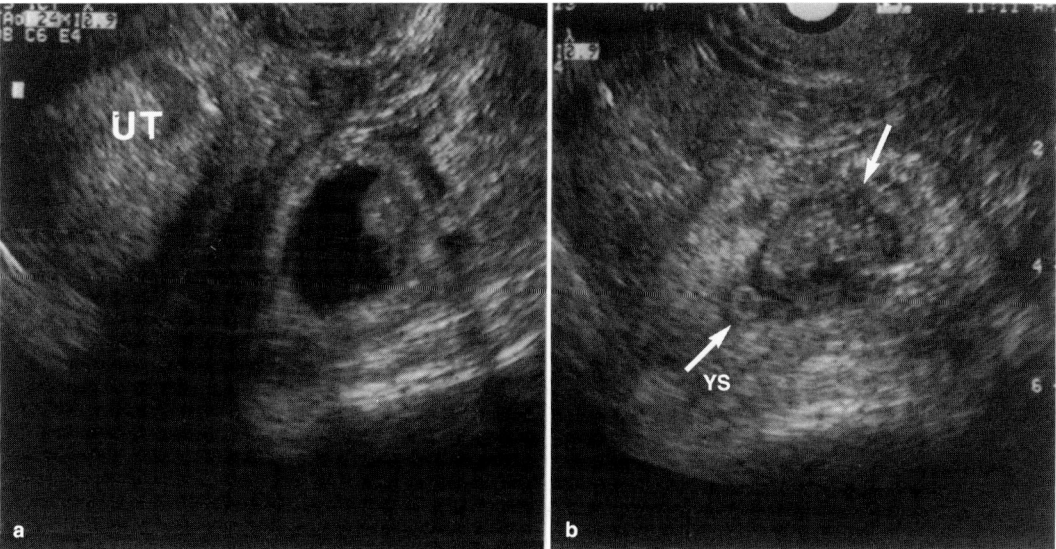

Figure 7 The embryonic and extraembryonic structures in a live, tubal ectopic pregnancy of 9 postmenstrual weeks. (a) 'Empty' uterus (UT) and left-sided tubal ring; (b) longitudinal section of the tubal ectopic pregnancy with the embryo (arrow) and yolk sac (YS)

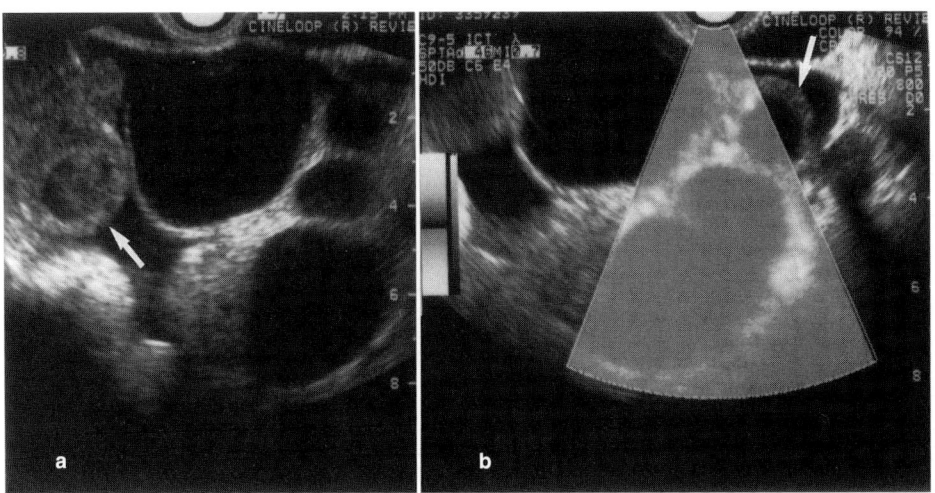

Figure 8 Illustration of the problem of detecting a tubal or ovarian pregnancy in a patient with hormone ovulation induction. (a) Gray-scale imaging showing the numerous ring-like structures in the left adnexa. (b) Even though the ring marked by an arrow raises the question of a 'tubal ring' of an ectopic pregnancy, all 'rings' were corpora lutea in this patient, who also had a normal intrauterine pregnancy of 6 postmenstrual weeks (power angiographic study)

Table 2 Performance characteristics of transvaginal sonographic criteria for diagnosis of ectopic pregnancy (data from reference 53)

Transvaginal sonography criterion*	Performance characteristics (%)			
	Sensitivity	Specificity	PPV	NPV
Adnexal embryo with heart beat	20.1	100	100	78.5
Adnexal mass containing yolk sac or embryo	36.1	100	100	82.2
Adnexal mass with echogenic rim ('tubal ring') or containing yolk sac or embryo	64.6	99.5	97.8	89.1
Any adnexal mass other than simple cyst or intraovarian lesion	84.4	98.9	96.3	94.8

PPV, positive predictive value; NPV, negative predictive value;
*based on average ectopic pregnancy prevalence rate of 25.5%

Several practical maneuvers should be mentioned which may be used to enhance the ability to arrive at the correct diagnosis. First is the use of the operator's abdominally placed second hand. In concert with the tip of the transvaginal probe used as an extension of an examining palpating finger, this enables movement of the structures to be examined into sight of the probe, and movement of others (e.g. bowel), interfering with the scan, out of sight. The second dynamic manoeuver is to test for pain by touching different structures under direct vision with the tip of the probe.

Cystic adnexal masses (ovarian cystadenoma, cystadenofibroma, endometrioma, teratoma) may raise differential diagnostic problems. So do pedunculated uterine fibroids and at times even perfectly round cross sections of bowel (which should be recognized in real time by its peristalsis) and various uterine malformations (bicornuate uteri, etc.).

The cul-de-sac

The sonographic examination of the cul-de-sac together with the clinical signs and symptoms will determine the urgency of the case almost regardless of the other sonographic findings (Figure 9). Fluid in the pelvis in a patient with the appropriate clinical

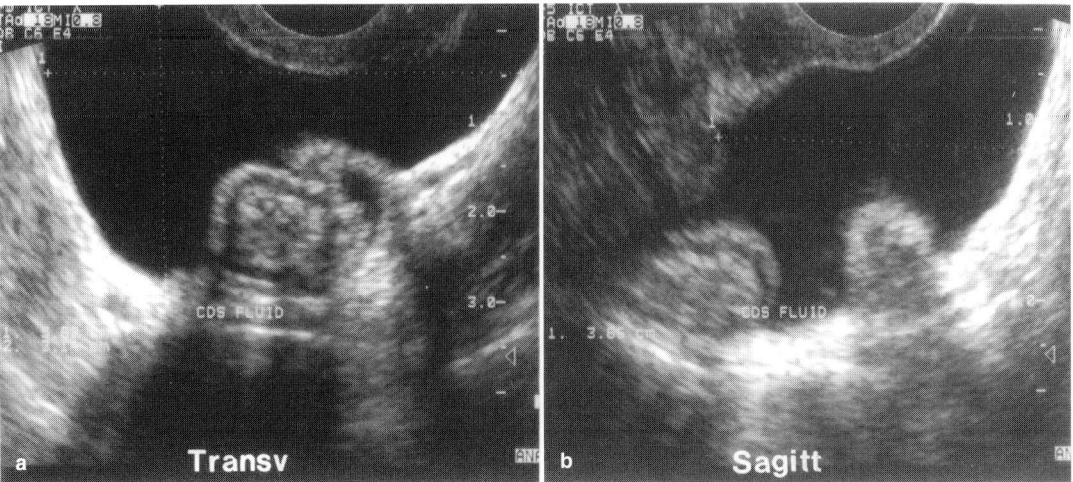

Figure 9 Cul-de-sac fluid is easy to visualize by transvaginal sonography. (a) Transverse section showing the fluid above the cross section of the rectum. The fluid measured 5.62×3.14 cm. (b) On the sagittal section, the depth of the fluid measured 3.86 cm. These measurements allow the estimation of the fluid volume in the pelvis, which in this case was about 44 ml (formula $(A \times B \times C) \times 0.523$)

history and a positive pregnancy test is a very strong indication of a ruptured or bleeding ectopic pregnancy such as a tubal abortion. Such a patient may need immediate attention. An exception may be a patient in whom hormonal superovulation was induced and previous scans revealed some pelvic fluid, explained as one of the consequences of ovarian hyperstimulation. If, on the other hand, there is no fluid in the cul-de-sac in a patient suspected of having an ectopic pregnancy, one can proceed to a more lengthy and more patient search. Also, no sonographic evaluation of a patient suspected of an ectopic pregnancy is complete without scanning the Morrison's space, between the liver and the right kidney (Figure 10a).

In teaching obstetrics and gynecology residents to perform TVS in the emergency suite, we always emphasize the point that a patient suspected of ectopic pregnancy in whom pelvic fluid was detected should not be discharged until a final diagnosis is established. Depending on the clinical status of the patient, this may be achieved by laparoscopy or by a second opinion rendered by an imaging specialist.

The literature reports that about 10–30% of patients with ectopic pregnancy demonstrate fluid in the cul-de-sac[49,54–57]. The diagnostic importance of sonolucent versus echogenic fluid containing particulate matter (blood?) will be touched upon later.

From a clinical point of view, there are several practical aspects of importance as to the presence or the absence of cul-de-sac fluid detected by TVS.

(1) The more fluid is seen, the higher the risk for finding a bleeding ectopic pregnancy.

(2) The chances of finding a ruptured and actively bleeding ectopic pregnancy or an actively bleeding tubal abortion are extremely low (almost zero) if no pelvic fluid is found.

(3) A large amount of fluid (in excess of 500 ml) will 'coat' the uterus from both sides and should even be visible by TAS in the Morrison's pouch between the liver and the right kidney (Figure 10b). One should not prolong the scanning time to establish the diagnosis of active bleeding by watching the increasing amount of fluid. TVS is not a replacement for regularly checking the vital signs of the patient.

(4) The most important statement about fluid in the cul-de-sac is the following: TVS is

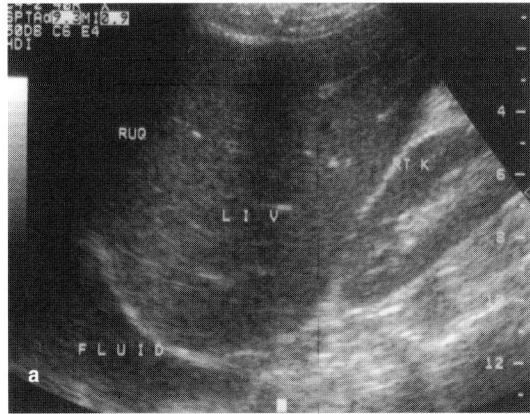

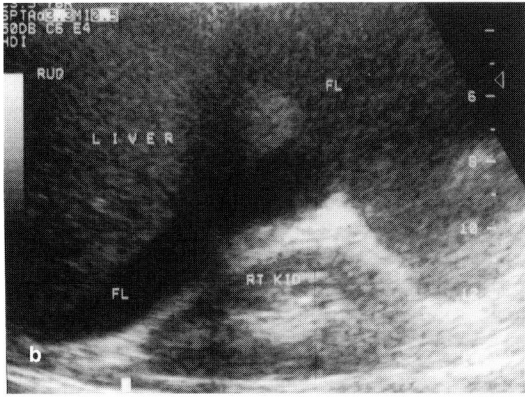

Figure 10 No sonographic evaluation for ectopic pregnancy is complete without scanning the Morrison's pouch, i.e. the space between the liver and the right kidney, along the anterior axillary line. (a) The normal appearance of the Morrison's pouch. No fluid is seen. (b) This picture shows fluid (FL) between the liver and right kidney. If such a picture is seen, one should assume that the amount of free fluid in the adnexa is over 500 ml

reliable enough to diagnose pelvic fluid; therefore, *culdocentesis is absolutely redundant.*

It is possible to evaluate the echogenicity of the pelvic fluid by gently touching and moving the fluid, at the same time slightly increasing the gains settings. The swirling motion of the particulate (cellular) matter of the fluid becomes evident. Typical echogenic fluid in the pelvis in a patient with clinical signs and symptoms of ectopic pregnancy is extremely unlikely to be other than blood. Echogenic fluid is more specific than sonolucent fluid, since it

correlates well with blood in the pelvis, which in turn is more likely to occur in extrauterine rather than intrauterine pregnancies[58,59]. Echogenic fluid, according to Nyberg and associates[58], increases the specificity of finding only a solid adnexal mass from 94 to 99%.

It is possible to estimate the approximate amount of pelvic fluid by simple gestalt; however, this requires experience. It seems more accurate to us to use the formula of volume = $(A \times B \times C) \times 0.523$, in which A, B and C represent the three dimensional measurements of the largest (and possibly only) pocket of pelvic fluid below the uterus. These can easily be measured on the transverse and sagittal images of the cul-de-sac fluid (Figure 9).

It seems extremely important (if possible) to differentiate sonographically between the bleeding of a tubal rupture and that of a tubal abortion. Tubal rupture is a dramatic occurrence accentuated by pain and deteriorating vital signs, in the presence of a low or significantly dropping hematocrit level. There is also a rapid increase in the amount of pelvic fluid. There is very little that TAS or TVS can add to the diagnosis in this patient. This patient should get swift surgical treatment.

However, the tubal abortion may present differently. It results from separation and expulsion of the products of conception through the fimbrial ostia into the pelvis. This tubal abortion may be associated at times with slow, and at other times with quite fast, bleeding into the pelvis. If there is a significant amount of bleeding, it is practically impossible to differentiate this from a ruptured ectopic pregnancy. If however, the amount of echogenic pelvic fluid is relatively small and stable in its quantity, and the patient's hematocrit and vital signs are stable, this patient may not need an invasive surgical approach. Such tubal abortion with minimal bleeding in a clinically stable patient, in spite of mild clinical symptoms of pain, may follow certain forms of non-surgical treatment such as simple follow-up, parenteral cytotoxic drugs (methotrexate, etoposide) and puncture injection of the ectopic gestation. In this case, close follow-up using TVS is imperative, to reassure both the patient and the doctor. The stable hematocrit and vital signs as well as a declining βhCG level are supporting factors in such cases. It is extremely important to understand that such a relatively silent tubal abortion does not represent the failure of the above-mentioned non-surgical treatment, unless significant and clinically recognizable bleeding takes place[60].

Other sites of implantation

About 5% of ectopic pregnancies implant in sites other than the tubes. At times these are more difficult to detect and some, owing to 'strategic' sites of implantation, may cause rupture, significant bleeding and higher morbidity and mortality than tubal gestations[61].

Cornual/interstitial pregnancy We acknowledge the controversy about the terms 'cervical' versus 'interstitial'. However, will deal with them as one sonographic entity. This ectopic pregnancy is located in the extreme cervical area of the uterus and at times it grows in the thinnest passage of the cervical area into the tube ('interstitial'). About 2% of all ectopic pregnancies are such. If left alone, these pregnancies will grow and rupture at seemingly late stages of development, causing significant bleeding and mortality[62]. Sonographically the cervical/interstitial pregnancy presents as a gestational sac containing embryonic/fetal and extraembryonic structures enveloped within a very thin (2–7 mm) myometrium[63–67] (Figure 11). The value of TVS in its detection is now unquestioned. It is necessary to demonstrate a lack of continuity of at least 1 cm between the endometrial echogenic line and the hyperechoic trophoblastic ring of the ectopic pregnancy. A special sonographic sign, the 'endometrial line', was proposed by Ackerman and colleagues[67]; this consists of the empty endometrial cavity line pointing directly towards the pregnancy in the cornual position.

Most cornual/interstitial ectopic pregnancies are treated by laparotomy and various surgical procedures (excision, suturing, etc.) in the involved cornual area of the uterus. Lately,

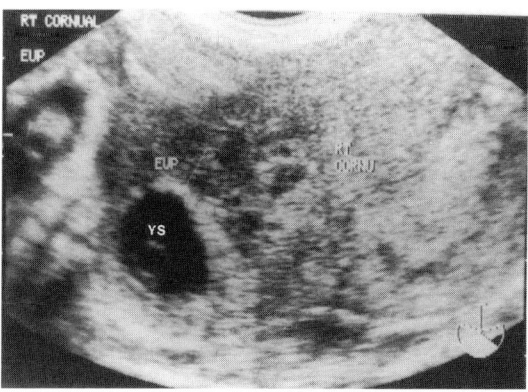

Figure 11 Right cornual ectopic pregnancy of 6 postmenstrual weeks showing the yolk sac (YS) in the chorionic sac surrounded by a very thin myometrial layer

TVS puncture and even conservative medical treatments of such ectopic pregnancies have been advocated[65,68–70]. Expectant management has also been described[65,71].

At times, it is difficult to differentiate a normal IUP in one of the horns of a bicornuate uterus (Figure 12) from a true cornual pregnancy.

Another variant of cervical/interstitial pregnancy is that found in a rudimentary horn. This is a pregnancy that is implanted in a blind horn of a bicornuate uterus with no possibility to 'drain' or to be extracted without surgery. Its appearance resembles that of a cornual pregnancy. The exact sonographic diagnosis is difficult to make; however, pre-rupture sonodiagnosis of such an ectopic pregnancy has been reported[72].

Cervical pregnancy Luckily, this type of ectopic pregnancy is quite rare. Owing to its potentially heavy blood loss, its diagnosis is complicated to manage. By TVS, its diagnosis is extremely simple (Figure 13). We stress again that the cervix is the first structure to look at, every time that TVS is performed. A stationary chorionic sac with fetal heart beats within fetal structures close to the external cervical os and at the level of or below the imaginary line between the two uterine arteries (easily seen with color Doppler) are prerequisites for the sonographic diagnosis. If a

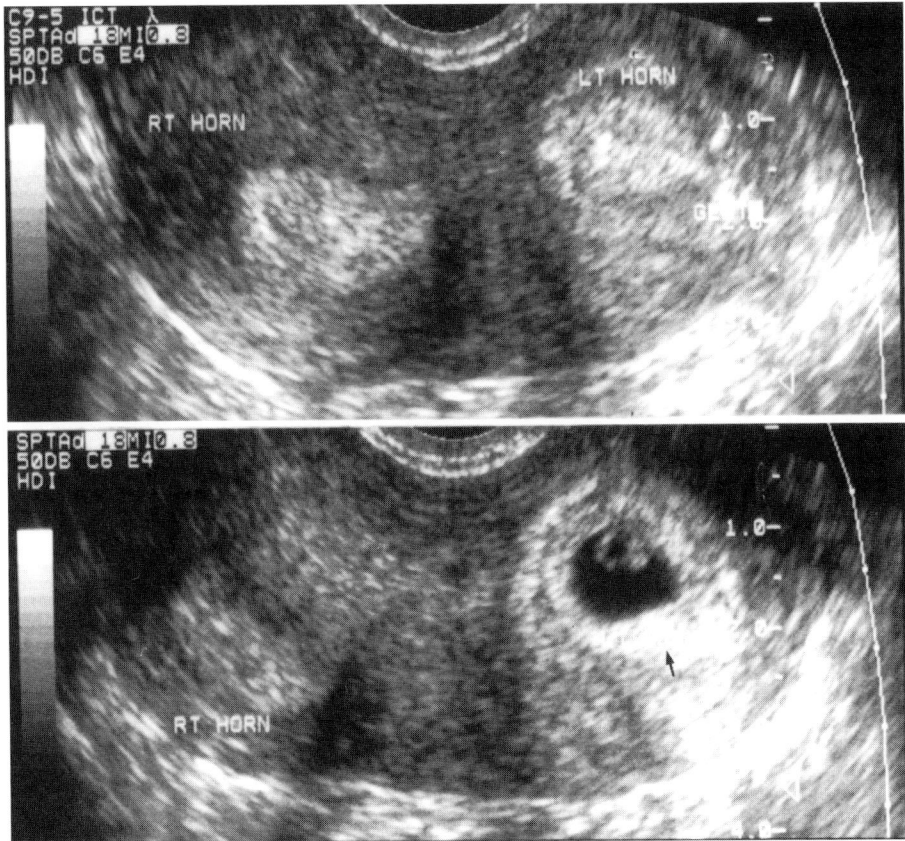

Figure 12 A normal, live, intrauterine pregnancy of 5 postmenstrual weeks and 5 days, as shown in the left horn of a bicornuate uterus. Upper panel: a higher horizontal section showing the two cavities highlighted by the hyperechoic decidua. Lower panel: the somewhat lower horizontal section passes through the decidua of the right horn and the intrauterine pregnancy in the left horn (arrow, the sac)

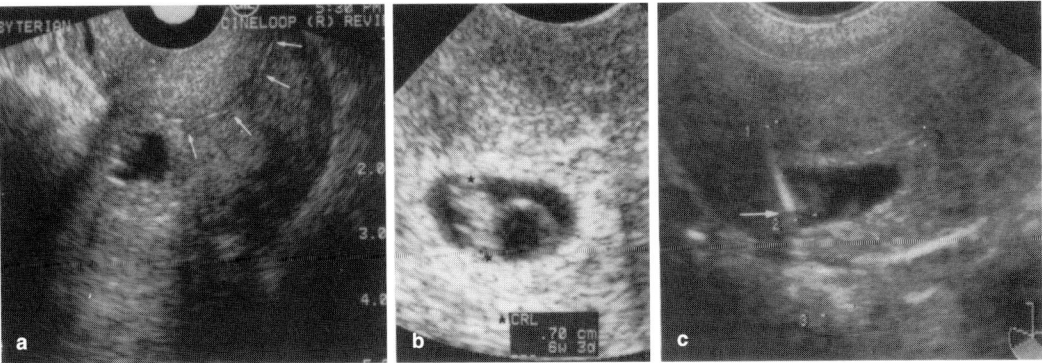

Figure 13 Cervical pregnancy at 6 postmenstrual weeks and 3 days. (a) Sagittal section. The distal part of the cervical canal is marked by small arrows. (b) The 0.7-cm crown–rump length of the embryo and the adjacent yolk sac. (c) This cervical pregnancy was injected with methotrexate. The tip of the needle is marked by an arrow

gestational sac with or without embryonic/fetal structures is seen within the cervix, but *it does not contain heart beats*, it should not be diagnosed as a cervical pregnancy. This rather represents products of conception 'running' through the cervical canal, on their way out, usually causing severe pain. A true live cervical pregnancy is painless. An intact gestational sac passing through the cervical canal will change its position in the cervical canal if it is observed over time. The true cervical pregnancy will remain stationary.

Color Doppler studies were suggested by our group[73]. These studies are geared towards an exact localization of the gestational sac. If the sac containing a live gestation is found at or below the level of the two uterine arteries (which in turn mark the level of the internal os), the pregnancy should be considered a cervical pregnancy.

Ovarian pregnancy The sonographic diagnosis of ovarian pregnancy is extremely difficult to establish. Similarly to the cervical ectopic pregnancy, ovarian pregnancy is also rare. Grimes and colleagues[74] calculated that the ratio of ovarian/tubal pregnancy was approximately 1 in 34 cases.

The sonographic diagnosis is based upon the findings of a hyperechoic trophoblastic ring detected within ovarian tissue, and the fact that it is impossible to separate the ectopic gestational sac from the ovary by both transabdominal pressure from the examiner's one hand and the transvaginal ultrasound probe (Figure 14). In spite of the diagnostic difficulties, transabdominal ultrasound detection of ovarian pregnancy has been published in the literature[75,76]. However, it seems that the primary diagnostic tool to diagnose an ovarian pregnancy is transvaginal sonography[73,77,78].

Abdominal pregnancy Ultrasound seems to be the most valuable diagnostic tool to localize this rare type of ectopic pregnancy. If the fertilized egg implants directly onto the peritoneal surface of the abdominal cavity, it is called primary abdominal pregnancy. If, however, an early tubal pregnancy dislodges and 'aborts' into the pelvis, adhering to the

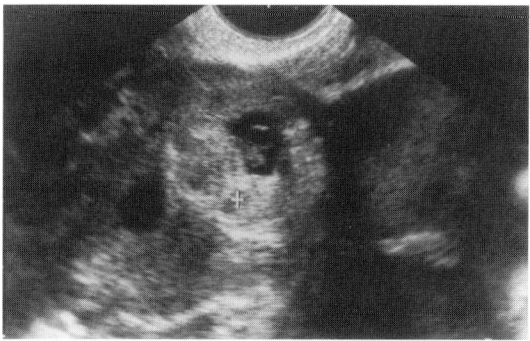

Figure 14 A live ovarian pregnancy of 6 postmenstrual weeks and 2 days. The patient underwent laparoscopic surgery. The diagnosis was confirmed by histology

peritoneal surface, it is termed secondary abdominal pregnancy through secondary nidation[79]. Regardless of the above-mentioned subdivision, the sonographic picture of the abdominal pregnancy is no different from that of any other ectopic pregnancy, i.e. showing a hyperechoic, ectopic gestational sac containing embryonic/fetal structures and extraembryonic structures with or without an active heart beat. At times, such a gestation may achieve a relatively advanced gestational age[80]. Oligohydramnios is the rule and there is no uterine mantle around the fetus[80,81].

Heterotopic pregnancy The term 'heterotopic pregnancy' is reserved for a simultaneously present intra- and extrauterine pregnancy, regardless of the location of the ectopic gestation (Figure 15). Traditionally, such combinations of pregnancies are rare and, in a general population not undergoing infertility treatments or artificial reproductive manipulations, the rate of 1 in 30 000 pregnancies is probably not exaggerated[82]. However, with the increase of infertility treatment rendered to patients with problems conceiving, the rate of heterotopic pregnancies has increased significantly, reaching 1 in 3000–4000[82–84].

The diagnosis can reliably be made by TAS and by TVS[85]. It should be remembered at all times, when dealing with a patient who has undergone treatment by assisted reproductive technologies, that these patients are at high risk for ectopic and for heterotopic

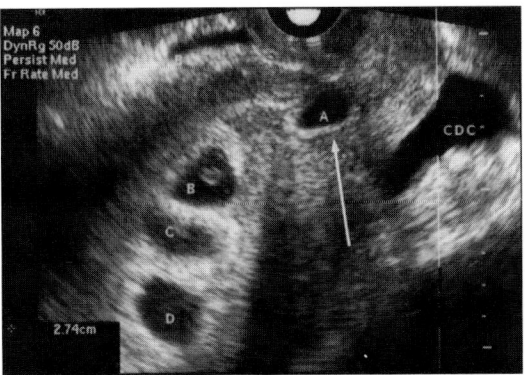

Figure 15 Heterotopic pregnancy. The quintuplet pregnancy (only four sacs shown on this plane) consisted of four intrauterine and one cervical (A) pregnancies. The sac with the embryo in the cervical position was injected at 7 postmenstrual weeks using the automated puncture device via the transvaginal route with potassium chloride. The other four fetuses were not reduced, at the request of the patient

pregnancies. There is a presence of multiple typical or atypical corpora lutea in patients with hormonal hyperstimulation with or without egg retrievals. The sonographic appearance of these bizarrely shaped corpora lutea present a difficult task for the sonographer/sonologist by masking an ectopic pregnancy. This task of finding a heterotopic pregnancy may further be complicated by the false sense of security produced by detecting an intrauterine pregnancy. The contribution of TVS in establishing the diagnosis of heterotopic pregnancy is beyond question. However, we cannot overemphasize the importance of a high degree of suspicion for heterotopic pregnancy in the high-risk population as part of the diagnostic process.

Color Doppler studies in ectopic pregnancies

The overwhelming majority of, if not all, ectopic pregnancies can be diagnosed by traditional gray-scale TVS. This fact is extremely important, since it will reassure those who own or operate only a good, reliable gray-scale ultrasound machine, and do not (yet) have color ultrasound or do not intend to buy such a machine in the very near future. This statement may not hold true if one regards the latest development in color Doppler studies, i.e. the power Doppler angiographic capability that was added in the last several years to the existing software packages of the machines. These issues will be touched upon later.

The task of Doppler equipment is to find the blood vessels around the trophoblastic ring and evaluate the flow profile with different quantitative or qualitative measurements. The physiological basis of the changes that may be observed in the case of ectopic pregnancy are those aimed at increasing the blood flow to the implanting blastocyst, regardless of whether it is implanted in the uterus or in an ectopic location. The result of this is a constantly decreasing impedance, with increasing velocity of flow to the developing gestation. As in the increased blood supply to the normal injured pregnancy, physiological vascular changes occur around any ectopic implantation with its surrounding ectopic trophoblast and ectopic placenta.

Even if we suspect an ectopic pregnancy implanted outside the uterine cavity, we should scan the endometrium around the cavity. Here a negative finding, i.e. the lack of a typical finding of a normally implanted pregnancy, may be of significance. A swollen and hyperechoic decidua and eventual pseudogestational sac will not demonstrate the typical and abundant periplacental and placental trophoblastic flow as perceived in a normal intrauterine gestation. It has been suggested that measuring velocities below 21 cm/s can be diagnostic for a pseudogestational sac and successfully rule out trophoblastic flow to a normal intrauterine pregnancy[86].

The second important area to concentrate on is the ovaries. First, the corpus luteum should be localized by traditional gray-scale scanning. Color Doppler studies will then be able to reveal the typical ring-like, color-rich, low-resistance, high-velocity flow (Figure 16).

If one finds the corpus luteum, one may make two assumptions. The first is that there may be more chances to help locate the expected ectopic pregnancy on the same side. Eighty-six per cent of the ectopic pregnancies were found to be on the same side of the corpus luteum[52]. The second assumption will hold up only in cases in which no hormonal superovulation took place. Under such an assumption, if a second color ring is found, this may be consistent with an abundant blood supply of the tubal ring (i.e. an ectopic/tubal pregnancy). It is our experience that one should not rely only upon measuring the resistance and the velocity of the flow, since the flow to both the corpus luteum and to any ectopic pregnancy (tubal, cornual or other) will be low and therefore entirely non-discriminatory.

Lastly, it is important to describe the findings of the color Doppler studies around or within the ectopic pregnancy itself. Color should be applied whenever a finding is in doubt and a suspicion of an ectopic pregnancy exists.

Lately, when the color power angiographic modality was added to the currently existing traditional color Doppler studies, we found that this modality offered valuable information (Figure 17). It usually provides, very quickly, a quite impressive picture, which consists of the sum of the absolute blood flow around a corpus luteum or an ectopic pregnancy. To remind the reader, the power amplitude modality enables us to observe the blood flow in a nondirectional manner, i.e. blood flow in every single vessel, regardless of its direction of flow and even sometimes of the lowest velocity, will show up assigned a single color. This provides a general and sensitive view of the vascularity around the targeted area[87].

There is, however, an important observation that should be used when applying color Doppler studies to an area that is suspected of containing an ectopic pregnancy. Ectopic pregnancies with a live embryo/fetus have higher βhCG levels and these will also demonstrate a higher quantity of color. This also will demonstrate what has been termed a 'hot flow pattern' in addition to a high diastolic flow, as opposed to ectopic pregnancies in which there is a long-standing embryonic demise in which less flow, therefore less color, will be seen[52]. We also found the color Doppler studies important in the follow-up of different kinds of non-live ectopic pregnancies managed expectantly or after puncture injections (Figure 18).

After a review of the literature and on the basis of our personal experience, it is clear that color Doppler studies are a convenient complement to the high-frequency transvaginal sonographic scanning modality in the diagnosis of ectopic pregnancies. As far as we are concerned, the diagnoses are facilitated and made more reliably, therefore it is reasonable to say that, even though color Doppler increases the diagnostic capabilities marginally, the diagnostic process is shortened significantly. The interested reader is referred to the literature to obtain additional and more detailed information[86-95].

TREATMENT OF THE ECTOPIC PREGNANCY

We here discuss some of the issues related to the treatment of the ectopic pregnancy, concentrating on those treatment modalities that rely heavily upon the use of ultrasound.

As stated before, ultrasonography, but mainly TVS, is found in every unit where diagnosis and treatment of each form of ectopic pregnancy is performed. The first-line diagnostic tool in the short- or long-term follow-up of the treated ectopic pregnancy is indeed TVS. Regardless of the treatment modality (i.e. surgical, medical, or puncture injection) of any kind of ectopic pregnancy, TVS will furnish the relevant information crucial to the subsequent management of the patients.

The role of TVS in patients with ectopic pregnancy treated with methotrexate has been evaluated by several authors[96-104]. It was stated that this is a reasonable treatment, but one has

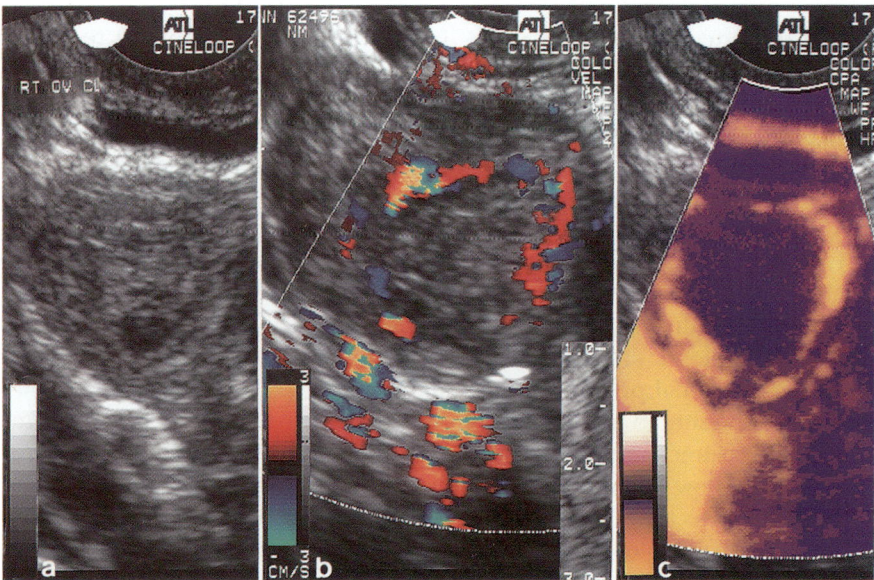

Figure 16 Scanning the corpus luteum in pregnancy. (a) Gray-scale scanning may overlook the almost uniformly echogenic corpus luteum (probably filled with blood clots). (b) Conventional color Doppler study showing the vascular ring. (c) Power color angiography of the corpus luteum, clearly showing its shape and confirming the diagnosis

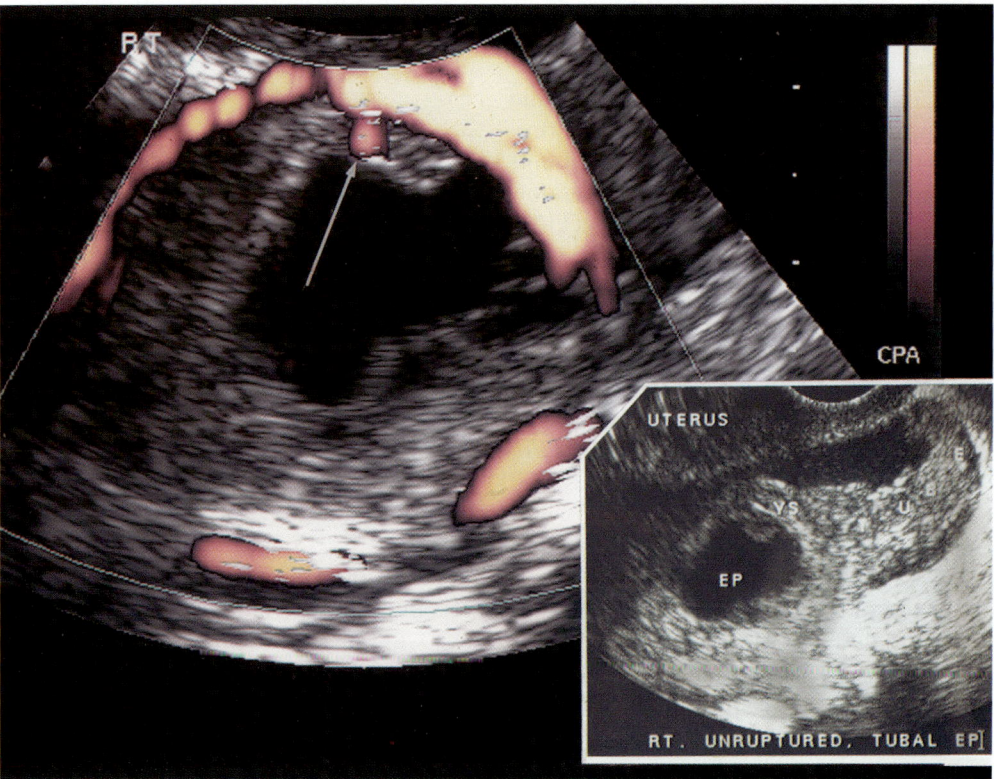

Figure 17 Power color angiographic study of a non-ruptured right tubal ectopic pregnancy. Note the vascular ring around the wall of the tube. Inset: the gray-scale image of the ectopic pregnancy

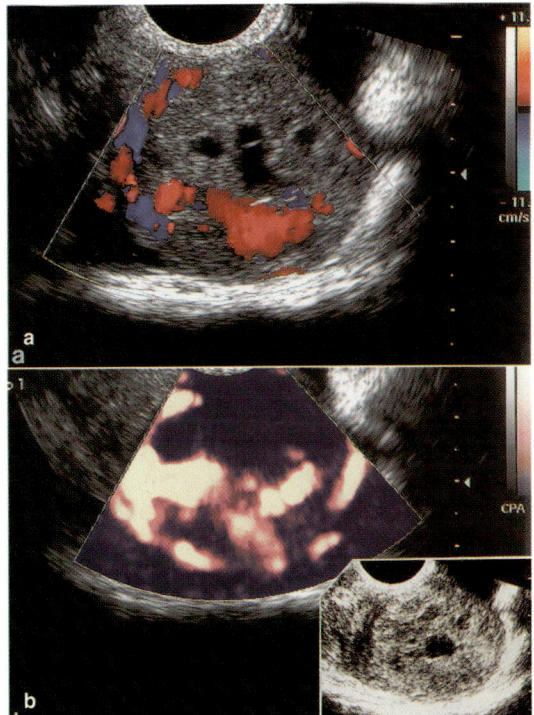

Figure 18 Non-live, right cornual ectopic pregnancy at 10 postmenstrual weeks, managed expectantly with several weekly follow-up scans. (a) Conventional color Doppler scan, showing the fluid around the lesion with features typical of flow seen surrounding gestational sacs containing an early fetal demise. (b) The right lower corner of this picture shows the gray-scale image of this cornual pregnancy. Using the power color angiographic feature of the machine, the intensive flow around the lesion becomes obvious. This flow diminished with time, after the acute stage of the disease was over

to understand the changing sonographic picture of the affected adnexal region as a result of such medical treatment.

It is less known that all of the existing forms of ectopic pregnancy, including heterotopic pregnancies, can be treated by sonographically directed puncture and injection of methotrexate or potassium chloride as the case may indicate. Historically, the first ectopic pregnancies injected were tubal gestations[105–123], followed by TVS-directed injection of cornual pregnancies[65,66] and finally the cervical pregnancies[73] and heterotopic pregnancies[85].

If the success rates of these puncture and injection-treated ectopic gestations are analyzed, it should be remembered that the reports are to be read carefully and critically. Results may vary according to patient selection, puncture route, needle gauge used, viability of the ectopic pregnancy (live versus non-live), operator experience and gestational age at the time of puncture. At times, additional parenteral methotrexate is (or was) used, which may further increase the variation in the reported results.

The overall results in successfully treating tubal ectopic pregnancies is about 75%. The success rates of puncture injections of cornual and cervical pregnancies treated up to or before 9 postmenstrual weeks are even higher.

With the use of the automated spring-loaded puncture device of Labotect (Göttingen, Germany), it is possible to achieve high accuracy in the placement of relatively thin needles. Our group has used this device successfully for the past 10 years. Our list of prerequisites for considering puncture injection treatment for any ectopic or heterotopic pregnancy is as follows.

(1) A compliant, stable asymptomatic patient capable of understanding the advantages and disadvantages as well as the possible complications of the procedure.

(2) A live, unruptured ectopic pregnancy and no active bleeding.

(3) A lesion of 4 cm or less.

(4) A pregnancy aged 8.5–9 postmenstrual weeks or less.

(5) The possibility of using the automated spring-loaded Labotect puncture device.

(6) A signed form, approved by the review board, granting informed consent.

Those engaging in such puncture procedures for the ectopic pregnancy should be familiar with several issues. There is quite a slow return of the hCG levels to normal. This may take several weeks, during which some pain and lower abdominal cramping may occur. In the specific cases of injected tubal ectopic pregnancies, this may be caused by the possible tubal abortion into the pelvis, with various amounts of bleeding[60]. These are usually not profuse bleedings. The patient's vital signs and hemoglobin levels as well as the amount of blood (fluid) visualized in the cul-de-sac by TVS should be checked before unnecessary surgical procedures are undertaken. Occurrences of pelvic pain may reveal themselves even several days after the puncture procedure.

Furthermore, the size of the injected region (tube, cornual area, cervix) may slowly increase for 1 or 2 weeks after the injection, before it slowly returns to the pre-injection size and then starts shrinking. Color flow studies will also reveal an increased quantity of color, owing to the abundant vascularity and the dilated venous spaces.

Our opinion is that puncture injections are a valid and reasonable alternative to a traditional surgical approach to the treatment. This is true if careful patient selection is kept in mind. Tubal pregnancies have so far benefited only in well-selected cases; however, we predict that the puncture injection treatment alternative for cornual and for cervical – and definitely for heterotopic – pregnancies has much to offer patients in terms of a less invasive procedure. This puncture procedure may replace and avoid a more complication-ridden and at times extremely 'bloody' surgical treatment. It may save patients a hysterectomy or future Cesarean sections.

CONCLUSIONS

The introduction of hCG testing and TVS has changed the diagnostic approach to the patient suspected of ectopic pregnancy. All of these changes occurred in the past decade. The real breakthrough of an early and accurate detection of the disease became almost generally accepted, and has been made available to the smallest medical centers, hospitals and even private offices. If, for some reason, this has not yet happened in your hospital/office, we advise considering the introduction of the TVS technique for work-up of the patient suspected of ectopic pregnancy, as soon as possible. Operating a simple device such as a vaginal ultrasound probe will not only make the diagnoses fast and reliable, but also save lives.

The only correct way to arrive at the diagnosis and the appropriate management plan is to combine the history, clinical science and symptoms, and the readily available transvaginal sonographic picture, as well as the level or a series of levels of hCG testing. The importance of a conscientious and extremely systematic scanning routine to find or rule out an ectopic pregnancy cannot be overstated. A transvaginal sonogram enables the selection of the adequate and proper as well as the least invasive treatment for expectant management of ectopic pregnancies. The reader should realize that TVS is important not only in diagnosing the ectopic pregnancy, but also in directing treatment by puncture injection of some selected or 'exotic' (i.e. heterotopic) cases of ectopic gestation. We are sure that shortening the diagnostic process is advantageous not only to the clinician but also to the patient.

References

1. Westrom, L. (1975). Effect of acute pelvic inflammatory disease on fertility. *Am. J. Obstet Gynecol.*, **121**, 707–13
2. Lavy, G., Diamond, M. P. and DeCherney, A. H. (1987). Ectopic pregnancy: its relationship to tubal reconstructive surgery. *Fertil. Steril.*, **47**, 543–56
3. Green, J. L. (1970). A 21-year survey of 654 ectopic pregnancies. *Am. J. Obstet. Gynecol.*, **106**, 1004–10

4. Corson, S. K. and Batzer, F. R. (1986). Ectopic pregnancy: a review of the etiologic factors. *J. Reprod. Med.*, **31**, 78–85

5. Sopelak, V. M. and Bates, G. B. (1987). Role of transmigration and abnormal embryogenesis in ectopic pregnancy. *Clin. Obstet. Gynecol.*, **30**, 210–16

6. Marchbanks, P. A., Annegers, J. F., Coulam, C. B. *et al.* (1988). Risk factors of ectopic pregnancy. A population based study. *J. Am. Med. Assoc.*, **259**, 1923–7

7. Davis, M. R. (1986). Recurrent ectopic pregnancy after tubal sterilization. *Obstet. Gynecol.*, **68**, 44S–45S

8. DeStefano, F., Peterson, H. B., Layde, P. M. and Rubin, G. L. (1982). Risk of ectopic pregnancy following tubal sterilization. *Obstet. Gynecol.*, **60**, 326–30

9. McCausland, A. (1980). High rate of ectopic pregnancy following laparoscopic tubal coagulation failures. *Am. J. Obstet. Gynecol.*, **136**, 97–101

10. Elias, S., LeBeau, M., Simpson, J. L., *et al.* (1981). Chromosome analysis of ectopic human conceptuses. *Am. J. Obstet. Gynecol.*, **141**, 698–703

11. Poland, B. J., Dill, F. J. and Styblo, C. (1976). Embryonic development in ectopic human pregnancy. *Teratology*, **14**, 315–21

12. Hodgson, B. J. and Talo, A. (1978). Spike bursts in rabbit oviduct: effects of estrogen and progesterone. *Am. J. Physiol.*, **234**, E439–43

13. Pulkkinen, M. O. and Talo, A. (1987). Tubal physiologic consideration in ectopic pregnancy. *Clin. Obstet. Gynecol.*, **30**, 164–72

14. Morris, J. M. and Wagnen, G. (1973). The use of postovulatory estrogens to prevent implantation. *Am. J. Obstet. Gynecol.*, **115**, 101–6

15. Gemzell, C., Guillome, J. and Wang, C. F. (1982). Ectopic pregnancy following treatment with human gonadotropins. *Am. J. Obstet. Gynecol.*, **143**, 761–5

16. Berry, S. M., Coulam, C. B., Hill, L. M., *et al.* (1985). Evidence of contralateral ovulation in ectopic pregnancy. *J. Ultrasound Med.*, **4**, 293–5

17. Walters, M. D., Eddy, C. and Pauerstein, C. J. (1987). The contralateral corpus luteum and tubal pregnancy. *Obstet. Gynecol.*, **70**, 823–6

18. Iffy, L. (1963). The role of premenstrual, post mid-cycle conception in the aetiology of ectopic gestation. *J. Obstet. Gynaecol. Br. Commonw.*, **70**, 966–71

19. Iffy, L. (1965). Embryological studies of time of conception in ectopic pregnancy and first trimester abortion. *Obstet. Gynecol.*, **26**, 490–8

20. Stoval, T. G. and Ling, F. W. (1933). *Extrauterine Pregnancy: Clinical Diagnosis and Management*, pp. 27–135. (New York: McGraw-Hill)

21. Timor-Tritsch, I. E., Greenridge, S., Admon, D. and Reuss, L. M. (1992). Emergency room use of transvaginal ultrasonography by obstetrics and gynecology residents. *Am. J. Obstet. Gynecol.*, **166**, 866–72

22. Kadar, N., DeVore, G. and Romero, R. (1981). Discriminatory hCG zone. Its use in sonographic evaluation for ectopic pregnancy. *Obstet. Gynecol.*, **58**, 156–61

23. Nyberg, D. A., Filly, R. A., Mahoney, B. S., *et al.* (1985). Early gestation: correlation of hCG levels and sonographic identification. *Am. J. Roentgenol.*, **144**, 951–4

24. Timor-Tritsch, I. E., Rottem, S. and Thaler, I. (1988). Review of transvaginal ultrasonography: description with clinical application. *Ultrasound Q.*, **6**, 1–32

25. Peisner, D. B., Timor-Tritsch, I. E., The discriminatory zone of β-hCG for vaginal probes. *J. Clin. Ultrasound*, **18**, 280–5

26. Fossum, G. T., Dvajan, V. and Kletzky, D. A. (1988). Early detection of pregnancy with transvaginal ultrasound. *Fertil. Steril.*, **49**, 788–91

27. Bernascheck, G., Ruaelstorfer, R. and Csaicsich, P. (1988). Vaginal sonography versus serum human chorionic gonadotropin in early detection of pregnancy. *Am. J. Obstet. Gynecol.*, **158**, 608–12

28. Matthews, C. P., Coulson, P. B. and Wild, R. A. (1986). Serum progesterone levels as an aid in the diagnosis of ectopic pregnancy. *Obstet. Gynecol.*, **68**, 390–4

29. Yeko, T. R., Gorrill, M. J., Hughes, L. H., *et al.* Timely diagnosis of early ectopic pregnancy using a single blood progesterone measurement. *Fertil. Steril.*, **48**, 1048–50

30. Buck, R. H., Joubert, S. M. and Normal, R. J. (1988). Serum progesterone in the diagnosis of ectopic pregnancy: a valuable test? *Fertil. Steril.*, **50**, 752–5

31. Gelder, M. S., Boots, L. R. and Younger, J. B. (1991). Use of a single random serum progesterone value as a diagnostic aid for ectopic pregnancy. *Fertil. Steril.*, **55**, 497–500

32. Stovall, T. G., Ling, F. W., Andersen, R. N. and Buster, J. E. (1992). Improved sensitivity and specificity of a single measurement of serum progesterone over serial quantitative beta-human chorionic gonadotropin in screening for ectopic pregnancy. *Hum. Reprod.*, **7**, 723–5

33. Stovall, T. G., Ling, F. W., Cope, B. J. and Buster, J. E. (1989). Preventing ruptured ectopic pregnancy with a single serum progesterone. *Am. J. Obstet. Gynecol.*, **160**, 1425–8

34. Stovall, T. G., Kellerman, A. L., Ling, F. W. and Buster, J. E. (1990). Emergency department

diagnosis of ectopic pregnancy. *Ann. Emerg. Med.*, **19**, 1098

35. Stovall, T. G., Ling, F. W., Carson, S. A. and Buster, J. E. (1992). Serum progesterone and uterine curettage in differential diagnosis of ectopic pregnancy. *Fertil. Steril.*, **57**, 456–7

36. Vermesh, M., Gvaczykowsky, J. W. and Sauer, M. V. (1990). Reevaluation of the culdocentesis in the management of ectopic pregnancy. *Am. J. Obstet. Gynecol.*, **162**, 411–13

37. Timor-Tritsch, I. E. and Rottem, S. (1987). Transvaginal sonographic study of the Fallopian tube. *Gynecol. Obstet.*, **70**, 424–8

38. deCrespigny, I. C. (1988). Demonstration of ectopic pregnancy by transvaginal ultrasound. *Br. J. Obstet. Gynaecol.*, **95**, 1253–6

39. Timor-Tritsch, I. E., Yeh, M. N., Peisner, D. B., *et al.* (1989). The use of transvaginal ultrasonography in the diagnosis of ectopic pregnancy. *Am. J. Obstet. Gynecol.*, **161**, 157–61

40. Cacciatore, B., Stenman, U.-H. and Ylostalo, P. (1989). Comparison of abdominal and vaginal sonography in suspected ectopic pregnancy. *Obstet. Gynecol.*, **73**, 770–4

41. Stiller, R. J., de Regt, R. H. and Blair, E. (1989). Transvaginal ultrasonography in patients at risk for ectopic pregnancy. *Am. J. Obstet. Gynecol.*, **161**, 930–3

42. Bateman, B. G., Nunley, W. C., Kolp, L. A., *et al.* (1990). Vaginal sonography findings and hCG dynamics of early intrauterine and tubal pregnancies. *Obstet. Gynecol.*, **75**, 421–7

43. Bohm-Velez, M., Mendelson, E. B. and Freimanis, M. G. (1990). Transvaginal sonography in evaluating ectopic pregnancy. *Semin. Ultrasound CT MR*, **11**, 44–58

44. Pellerito, J. S. and Taylor, K. J. W. (1994). Ectopic pregnancy. In Copel, J. A. and Reed, K. L. (eds.) *Doppler Ultrasound in Obstetrics and Gynecology*, p. 41. (New York: Raven Press)

45. Turetsky, D. B., Alexander, A. A. and Linden, S. S. (1991). Pseudogestational sac or ectopic pregnancy stimulating intrauterine pregnancy with transvaginal sonography. *J. Clin. Ultrasound*, **19**, 120–3

46. Ackerman, T. E., Levi, C. S., Lyons, E. A., Dashefsky, S. M., Lindsay, D. J. and Holt, S. C. (1993). Decidual cyst: endovaginal sonographic sign of ectopic pregnancy. *Radiology*, **189**, 727–31

47. Timor-Tritsch, I. E., Yeh, M. N., Peisner, D. B., Lesser, K. B. and Slavik, T. A. (1989). The use of transvaginal ultrasonography in the diagnosis of ectopic pregnancy. *Am. J. Obstet. Gynecol.*, **161**, 157–61

48. Cacciatore, B., Stenman, U.-H. and Ylostalo, P. (1989). Comparison of abdominal and vaginal sonography in suspected ectopic pregnancy. *Obstet. Gynecol.*, **73**, 770–4

49. Stiller, R. J., de Regt, R. H. and Blair, E. (1989). Transvaginal ultrasonography in patients at risk for ectopic pregnancy. *Am. J. Obstet. Gynecol.*, **161**, 930–3

50. Warren, W. B., Timor-Tritsch, I. E., Peisner, D. B., Raju, S. and Rosen, M. G. (1989). Dating of the early pregnancy by sequential appearance of embryonic structures. *Am. J. Obstet. Gynecol.*, **161**, 747–53

51. Timor-Tritsch, I. E., Warren, W. B., Peisner, D. B. and Pirrone, E. (1989). First trimester midgut herniation: a high frequency transvaginal sonographic study. *Am. J. Obstet. Gynecol.*, **161**, 831–3

52. Pellerito, J. S., Taylor, K. J. W., Quedens-Case, C., *et al.* (1992). Ectopic pregnancy: evaluation with endovaginal color flow imaging. *Radiology*, **183**, 407–11

53. Brown, D. L. and Doubilet, P. M. (1994). Transvaginal sonography for diagnosing ectopic pregnancy: positivity criteria and performance characteristics. *J. Ultrasound Med.*, **13**, 259–66

54. Romero, R., Copel, J. A., Kadar, N., *et al.* (1985). Value of culdocentesis in the diagnosis of ectopic pregnancy. *Obstet. Gynecol.*, **65**, 319–22

55. Fleischer, A. C., Pennell, R. G., McKee, M. S., *et al.* (1990). Ectopic pregnancy: features at transvaginal sonography. *Radiology*, **174**, 375–8

56. Timor-Tritsch, I. E., Peisner, D. B. and Monteagudo, A. (1991). Transvaginal sonography in the diagnosis of ectopic pregnancy. In Grunfeld, L. (ed.) *Ultrasonography in Reproductive Medicine. Infertil. Reprod. Med. Clin. North Am.*, **2**, 727–39

57. Rottem, S., Thaler, I. and Timor-Tritsch, I. E. (1991). Classification of tubal gestation by transvaginal sonography. *Ultrasound Obstet. Gynecol.*, **1**, 197–201

58. Nyberg, D. A., Hughes, M. P., Mack, L. A. and Wang, K. Y. (1991). Extrauterine findings of ectopic pregnancy of transvaginal US: importance of echogenic fluid. *Radiology*, **178**, 823–6

59. Jeffrey, R. B. and Laing, F. C. (1982). Echogenic clot: a useful sign of pelvic hemoperitoneum. *Radiology*, **145**, 139–41

60. Carson, S. A. and Buster, J. F. (1993). Ectopic pregnancy. *N. Engl. J. Med.*, **329**, 1174–81

61. Bayless, R. B. (1987). Nontubal ectopic pregnancy. *Clin. Obstet. Gynecol.*, **30**, 191–9

62. Dorfman, S. F., Grimes, D. A., Cates, W. Jr, *et al.* (1984). Ectopic pregnancy mortality. United States, 1979 to 1980: clinical aspects. *Obstet. Gynecol.*, **64**, 386–90

63. Jafri, S. Z., Loginsky, S. J., Bouffard, J. A. and Selis, J. E. (1987). Sonographic detection of

interstitial pregnancy. *J. Clin. Ultrasound*, **15**, 253–7

64. Sherer, D. M., Allen, T., Singh, G. S. and Woods, J. R. Jr. (1990). Transvaginal sonographic diagnosis of an unruptured interstitial pregnancy. *J. Clin. Ultrasound*, **18**, 582–5

65. Timor-Tritsch, I. E., Monteagudo, A., Matera, C. and Veit, C. R. (1992). Sonographic evaluation of cornual pregnancies treated without surgery. *Obstet. Gynecol.*, **79**, 1044–9

66. Timor-Tritsch, I. E., Monteagudo, A. and Lerner, J. P. (1996). A 'potentially safer' route for puncture and injection of cornual ectopic pregnancies. *Ultrasound Obstet. Gynecol.*, **7**, 353–5

67. Ackerman, T. E., Levi, C. S., Dashefsky, S. M., Holt, S. C. and Lindsay, D. J. (1993). Interstitial line: sonographic finding in interstitial (cornual) ectopic pregnancy. *Radiology*, **189**, 83–7

68. Fernandez, H., Baton, C., Leelaider, C. and Frudman, R. (1991). Conservative management of ectopic pregnancy: prospective randomized clinical trial of methotrexate versus prostaglandin sulpostone by combined transvaginal and systemic administration. *Fertil. Steril.*, **55**, 746–50

69. Oelsner, G., Admon, D., Shalev, E., *et al.* (1993). A new approach for the treatment of interstitial pregnancy. *Fertil. Steril.*, **59**, 924–5

70. Shalev, E., Romano, S. and Bustan, M. (1989). Interstitial pregnancy – successful treatment with methotrexate. *Isr. J. Med. Sci.*, **25**, 239–40

71. Zalel, Y., Caspi, B. and Insler, V. (1994). Expectant management of interstitial pregnancy. *Ultrasound Obstet. Gynecol.*, **4**, 238–40

72. Holden, R. and Hart, P. (1983). First trimester rudimentary horn pregnancy: prerupture ultrasound diagnosis. *Obstet. Gynecol.*, **61**, 56S

73. Timor-Tritsch, I. E., Monteagudo, A., Mandeville, E. O., *et al.* (1994). Successful management of viable cervical pregnancy by local injection of methotrexate guided by transvaginal sonography *Am. J. Obstet. Gynecol.*, **170**, 737–9

74. Grimes, H. G., Nosal, R. A. and Gallagher, J. C. (1983). Ovarian pregnancy: a series of 24 cases. *Obstet. Gynecol.*, **61**, 174–80

75. Hallatt, J. G. (1982). Primary ovarian pregnancy: a report of twenty-five cases. *Am. J. Obstet. Gynecol.*, **143**, 55–60

76. Athey, P. A., Jayson, H. T., Estrada, R. and Watson, A. B. Jr. (1990). Sonographic findings in primary ovarian pregnancy. *J. Clin. Ultrasound*, **18**, 730–2

77. Malinger, G., Achiron, R., Treschan, O. and Zakut, H. (1988). Ovarian pregnancy – ultrasonographic diagnosis. *Acta Obstet. Gynecol. Scand.*, **67**, 561–3

78. Russell, J. B. and Cutler, L. R. (1989) Transvaginal ultrasonographic detection of ovarian pregnancy with laparoscopic removal: a case report. *Fertil. Steril.*, **51**, 1055

79. Bayless, R. B. (1987). Non-tubal ectopic pregnancy. In DeCherney, A. H. (ed.). *Ectopic Pregnancy. Clin. Obstet. Gynecol.*, **30**, 191–9

80. Hertz, R. H., Timor-Tritsch, I. E., Sokol, R. J. and Zador, I. (1977). Diagnostic studies and fetal assessment in advanced extrauterine pregnancy. *Obstet. Gynecol.*, **50**, 63–5

81. Stanley, J. H., Horger, E. O. III, Fagan, C. J., *et al.* (1986). Sonographic findings in abdominal pregnancy. *Am. J. Roentgenol.*, **174**, 1043–6

82. Reece, E. A., Petrie, R. H., Sirmans, M. F., Finster, M. and Todd, W. D. (1983). Combined intrauterine and extrauterine gestations: a review. *Am. J. Obstet. Gynecol.*, **146**, 323–30

83. Bello, G. V., Schonholz, D., Moshirpur, J., Jeng, D.-Y. and Berkowitz, R. L. (1986). Combined pregnancy: The Mount Sinai experience. *Obstet. Gynecol. Surv.*, **41**, 603–13

84. Tal, J., Haddad, S., Gordon, N. and Timor-Tritsch, I. E. (1996). Heterotopic pregnancy after ovulation induction and assisted reproductive technologies: a literature review from 1971 to 1993. *Fertil. Steril.*, **66**, 1–11

85. Monteagudo, A., Tarricone, N. J., Timor-Tritsch, I. E. and Lerner, J. P. (1996). Successful transvaginal ultrasound-guided puncture and injection of a cervical pregnancy in a patient with simultaneous intrauterine pregnancy and a history of a previous cervical pregnancy. *Ultrasound Obstet. Gynecol.*, **8**, 381–6

86. Dillon, E. H., Feycock, A. L. and Taylor, K. J. W. (1990). Pseudogestational sacs: Doppler US differentiation from normal or abnormal intrauterine pregnancies. *Radiology*, **176**, 359–64

87. Taylor, K. J. W., Ramos, I. M., Feycock, A. L., *et al.* (1989). Ectopic pregnancy duplex Doppler evaluation. *Radiology*, **173**, 93–6

88. Taylor, K. J. W. and Meyer, W. R. (1991). New technologies in the diagnosis of ectopic pregnancy. *Obstet. Gynecol. Clin. North Am.*, **18**, 39–54

89. Emerson, D. S., Cartier, M. S., Altieri, L. A., *et al.* (1992). Diagnostic efficacy of endovaginal color Doppler flow imaging in an ectopic pregnancy screening program. *Radiology*, **183**, 413–20

90. Jurkovic, D., Bourne, T. H., Jauniaux, E., *et al.* (1992). Transvaginal color Doppler study of blood flow in ectopic pregnancies. *Fertil. Steril.*, **57**, 68–73

91. Kirchler, H. C., Kolle, D. and Schwegel, P. (1988). Changes in tubal blood flow in

evaluating ectopic pregnancy. *Ultrasound Obstet. Gynecol.*, **2**, 283–8

92. Tekay, A. and Jouppila, P. (1992). Color Doppler flow as an indicator of trophoblastic activity in tubal pregnancies detected by transvaginal ultrasound. *Obstet. Gynecol.*, **80**, 995–9

93. Kurjak, A., Zalud, I. and Volpe, G. (1990). Conventional B-mode and transvaginal color Doppler in ultrasound assessment of ectopic pregnancy. *Acta Med. Jugosl.*, **44**, 91–103

94. Atri, M. (1993). Ectopic pregnancy: evaluation with endovaginal color Doppler flow imaging. *Radiology*, **187**, 19; discussion 21–2

95. Brown, D. L. (1993). Diagnosis of ectopic pregnancy with endovaginal color Doppler US. *Radiology*, **187**, 20–4

96. Rodi, I. A., Sauer, M. V., Gorrill, M. J., *et al.* (1986). The medical treatment of unruptured ectopic pregnancy with methotrexate and citrovorum rescue: preliminary experience. *Fertil. Steril.*, **46**, 811–13

97. Sauer, M. V., Gorrill, M. J., Rodi, I. A., *et al.* (1987). Nonsurgical management of unruptured ectopic pregnancy: an extended clinical trial. *Fertil. Steril.*, **48**, 752–5

98. Stovall, T. G., Ling, F. W. and Buster, J. E. (1987). Outpatient chemotherapy of unruptured ectopic pregnancy: an extended clinical trial. *Fertil Steril.*, **48**, 752–5

99. Stovall, T. G., Ling, F. W. and Buster, J. E. (1990). Reproductive performance after methotrexate treatment of ectopic pregnancy. *Am. J. Obstet. Gynecol.*, **162**, 1620–4

100. Brown, D. L., Felker, R. E., Stovall, T. G., *et al.* (1991). Serial endovaginal sonography of ectopic pregnancies treated with methotrexate. *Obstet. Gynecol.*, **77**, 406–9

101. Stovall, T. G., Ling, F. W., Gray, L. A., *et al.* (1991). Methotrexate treatment of unruptured ectopic pregnancy. *Obstet. Gynecol.*, **77**, 754–7

102. Stovall, T. G., Ling, F. W. and Gray, L. A. (1991). Single-dose methotrexate for treatment of ectopic pregnancy. *Obstet. Gynecol.*, **77**, 754–7

103. Schiff, E., Shaler, E., Bustan, M., *et al.* (1992). Pharmacokinetics of methotrexate after local tubal injection for conservative treatment of ectopic pregnancy. *Fertil. Steril.*, **57**, 688–90

104. Ransom, M. X., Garcia, A. J., Bohrer, M., *et al.* (1994). Serum progesterone as a predictor of methotrexate success in the treatment of ectopic pregnancy. *Obstet. Gynecol.*, **83**, 1033–7

105. Timor-Tritsch, I. E., Peisner, D. B. and Monteagudo, A. (1991). Transvaginal sonography in the diagnosis of ectopic pregnancy. In Grunfeld, L. (ed.). *Ultrasonography in Reproductive Medicine. Infertil. Reprod. Med. Clin. North Am.*, **2**, 727–39

106. Feichtinger, W. and Kemeter, P. (1987). Conservative treatment of ectopic pregnancy by transvaginal aspiration under sonographic control and methotrexate injection. *Lancet*, **1**, 381

107. Timor-Tritsch, I. E., Baxi, L. and Peisner, D. B. (1989). Transvaginal salpingocentesis: a new technique for treating ectopic pregnancy. *Am. J. Obstet. Gynecol.*, **160**, 459–61

108. Menard, A., Crequat, J., Mandelbrot, L., Hauuy, J.-P. and Madelenat, P. (1990). Treatment of unruptured tubal pregnancy by local injection of methotrexate under transvaginal sonographic control. *Fertil. Steril.*, **54**, 47–50

109. Aboulghar, M. A., Mansour, R. T. and Serour, G. I. (1990). Transvaginal injection of potassium chloride and methotrexate for the treatment of tubal pregnancy with a live fetus. *Hum. Reprod.*, **5**, 887–8

110. Feichtinger, W. and Kemeter, P. (1989). Treatment of unruptured ectopic pregnancy by needling of sac and injection of methotrexate or PGE2 under transvaginal sonography control: report of 10 cases. *Arch. Gynecol. Obstet.*, **246**, 85–9

111. Robertson, D. E., Smith, W. and Moye, M. A. H. (1987). Reduction of ectopic pregnancy by injection under ultrasound control. *Lancet*, **1**, 974–5

112. Robert, D. E., Smith, W. and Craft, I. (1987). Reduction of ectopic pregnancy by ultrasound methods. *Lancet*, **2**, 1524–5

113. Leeton, J. and Davison, G. (1988). Nonsurgical management of unruptured tubal pregnancy with intra-amniotic methotrexate: preliminary report of two cases. *Fertil. Steril.*, **50**, 167–9

114. Timor-Tritsch, I. E., Peisner, D. B. and Monteatgudo, A. (1991). Puncture procedures utilizing transvaginal ultrasonic guidance. *Ultrasound Obstet. Gynecol.*, **1**, 144–50

115. Fernandez, H., Baton, C., Lelaidier, C. and Frydman, R. (1991). Conservative management of ectopic pregnancy: prospective randomized clinical trial of methotrexate versus prostaglandin sulpostrone by combined transvaginal and systemic administration. *Fertil. Steril.*, **55**, 746–50

116. Tulandi, T., Bret, P. M., Atri, M. and Senterman, M. (1991). Treatment of ectopic pregnancy by transvaginal intratubal methotrexate administration. *Obstet. Gynecol.*, **77**, 627–43

117. Popp, L. W., Mettler, L., Weisner, H., Mecke, I., Freys, I. and Semm, K. (1991). Ectopic pregnancy treatment using pelviscopic or vaginosonographically guided intrachorionic injection of methotrexate. *Ultrasound Obstet. Gynecol.*, **1**, 136–43

118. Shalev, E., Zalel, Y., Bustan, M. and Weiner, E. (1991). Ectopic pregnancy: sonographically guided transvaginal reduction. *Ultrasound Obstet Gynecol.*, **1**, 127–31

119. Venezia, R., Zangara, C., Comparetto, G. and Cittadini, E. (1991). Conservative treatment of ectopic pregnancies using a single echo-guided injection of methotrexate into a gestational sac. *Ultrasound Obstet. Gynecol.*, **1**, 132–5

120. Jehng, C. H., Ng, K. Y., Jou, H. J., Jenh, A. L. and Lien, Y. R. (1992). Successful treatment of two viable tubal pregnancies by two-step local injection. *J. Formos Med. Assoc.*, **91**, 823–7

121. Atri, M., Bret, P. M., Tulandi, T. and Senterman, M. K. (1992). Ectopic pregnancy: revolution after treatment with transvaginal methotrexate. *Radiology*, **185**, 749–53

122. Bider, D., Oelsner, G., Admon, D., *et al.* (1992). Unsuccessful methotrexate treatment of a tubal pregnancy with a live embryo. *Eur. J. Obstet. Gynecol. Reprod. Med.*, **46**, 154–7

123. Caspi, B., Barash, A., Friedman, A., Appelman, Z., Pausky, M. and Borenstein, R. (1992). Aspiration of ectopic pregnancy under guidance of vaginal ultrasonography. *Eur. J. Obstet. Gynecol. Reprod. Biol.*, **46**, 51–2

Ultrasound-guided administration of methotrexate in ectopic pregnancies

20

H. Fernandez

INTRODUCTION

Early diagnosis of ectopic pregnancy has become a reality. With knowledge of its risk factors[1] (history of salpingitis, *Chlamydia trachomatis*, tubal surgery, previous ectopic pregnancy, cigarette smoking, and pregnancy during contraceptive use or after ovarian stimulation), and with assays of human chorionic gonadotropin (hCG) and plasma progesterone, and transvaginal ultrasonography, ectopic pregnancy can be diagnosed early, sometimes even before any clinical symptoms appear. Its treatment strategy has thus been transformed, for it can now be diagnosed before any emergency exists and even, 95% of the time, without laparoscopy.

This progress in ectopic pregnancy management has occurred at the same time as an increase in its incidence, which one regional registry in France now assesses at 2% of births[2]. Laparoscopy remains the treatment of choice and represents a major step forward from laparotomy, due to the reduced duration of hospitalization and of total recovery, and also due to the cost reduction. Nonetheless, other possible treatments have been developed since the early 1980s. The principal alternatives to a surgical approach are expectant management[3–5] and systemic (oral, intramuscular or intravenous)[6–9] or *in situ* (by injection during laparoscopy or ultrasonography)[10–12] medical treatment. Whatever therapeutic approach is used, subsequent fertility is primarily linked to the patient age and history of infertility, more than to the treatment proposed for the current ectopic pregnancy[13].

ULTRASOUND DIAGNOSIS OF ECTOPIC PREGNANCY

The improvement of ultrasound scanners and probes and the availability of endovaginal ultrasound probes have modified the approach to diagnosing ectopic pregnancy. At the same time, plasma assays of hCG and progesterone allow early detection of conception and monitoring of its development. Nonetheless, only with ultrasound can the pregnancy be precisely localized. It is thus essential for the ultrasonographer to know the laboratory results before performing an examination.

Comparison of the clinical, laboratory and ultrasound findings usually reveals one of three principal situations. Diagnosis of a barely-developed ectopic pregnancy is the most common situation and leads to an early ultrasonographic diagnosis, before the period when complications normally develop[14]. Diagnosis of a developed ectopic pregnancy has become easy and reliable. Diagnostic uncertainty in situations that may turn dangerous has become quite rare: when a highly developed ectopic pregnancy can be presumed (advanced term, high hCG level, suspected fissuration), ultrasound will only in exceptional cases fail to reach a conclusion at the first examination. Doubt and a 'wait-and-see' attitude are also possible. False-positives and false-negatives are both uncommon: doubt or diagnostic error usually occurs when there are no or only mild symptoms. If no symptoms are potentially worrisome in the short term, an experienced ultrasonographer may reasonably suggest repeating the blood and ultrasound examinations in another 48 h, thereby avoiding an unnecessary diagnostic laparoscopy. This expectant attitude is essential in the current diagnostic strategy and therapeutic management of ectopic pregnancy. It is only possible, however, after a thorough analysis of the file, by both the clinician and the ultrasonographer.

The ultrasonographic signs that result in a diagnosis of ectopic pregnancy involve the analysis of five points.

Non-visualization of an intrauterine gestational sac

In most cases, the absence of an intrauterine gestational sac is expected in sub-pubic trans-abdominal ultrasonography, then verified with transvaginal ultrasonography, especially for uterine retroversion. One basis for suspecting ectopic pregnancy is the failure to visualize a gestational sac at appropriate hCG levels: for a normally developing intrauterine pregnancy, the threshold is usually considered to be between 350 and 1000 mIU/ml. When the level is below 350 mIU/ml, a developing gestational sac can be seen only rarely; above 1000 mIU/ml, it can almost always be found. At the intermediate levels, a follow-up blood test and an ultrasound examination 48 h later resolve most questions. A non-developing gestational sac, either intra- or extrauterine, may have a very different threshold of visualization. In a non-developing pregnancy, a 5-mm ectopic sac can easily be associated with an hCG level below 100 mIU/ml. Conversely, but rarely, a non-developing intrauterine gestational sac associated with an hCG level of 2000 mIU/ml can have a central cavity that is hardly visible (less than 2 mm).

Decidua

The appearance of the endometrium must be considered in conjunction with the trend of the hCG titers. The presence or absence of an intrauterine decidua is a valuable sign in diagnosing silent ectopic pregnancy. If the endometrium is very thin (decidua already expelled), the failure of the hCG level to fall is a diagnostic argument almost pathognomonic for ectopic pregnancy: no intrauterine trophoblast can persist after expulsion of the decidua. Conversely, if it has not been expelled (that is, if the endometrium remains thick and echogenic), neither the lack of any decline in the hCG level nor its persistence at a level below 1000 mIU/ml can any longer be considered a diagnostic argument, because a non-developing intrauterine gestational sac too small to be visualized sonographically (coelom less than 1 or 2 mm), but biologically active, may well be implanted in the decidua.

Corpus luteum and active ovary

The identification of the corpus luteum (almost always visible) and of the exact limits of the ovary is an essential stage in diagnosing ectopic pregnancy, since such pregnancies are usually located in the vicinity of the corpus luteum. Corpora lutea of pregnancy can have various aspects. Those that are cystic and of medium or large size usually present no diagnostic problems. Small ones (less than 15 mm), often echogenic and heterogeneous, can cause more problems (failure to recognize them or confusing them with either an ectopic pregnancy or a hematosalpinx). In practice, an experienced ultrasonographer should recognize these small corpora lutea by a meticulous identification of the ovarian parenchyma and the ovarian edges. In difficult cases, transvaginal ultrasound and a Doppler color study of the vascularization of the corpus luteum can be useful (Figure 1).

Abnormal adnexal mass

Once the active ovary and corpus luteum have been identified, extensive analysis of the ipsilateral adnexa allows a diagnosis in almost 95% of cases. An ectopic pregnancy is usually a mass very close to the ovary, protruding beyond the oval contours of the ovary. The main axis of this mass can range from 3 to 40 mm. Its aspect is a typical gestational sac, made up of an echogenic crown centered by an anechoic gap. Visualization of the yolk sac, or even the embryo, guarantees the specificity of the diagnosis, even for a very tiny gestational sac. An echogenic heterogeneous mass corresponds to a hematosalpinx. It is most echogenic and heterogeneous when newest. Frequently there is an association of an ectopic gestational sac inside the hematosalpinx: a lacunary or heterogeneous minimal image, less than 10 mm, sonographically unspecific (Figures 2, 3, 4 and 5).

Hematocele and hemoperitoneum

A hemoperitoneum is usually easily identified behind the uterus, a location that facilitates the assessment of its volume in relation to the level of the posterior uterine wall. The hematocele is visualized as an echogenic mass, often heterogeneous, at a distance from the ovary or behind the isthmus[15].

Conclusions from the ultrasound examination

The diagnostic procedures described above allow the diagnosis of a patent or presumptive ectopic pregnancy in 70% of cases. Moreover, the short-term development can usually be reliably judged from the beginning. It is thus easier to define the ultrasonographic criteria for low-risk development.

Early in gestation, if the ultrasonographer is certain that all the adnexa have been examined (in particular the upper peri-ovarian regions) and no abnormal mass has been visualized, a potentially dangerous hematosalpinx should not have been missed. Thus, when the diagnosis of ectopic pregnancy is not obvious at the first examination, it is reasonable, depending on the clinical and laboratory test results, to suggest a follow-up assessment 48 h later. On the other hand, some findings require extreme caution. Among the unfavorable ultrasonographic signs, hemoperitoneum, hematosalpinx and large hematoceles have become relatively rare.

The short-term prognosis depends on other factors and, in particular, on the location of the pregnancy in relation to the ovary. An ectopic pregnancy at a distance from the ovary

may be located in the isthmus and can become acute. The appearance of the hematosalpinx (volume, shape and position) should be represented in a diagram, to facilitate early screening of any deterioration, especially when the treatment strategy is non-invasive (expectant management or medical treatment). During transvaginal ultrasound, acute pain on pressure to the adnexal zone where the pregnancy is localized may suggest rapid growth of the ectopic gestational mass and thus the need for caution. The appearance of the gestational sac provides additional elements from which the short-term risks of dangerous development can be assessed: the volume of the gestational sac and the presence of an embryo, with or without cardiac activity.

Analysis with pulsed or color Doppler does not seem to contribute to diagnosis, except for visualizing the corpus luteum, specifying the adnexal topography, and assessing trophoblastic vascularization. Doppler velocimetry around the ampullae mainly shows the functional activity of the corpus luteum. Integrating information from the Doppler velocimetry into the diagnostic algorithm is therefore difficult. Moreover, changes in the peritrophoblastic vascularization are often the first signs of involution of an ectopic pregnancy. There remain, nonetheless, some diagnostic problems[16]. The existence of a pregnancy may not be recognized, although this has become extremely rare since hCG assays have become routine in gynecologic contexts. Alternatively, a heterotopic pregnancy may be present, since ultrasound imaging after ovarian stimulation and oocyte retrieval (for *in vitro* fertilization) can make analysis of its signs difficult. When the pelvis is scarred and has adhesions, diagnosis of an ectopic pregnancy is difficult and necessitates a deliberate search, using an abdominal probe, for an ectopic pregnancy located high in the pelvis.

All of the ultrasound diagnostic signs described here must be considered in the pretreatment assessment, so that the alternatives to standard surgical treatment can be discussed. Thus, envisaging medical treatment by an *in situ* injection must take into account the following elements: the accessibility of the gestational sac

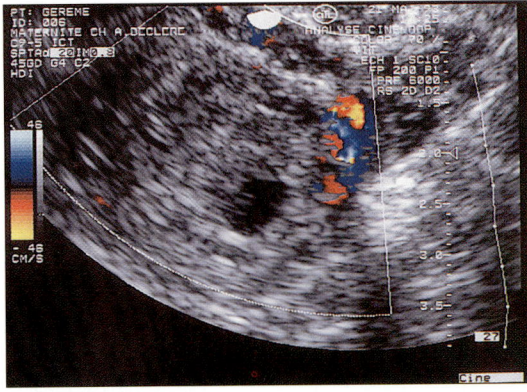

Figure 1 Ectopic pregnancy located in the vicinity of the corpus luteum. Color Doppler facilitates detection of the peritrophoblastic flow and corpus luteum vascularization

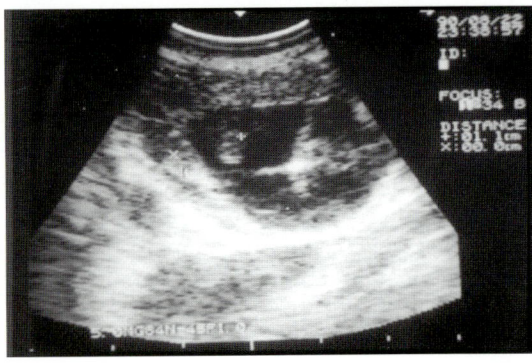

Figure 4 Twin ectopic pregnancy resulting from in vitro fertilization/embryo transfer treatment. Two hyperechogenic tubal rings and embryonic echoes are imaged side by side

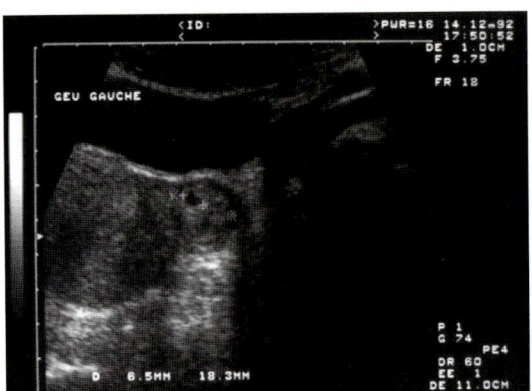

Figure 2 Transabdominal scan of the interstitial pregnancy: note ring-like structure attaching the uterine border

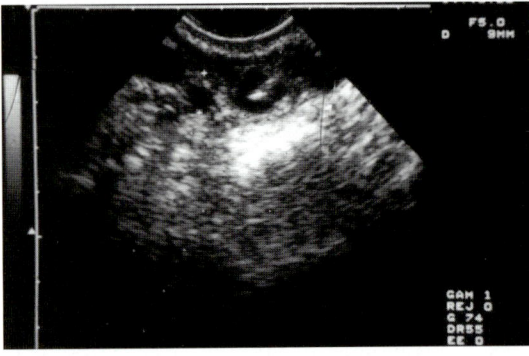

Figure 5 Typical picture of tubal abortion. Note the intact tubal ring containing embryonic echo and ipsilateral ovary. Note that although there may be slow bleeding through the fimbria there is no rupture of the tubal ring and the echogenicity of the ovary is lower than that of the tubal ring. Laparoscopy confirmed the diagnosis

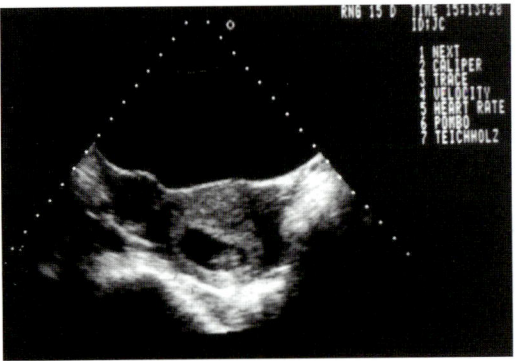

Figure 3 Two ring-like structures: the left one has echogenic content and corresponds to corpus luteum, while the right one is more elongated and contains embryonic echo

to puncture (for aspiration and injection), the appearance and volume of both the gestational sac and the hematosalpinx, any pain from pressure during the trans vaginal ultrasonography, and any pelvic effusion. These principal ultrasonographic signs are thus included in scores for pretreatment decision-making.

MEDICAL TREATMENT OF ECTOPIC PREGNANCY

Indications for medical treatment

Adoption of a treatment strategy that includes non-surgical treatment implies early diagnosis. Clinical conditions, the results of hCG

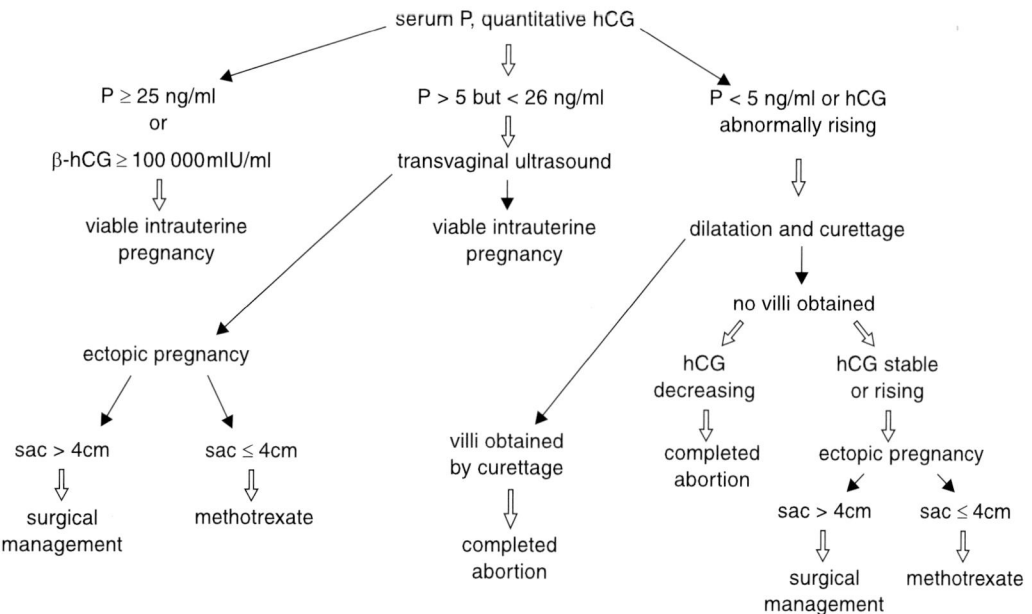

Figure 6 Algorithm for the diagnosis of unruptured ectopic pregnancy without laparoscopy. P, progesterone; hCG, human chorionic gonadotropin. From reference 17, with permission

Table 1   The pretherapeutic predictive score

	Score		
Variable	1	2	3
Gestational age (days)	> 49	≤ 49	≤ 42
Level of hCG (mIU/ml)	≤ 1000	≤ 5000	> 5000
Progesterone (ng/ml)	≤ 5	≤ 10	> 10
Abdominal pain	none	induced	sponta-neous
Hematosalpinx (cm)	≤ 1	≤ 3	> 3
Hemoperitoneum (cm³)	≤ 10	≤ 100	> 100

hCG, human chorionic gonadotropin

and plasma progesterone assays, and the ultrasonography findings are the foundation for diagnostic and therapeutic algorithms. Carson and Buster[17] have proposed a decision tree for the early diagnosis of an unruptured ectopic pregnancy, to select patients who might benefit from a medical approach. This algorithm (Figure 6) is based upon hCG and plasma progesterone measurements, transvaginal ultrasound findings, and a uterine curettage that can be performed on an outpatient basis and investigates chorionic villi.

We have proposed a score (Table 1) that integrates the clinical, laboratory and ultrasound elements and uses six variables: gestational age, the concept of pelvic pain, the size of the hematosalpinx, the volume of the hemoperitoneum, and the initial levels of hCG and progesterone. Each variable is scored from 1 to 3. For scores of 12 or less, the success rate for medical treatment is greater than 90%. For scores 12 or less, the failure rate is nearly 50%[18]. The pragmatic use of these scores allows us to define a population of women who appear to have a probability of success with medical treatment equivalent to that observed after conservative laparoscopic treatment. Nonetheless, *in situ* medical treatment ought not to be recommended when the hCG level is greater than 10 000 mIU/ml or an embryo is visualized, for the success rate is then only 50%. Nonetheless, even when the failure rate is high, this treatment may nonetheless be indicated for a few ectopic locations – interstitial, angular, cervical or ovarian – since in these cases medical treatment may still be less traumatic than laparotomy.

Table 2   Treatment of ectopic pregnancy by ultrasound-guided *in situ* injection of methotrexate

Study	No. of cases	No. of successes	Tubal permeability	Intrauterine pregnancy	Recurrence of ectopic pregnancies
Feichtinger and Kemeter (1987)[19]	8	8			
Mottla *et al.* (1992)[20]	7	4			
Tulandi *et al.* (1992)[10]	40	28			7.1% (2/28)
Fernandez *et al.* (1993)[11]	100	83	72/80	34/58	8.8% (3/34)
Darai (1994)[12]	100	78	13/26	21/75	28.6% (6/21)
Total	255	201 (78.8%)	106 (80.2%)	55/133 (41.3%)	

Ultrasound-guided medical treatment: procedures and results

Feichtinger and Kemeter[19] reported the first treatment by local injection of an ectopic pregnancy; they used the technique of ultrasound-guided endovaginal aspiration, originally proposed for retrieving oocytes during *in vitro* fertilization (IVF) procedures. The amniotic sac, identified ultrasonographically, is first punctured, emptied, and then injected. This technique requires that the ectopic pregnancy be directly and indisputably visualized by transvaginal ultrasound, which is the case 90–95% of the time. The results of the principal series in which ectopic pregnancies were treated by ultrasound-guided *in situ* injections[10–12,19,20] are presented in Table 2. In our series, when we consider only those scores below or equal to 12[11], the overall success rate of 83% increases to 93%[11].

Contraindications and indications for ultrasound-guided medical treatment by methotrexate

Contraindications

The contraindications for methotrexate treatment are related to the properties of methotrexate and to the clinical form of the ectopic pregnancy. Thus, patients are excluded from treatment protocols if they present thrombopenia lower than $100 \times 10^9/l$, any blood coagulation anomalies, elevated creatinine levels (creatinemia), or elevated levels of hepatic enzymes. Before any methotrexate treatment, therefore, a blood count, serum electrolyte analysis, and liver-enzyme assays must be performed. Patients are excluded if their clinical picture suggests intraperitoneal bleeding or signs indicating substantial trophoblast activity, including a pretreatment score greater than 13, an initial hCG level greater than 10 000 mIU/ml, a hematosalpinx larger than 4 cm, or any embryonic cardiac activity. There is, however, no definitive consensus on this last point. The success rate for this treatment when there is cardiac activity only rarely exceeds 50%[11]; indeed, in the trial of Stovall and Ling[21] it was only 14.3%.

Indications

Methotrexate treatment appears to be indicated, essentially, for an asymptomatic or only slightly symptomatic ectopic pregnancy that has been diagnosed by ultrasound.

In principal, only one injection is performed, and a secondary intramuscular injection is proposed only when the hCG level does not fall according to the normal pattern (Table 3).

Monitoring after methotrexate treatment

Post-treatment development must be monitored. After ultrasound aspiration of the ectopic sac, hCG is assayed on the 2nd, 5th and 10th days, and then every 10 days until it returns to normal, a process that takes, on average, 28 days.

During the 1st week, the hCG level increases and only returns to its value at the moment of the injection at around the 8th day (Figure 7). This peak may be as much as 25 to 40% higher than the initial hCG level. Two phenomena explain this rise: the methotrexate initially

Table 3 Success and reproductive performance following single-dose methotrexate for unruptured ectopic pregnancy

Study	n	Resolved without surgery	Second dose required	Tubal patency	Subsequent fertility		
					Nb	IUP	EP
Stovall and Ling (1993)[21]	120	113	4	51/62	49	34	5
Glock et al. (1994)[9]	35	30	2	10/13	15	5	0
Fernandez et al. (1993)[11]	100	83	28	72/80	58	34	3
Henry and Gentry (1994)[22]	61	52	16	—	—	—	—
Total	228	205 (90%)	22 (10%)	61/75 (81%)	64	39 (61%)	5 (8%)

Nb, Live birth + EP + miscarriage; IUP, intrauterine pregnancy; EP, ectopic pregnancy

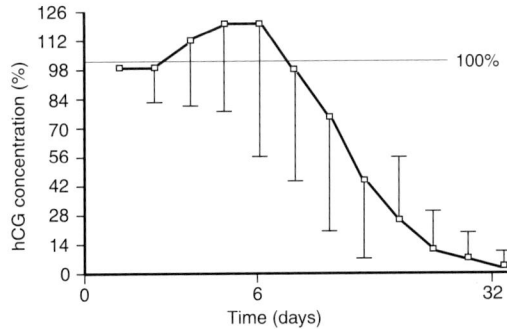

Figure 7 Evolution of human chorionic gonadotropin (hCG) levels after methotrexate treatment of ectopic pregnancy. 100% = Level of hCG at injection. Bars represent SEM

accelerates the metabolism of hCG, and death of trophoblastic cells increases its systemic release. Knowing this, we can avoid excessive intervention during the 1st week, based solely on the non-decline of hCG. As we have seen, only if it changed in a pattern different from that of the reference curve would a supplemental intramuscular injection of methotrexate be indicated as rescue therapy. It can only be considered if the patient remains asymptomatic and if the ultrasound monitoring, which is indicated only in this situation, shows neither any change in the volume of the gestational sac or the hematosalpinx nor the appearance or increase of a hemoperitoneum. As part of the immediate after-effects, abdominal pain suggesting tubal rupture may occur, as late as 6 or 7 days after the methotrexate administration. This pain is observed in 33–59% of cases[9–21]. In these situations, an ultrasound examination is necessary to determine if the size of the hematosalpinx

has changed or a hemoperitoneum has developed, or, if the image is unchanged, to confirm that the pain is probably an expression of necrosis as the pregnancy resolves. Follow-up studies comparing the hCG decrease and the ultrasound image show no correlation at all. Atri and colleagues[23] have shown, in 25 patients after medical treatment, an increase in the size and vascularization of the pregnancy. Brown and associates[24] have also confirmed the absence of correlation between hCG levels and ultrasound findings. These studies show that a routine ultrasound examination after medical treatment is not necessary.

Side-effects of methotrexate treatment

The principal side-effects are hepatic cytolysis, stomatitis, gastroenteritis, and lung and bone marrow disorders. The incidence of such effects is 21% when methotrexate is administered intramuscularly and 2% when it is administered locally[25]. Nonetheless, a single dose seems to reduce the risk of side-effects[8–10], although Glock and colleagues observed them in 34% of cases[9]. No specific pathologic lesions have been observed, either in animal studies of rats and rabbits, or in a histologic study based on salpingectomies performed after methotrexate injection[26–28].

Methotrexate: *in situ* or intramuscular?

Pharmacokinetic studies of methotrexate that compare ultrasound-guided local administration with intramuscular administration show that the maximum plasma concentration and area below the curve are similar for both

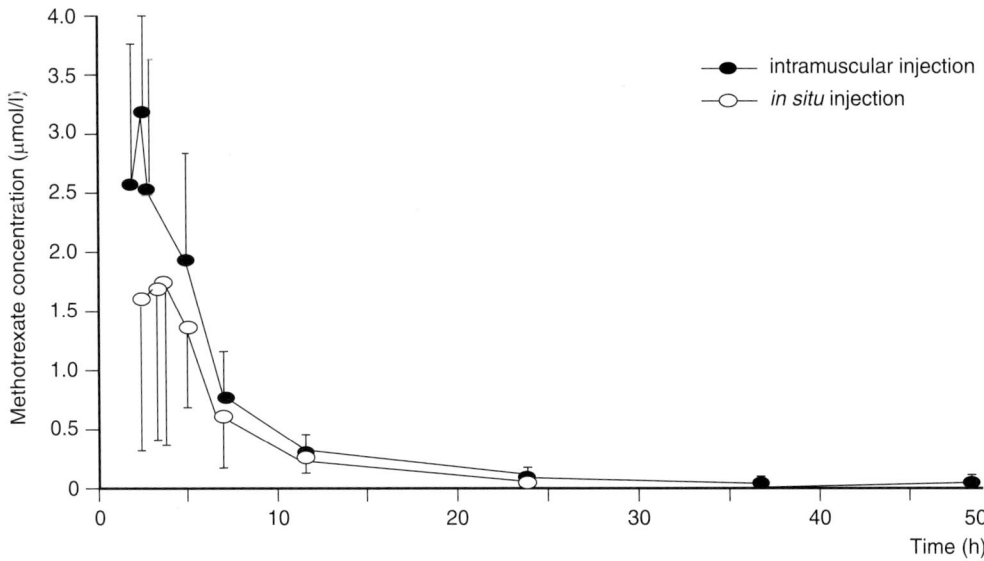

Figure 8 Methotrexate pharmacokinetics after intramuscular and *in situ* injection of 1 mg/kg methotrexate for the treatment of ectopic pregnancy

types of injection. A prospective study[29] has confirmed that ultrasound-guided local injection yields results equivalent to those of intramuscular injections, at the same time as it reduces the number of side-effects. This study comprised four patient groups treated by different routes of administration and different doses. The analysis by route of administration shows a sharper slope for the area under the curve after ultrasound-guided injection, because of the reduction in the bioavailability of methotrexate (Figure 8). Apparently, the trophoblast captures the methotrexate, temporarily removing it from the hepatic metabolism. This phenomenon may explain the reduced toxicity associated with local administration. This study confirmed that after 24 h only a residual blood concentration of methotrexate could be found, ranging between 1×10^{-8} and 1×10^{-7} mol/l. Thus the 'rescue' treatment by folinic acid (citrovorum factor) recommended in early treatment protocols serves no purpose. Based upon this and other studies, we recommend a dose of 1 mg/kg or 50 mg/m^2. In a clinical trial (unpublished data) comparing the efficacy of local and systemic treatment (30 patients in each group), the success rate was significantly higher in the group with the ultrasound-guided administration (92% compared with 81%) ($p < 0.05$).

Other medical treatments administered with ultrasound guidance

After methotrexate, prostaglandins are the most frequently used substances for medical treatment of ectopic pregnancy. Three types of prostaglandins are commonly used: type F2α (1–3 mg), E2 analogs (500–1500 mg), or 15-methyl-PgF2α (150 mg). The F2α prostaglandins are usually preferred because of their longer half-life; they are injected into the ectopic pregnancy, either laparoscopically or by ultrasound guidance, or into the corpus luteum. Nonetheless, because of secondary cardiovascular effects and a lesser efficacy, methotrexate is to be preferred[30].

Potassium chloride is injected intra-tubally with ultrasound guidance. It is less effective than either methotrexate or the prostaglandins, but appears to be the best recourse for medical treatment of heterotopic pregnancies, especially those that are cornual[31,32], since the potassium chloride is not toxic to the associated intrauterine embryo.

The other medical treatments that have been proposed, namely hyperosmolar glucose, actinomycin D and RU 486, are primarily used laparoscopically or orally and have shown an efficacy similar to that of expectant management.

CONSERVATIVE LAPAROSCOPIC TREATMENT COMPARED WITH MEDICAL TREATMENT

Two clinical trials have compared conservative laparoscopic treatment with local injection of methotrexate, administered laparoscopically. O'Shea and colleagues[33] obtained success rates of 87.5% among 24 patients treated conservatively and 89.7% among the 29 patients who received a local injection. A trial by Mottla and associates[20] was stopped early because of the poor results observed after medical treatment. Fernandez and colleagues[34] have reported a prospective randomized trial comparing conservative laparoscopic treatment and ultrasound-guided puncture. The first published series showed, in both groups, 19 successes among 20 patients. A subsequent series, containing 50 patients in each group (unpublished data) found 47 successes in each group. Since the inclusion criteria were identical, there does not appear to be any difference in the results when the indications are the same.

Nonetheless, a major problem with this type of therapeutic trial is that the absence of a large series can reduce the statistical power.

In a retrospective study, Yao and colleagues[35] examined the direct medical costs of 40 patients treated with methotrexate and 40 treated with laparoscopic surgery. The direct cost per patient took into account the failure rate, the need for secondary treatment, and the follow-up: it was significantly lower in the methotrexate group (Can\$ 880 ± 60 compared with Can\$ 1840 ± 150). For the 90% success rate observed with ultrasound-guided medical treatment after specific indications, Can\$ 131 055 is thus saved for each 100 patients treated with methotrexate.

CONCLUSIONS

Even though laparoscopy remains the standard treatment, 30 to 40% of patients with an ectopic pregnancy diagnosed by ultrasound can benefit from medical treatment. Even though early series show a similar success rate for local and systemic treatments, studies not yet published seem to show better results with the ultrasound-guided administration, which can be practiced on an outpatient basis and without anesthesia, but which requires a month of follow-up to monitor hCG levels. Indications for such treatments appear to be ectopic pregnancies that are considered inactive, based upon the hCG and progesterone assays and the ultrasound findings.

References

1. Coste, J., Spira, N. and Fernandez, H. (1991). Increased risk of ectopic pregnancy with cigarette smoking. *Am. J. Public Health*, **81**, 199–201
2. Coste, J., Job-Spira, N., Aublet-Cuvelier, B., Germain, E., Bouyer, J., Fernandez, H. and Pouly, J. L. (1994). Incidence of ectopic pregnancy. First results of a population-based register in France. *Hum. Reprod.*, **9**, 742–5
3. Fernandez, H., Rainhorn, J. D., Papiernik, E., Bellet, D. and Frydman, R. (1988). Spontaneous

resolution of ectopic pregnancy. *Obstet. Gynecol.*, **71**, 171–4
4. Ylostalo, P., Cacciatore, B., Sjoberg, J., Kaariainen, M., Tenhunen, A. and Stenman, U. H. (1992). Expectant management of ectopic pregnancy. *Obstet. Gynecol.*, **80**, 345–8
5. Shalev, E., Peleg, D., Tsabari, A., Romano, S. and Bustan, M. (1993). Spontaneous resolution of ectopic tubal pregnancy: natural history. *Fertil. Steril.*, **63**, 15–19

6. Ory, S. J., Villanneuva, A. L., Sand, P. K. and Tamura, R. K. (1986). Conservative treatment of ectopic pregnancy with methotrexate. *Am. J. Obstet. Gynecol.*, **154**, 1299

7. Pastner, B. and Kenigsberg, G. D. (1998). Successful treatment of persistant ectopic pregnancy with oral methotrexate therapy. *Fertil. Steril.*, **50**, 982

8. Stovall, T. G., Ling, F. W. and Gray, L. A. (1991). Methotrexate treatment of unruptured pregnancy: a report of 100 cases. *Obstet. Gynecol.*, **77**, 749–53

9. Glock, J., Johnson, J. and Brumsted, R. (1994). Efficacy and safety of single dose systemic methotrexate in the treatment of ectopic pregnancy. *Fertil. Steril.*, **62**, 716–21

10. Tulandi, T., Atri, M., Bret, P., Falcone, T. and Khalife, S. (1992). Transvaginal intratubal methotrexate treatment of ectopic pregnancy. *Fertil. Steril.*, **58**, 98–100

11. Fernandez, H., Benifla, J. L., Lelaidier, C., Baton, C. and Frydman, R. (1993). Methotrexate treatment of ectopic pregnancy: 100 cases treated by primary transvaginal injection under sonographic control. *Fertil. Steril.*, **59**, 773–7

12. Darai, E., Benifla, J. L., Naouri, M., Pennehouat, G., Guglielmina, J. N., Deval, B., Filippini, F., Crequat, J. and Madelenat, P. (1995). Transvaginal intratubal methotrexate treatment of ectopic pregnancy. Report of 100 cases. *Hum. Reprod.*, **11**, 420–4

13. Job-Spira, N., Bouyer, J., Pouly, J. L., Germain, E., Coste, G. and Fernandez, H. (1996). Fertility after ectopic pregnancy. First results of a population-based cohort study in France. *Hum. Reprod.*, **11**, 99–104

14. Maymon, R., Shulman, A. and Maymon, B. B. (1992). Ectopic pregnancy, the new gynecological epidemic disease: review of the modern work-up and the nonsurgical treatment option. *Int. J. Fertil.*, **37**, 146–64

15. Nyberg, D. A., Hugues, M. P., Mack, L. A. and Wang, K. Y. (1991). Extrauterine findings of ectopic pregnancy of transvaginal ultrasound: importance of echogenic fluid. *Radiology*, **178**, 823–6

16. Parvey, H. R. and Maklad, N. (1993). Pitfalls in the transvaginal sonographic diagnosis of ectopic pregnancy. *J. Ultrasound Med.*, **12**, 139–44

17. Carson, S. A. and Buster, J. E. (1993). Ectopic pregnancy. *N. Engl. J. Med.*, **329**, 1174–80

18. Fernandez, H., Lelaidier, C., Thouvenez, V. and Frydman, R. (1991). The use of a pretherapeutic, predictive score to determine inclusion criteria for the non-surgical treatment of ectopic pregnancy. *Hum. Reprod.*, **6**, 995–8

19. Feichtinger, W. and Kemeter, P. (1987). Conservative treatment of ectopic pregnancy by transvaginal aspiration under sonographic control and methotrexate injection. *Lancet*, **1**, 381

20. Mottla, G. L., Rulin, M. C. and Guzick, D. S. (1992). Lack of resolution of ectopic pregnancy by intratubal injection of methotrexate. *Fertil. Steril.*, **5**, 685–7

21. Stovall, T. G. and Ling, F. W. (1993). Single-dose methotrexate: an expanded clinical trial. *Am. J. Obstet. Gynecol.*, **168**, 1759–65

22. Henry, M. A. and Gentry W. L. (1994). Single injection of methotrexate for treatment of ectopic pregnancies. *Am. J. Obstet. Gynecol.*, **171**, 1584–7

23. Atri, M., Bret, P. M., Tulandi, T. and Senterman, M. K. (1992). Ectopic pregnancy: evolution after treatment with transvaginal methotrexate. *Radiology*, **185**, 749–53

24. Brown, D. L., Felker, R. E., Stovall, T. H., Emerson, D. S. and Ling, F. W. (1991). Serial endovaginal sonography of ectopic pregnancies treated with methotrexate. *Obstet. Gynecol.*, **77**, 406–9

25. Kooi, S. and Kock, H. C. L. V. (1992). A review of the literature on nonsurgical treatment in tubal pregnancies. *Obstet. Gynecol. Surv.*, **47**, 739–49

26. Perrotez, C., Gebauer, C., Menard, A., Guyard, B., Michaud, P., Madelenat, P. and Feldmann, G. (1991). Toxic effects of methotrexate injected into the uterine horn of pregnant female rats. *Hum. Reprod.*, **6**, 180–3

27. Lecuru, F., Querleu, D., Bucher-Bouverne, B. and Subtil, D. (1992). The effect of tubal injection of methotrexate on fertility in the rabbit. *Fertil. Steril.*, **81**, 422–4

28. Kooi, S., Van Etten, E. and Koch, H. (1992). Histopathology after treatment with methotrexate for a tubal pregnancy. *Fertil. Steril.*, **57**, 341–5

29. Fernandez, H., Bourget, P., Ville, Y., Lelaidier, C. and Frydman, R. (1994). Treatment of unruptured tubal pregnancy with methotrexate: pharmacokinetic analysis of local versus intramuscular administration. *Fertil. Steril.*, **62**, 943–7

30. Lindblom, B., Hahlin, M., Lundorff, P. and Thorburn, J. (1990). Treatment of tubal pregnancy by laparoscope-guided injection of prostaglandin F2α. *Fertil. Steril.*, **54**, 404–8

31. Fernandez, H., Lelaidier, C. and Doumerc, S. (1993). Non-surgical treatment of heterotopic pregnancy: a report of six cases. *Fertil. Steril.*, **60**, 428–32

32. Fernandez, H., de Ziegler, D. and Bourget, P. (1991). The place of methotrexate in the management of interstitial pregnancy. *Hum. Reprod.*, **6**, 302–6

33. O'Shea, R. T., Thompson, G. R. and Harding, A. (1994). Intra-amniotic methotrexate versus CO_2 laser laparoscopic salpingotomy in the management of tubal ectopic pregnancy. A prospective randomized trial. *Fertil. Steril.*, **62**, 876

34. Fernandez, H., Pauthier, S., Doumerc, S., Lelaidier, C., Olivennes, F., Ville, Y. and Frydman, R. (1995). Ultrasound-guided injection of methotrexate versus laparoscopic salpingotomy in ectopic pregnancy. *Fertil. Steril.*, **63**, 25–9

35. Yao, M., Tulandi, T., Kaplow, M. and Smith, A. P. (1996). A comparison of methotrexate versus laparoscopic surgery for the treatment of ectopic pregnancy: a cost analysis. *Hum. Reprod.*, **11**, 2762–6

Interventional ultrasound in human reproduction

21

S. Kupesic and A. Kurjak

INTRODUCTION

Laparoscopy was a logical method of oocyte retrieval in first reports of successful *in vitro* fertilization (IVF)[1-5]. The main disadvantage of this method was that follicles located deep in the ovary were not directly visualized, and the same problem applied to ovaries buried in adhesions[6]. Furthermore, it required general anesthesia and was associated with increased operative morbidity and/or mortality. Particularly, abdominal insufflation with carbon dioxide led to subtle and transient changes of pH, which may have had deleterious effects on the oocytes. During the early 1980s, the first generation of real-time sector scanners became available, offering better resolution and allowing ultrasound-guided percutaneous aspiration of oocytes.

TRANSABDOMINAL OOCYTE RECOVERY

Lenz and colleagues[7] were the first to describe the technique of ultrasound-guided oocyte retrieval. The use of various analgesics and tranquilizers made the procedure pain-free and ensured patient acceptability[8]. The use of general anesthesia should be avoided since it can lead to hyperprolactinemia, which may adversely affect the microenvironment of the oocyte[9]. Early reports described the use of linear array transducers[10], while most operators find sector scanners more suitable. High-resolution transducers have a detachable biopsy guide accompanied by the appropriate software facility. Most authors report the use of a 16-gauge needle with an inner diameter of 1.1 mm[10,11]. Teflon coating of the needles can reduce adhesion to the oocytes, while sharp cutting allows adequate penetration through ovarian tissue with minimal force or pain. The sonographer's end of the needle fits into the teflon tubing, which is attached to a large syringe containing the heparinized warm culture medium for flushing the follicle. Flushing the follicles after aspiration enables operators to achieve a satisfactory oocyte recovery rate per punctured follicle[9]. Flushing channels are constructed either parallel or concentric to the aspiration needle. Manual suction with a 5-ml syringe was used during the first attempts, but since uncontrolled pressure during the aspiration procedure may lead to fracture of the zona pellucida, operators introduced controlled mechanical suction via a foot pump, producing a maximum pressure of 80–100 mmHg[12]. Other necessary equipment includes a comfortable table for the patient, sterile sheets and a cover for the ultrasound transducers, sterile ultrasound gel and a waterbath or heater. Each patient should be counseled and carefully prepared. A wide variety of induction protocols are used to initiate growth of multiple follicles, while a combination of both endocrinologic and ultrasonographic data is employed for timing the administration of human chorionic gonadotropin (hCG). Before entering the procedure an ultrasound scan is recommended. The aim of this scan is to define the number and size of available follicles and compare them with the data obtained on the day of hCG administration. The patient should be instructed to drink 2 l of fluid 1 h before the expected procedure. In some cases catheterization and instillation of Hartmann's solution is performed. However, the operator should be aware of a risk of introducing infection and provoking bladder irritability. An adequately full bladder allows clear visualization of the ovarian follicles and prevents interposition of the bowel between the abdominal wall and the ovary. Most programs use a combination of a tranquilizer and an analgesic, while local anesthesia is usually given at the needle insertion site. As alternatives, epidural, spinal or general anesthesia may be used. After cleaning the lower abdomen with antiseptic fluid, sterile sheets are placed to margin the operating area. The transducer is covered with a sterile ultrasound gel and then wrapped around by a sterile bag or envelope. A sterile and transparent plastic sheet is placed over the keyboard of the ultrasound equipment. The needle is inserted either using the free hand technique or through a biopsy guide directly into the bladder. After passing the posterior bladder wall and ovarian capsule, the position of the needle tip is adjusted to the middle of the proximal follicle. The follicular fluid is aspirated, and the collapsed follicle may be flushed with a similar volume of the medium. In the same manner all the follicles are systematically aspirated without withdrawal from the ovary. The operator should be aware that inadequate bladder filling and the presence of pelvic adhesions may alter the ovarian position, while obesity and scar tissue can cause poor visualization of pelvic organs. After completion of the procedure the patient is allowed to empty the bladder and is usually discharged within 2 h.

PERURETHRAL OOCYTE RECOVERY UNDER SONOGRAPHIC CONTROL

Gleicher and colleagues[13] were the first to report ultrasound-directed follicle aspiration while scanning transabdominally through the bladder. A speculum was introduced into the vagina, and a needle was inserted through the vaginal fornix into the ovary. Parsons and associates[14] and Dellenbach and colleagues[15] developed the perurethral technique for collection of oocytes. The programs were conducted on an outpatient basis, keeping the

costs down. The patient was placed in the lithotomy position with the operator standing on her right, the ultrasound machine on her left, and the assistant sitting between the legs[16]. A solution of cetrimide and clorhexidine was used for vulvar toilet. The needle tip was placed in the side hole of a Foley catheter 14 and was inserted into the bladder via the urethra. The patient's bladder was then filled with Hartmann's solution, the catheter balloon was inflated, and the needle tip was disengaged from the catheter. After visualization of the needle tip by ultrasound, the operator guided it through the posterior wall of the bladder into the nearest follicle. Follicles were aspirated and flushed in order, and after all of them had been emptied, the needle was withdrawn, the bladder was emptied, and the catheter removed. The patient was encouraged to drink and void urine before leaving the hospital. The overall complication rate was minimal, while no patient developed urinary or pelvic infections after the procedure. Booker and colleagues[17] compared the perurethral route with the transvaginal route in a prospective randomized study. Significantly more follicles could be visualized with the transvaginal probe than with the transabdominal probe. However, there was no difference in the number of oocytes retrieved. The mean times of the procedures were similar, as well as the fertilization rates, embryo transfer rates and pregnancy rates. Therefore, the authors concluded that the perurethral and transvaginal routes for ultrasound-directed follicle aspiration are equally efficient.

TRANSVAGINAL OOCYTE RETRIEVAL

Experience has shown that the transvaginal technique using needle-guidance is superior to all other ultrasound-guided techniques[18]. The proximity of the transducer to the pelvic organs makes possible the use of high-frequency probes, thereby enhancing the resolution and clinical efficiency. The elastic vault of the vagina allows approximation of the ovaries by increased pressure of the tip of the probe.

Since there is no need for a full urinary bladder, pelvic anatomy is undistorted and the ovaries are kept beyond the focal zone of the transducer. Obesity or adhesions do not inhibit the visualization of the follicles and are not contraindications for this technique.

Standardized programmed stimulation is monitored by transvaginal sonography[19]. Additional information may be obtained by hormonal estimation and color Doppler studies[20-22] of the ovarian and uterine circulations. The entire treatment is carried out in an outpatient setting. The patient is placed on a gynecological table in the lithotomy position. Although anesthesia and sedative analgesia have been abandoned in about 50% of IVF programs[23], sedative medication (consisting of flunitrazepam, droperidol and pentazocine) may be used. Since the mean duration of the oocyte retrieval is 10 min, most patients tolerate the procedure easily. However, the operator should be aware of possible hypotonic reactions and discomfort experienced by some patients. Before inserting the probe into the cover, the operator should apply the ultrasonic coupling gel. The cover (a sterile condom, surgical rubber glove or specially-produced rubber cover) is stretched over the gel to expel the air from the tip of the probe. This can prevent artifacts during the procedure. The gel or lubricant should not be used while inserting the probe because of spermicidal action and reported embryotoxicity[24]. Instead, one can use a physiologic saline or culture medium. Sterile needle guides are used for transvaginal puncture of the follicles. The keyboard of the ultrasound machine is covered with a sterile cover which enables the operator to make any readjustment under sterile conditions. The patient's legs and perigenital area are then covered using sterile drapes. After cleaning the vagina with isotonic saline or culture medium the vaginal probe is inserted into the vagina.

To prevent potential risks of the puncture procedures, an automatic puncturing device has been developed. This device contains a mobile metal tube, the needle carrier, into which the aspiration needle is inserted and locked by a twisting movement[18]. Before

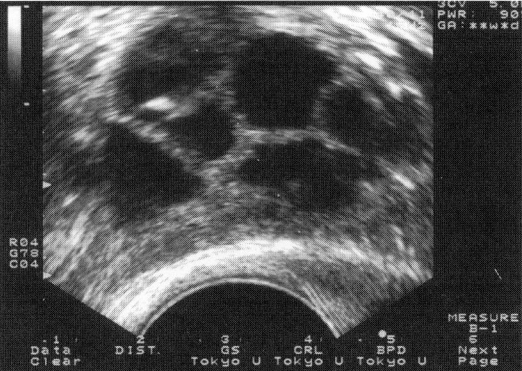

Figure 1 Transvaginal oocyte retrieval. The needle guide is attached to the probe, and a dotted guideline passes through the largest diameter of the ovary. The suction begins when the needle tip reaches the follicle

inserting the probe with a puncture device into the vagina, the device should be loaded and secured. After insertion, a detailed ultrasound examination is performed to locate the uterus and the ovaries. The probe is directed, allowing the biopsy vector to be placed at the central part of the nearest follicle, indicating the direction of the needle (Figure 1). The operator measures the distance on the biopsy vector on the screen and 'shoots' the follicle, either automatically (using the depth-limiting screw) or manually. After the needle is rapidly advanced into the follicle, the operator begins suction through the tubing connected to the suction pump. As the follicular fluid is aspirated one can see the follicle collapsing, while follicular fluid is pulled into the collecting chamber[18]. A flushing procedure may be used to improve the rate of oocyte aspiration. A flushing medium that contains heparin is injected through the tubing or using an automated flushing system. All the follicles along the same line are aspirated without withdrawing the needle. Feichtinger and colleagues[25] reported a low incidence of complications while using the transvaginal technique for oocyte recovery. Iliac veins were confused for a follicle and were mistakenly punctured in 2.4% of all cases. Bleeding into the pouch of Douglas was detected on the ultrasound screen, and stopped spontaneously in all cases.

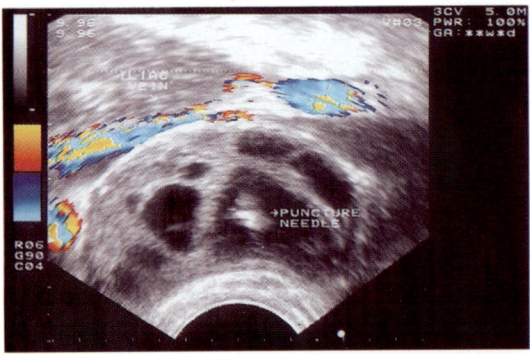

Figure 2 Demonstration of transvaginal oocyte retrieval using color Doppler. The dotted guideline passes through one of the ovarian follicles. A needle is inserted with the needle tip inside the proximal follicle, and aspiration begins. Color Doppler facilitates the visualization of the iliac vessels

An observation was made that filling the bladder may exert pressure on the site, and therefore stop the bleeding. Color Doppler can easily prevent such a complication, since iliac vessels are easily visualized using this technique (Figure 2). Bleeding from the vaginal vault is easily detectable and can be stopped by compression. Pelvic inflammatory disease (PID) is a rare complication of transvaginal follicle aspiration, reported in 0.14% of patients[25]. The infections are mostly caused by infected semen, and occur in patients with a positive history of PID.

GAMETE AND ZYGOTE INTRAFALLOPIAN TRANSFER

The gamete intrafallopian transfer (GIFT) procedure was developed to eliminate certain barriers to sperm transport and to eliminate the failure of the Fallopian tube to capture an egg at the time of ovulation[26]. These patients undergo ovulation induction and ultrasound monitoring. Laparoscopy is carried out to obtain the oocytes, and after identification in the laboratory, they are taken into a catheter which contains 100 000 sperm separated by the swim-up technique[26]. The transfer catheter is then guided into the upper outer third of the Fallopian tube and the contents are gently discharged. This technique brings the sperm and the oocytes into proximity and eliminates many of the barriers that might impede sperm transport and fusion[27]. Since fertilization takes place in its natural location the reported success rate is up to 26.5% deliveries per retrieval[28].

In zygote intrafallopian transfer (ZIFT), oocytes are obtained by vaginal aspiration, fertilized *in vitro*, and then 1 day later at the pronuclear stage placed in the Fallopian tubes by the GIFT technique[29]. The technique of transvaginal aspiration for the ZIFT procedure is the same as reported for IVF. The overall success rate seems to be the same as for GIFT and IVF procedures. The disadvantages of GIFT and ZIFT are that they cannot be used in cases of tubal damage, and that they require anesthesia and operating room facilities. Furthermore, they cannot be used in cases of male infertility when it is important to know whether fertilization has taken place. Modifications of GIFT and ZIFT include transcervical cannulation of the Fallopian tube with injection of the gametes or embryos into the tube. Accordingly, the cost of the procedure and risks are significantly decreased, while pregnancy rates remain at the same level.

EMBRYO TRANSFER

Intrauterine embryo transfer is a critical last step in the process of *in vitro* fertilization. Inaccurate placement of the embryos within the uterus may be an important factor causing unsuccessful implantation. Therefore, ultrasound-guided embryo transfer could have significant advantages over the more common 'blind' transfer[30]. Hurley and colleagues[31] used transvaginal sonographic guidance for intrauterine embryo transfer with a transcervical catheter in 94 patients. A culture medium containing the embryos was subsequently injected by air bubbles, which ensured accurate placement of the embryos within the uterus. This method was particularly helpful in six cases in which the catheter coiled in the region of the internal cervical os, despite the operator's impression that the catheter had

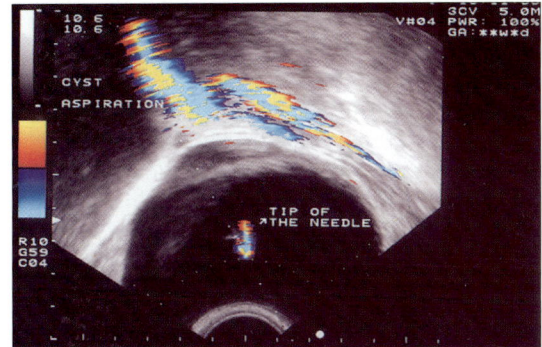

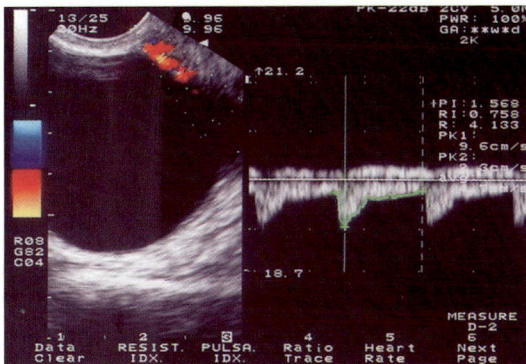

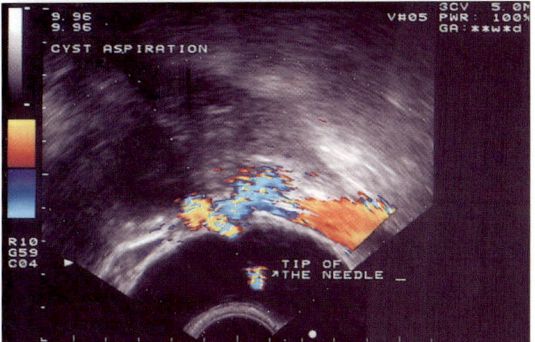

Figure 4 A transvaginal ultrasound scan of a solitary anechoic ovarian cyst. Color Doppler imaging demonstrates pericystic flow with a high resistance index (0.75)

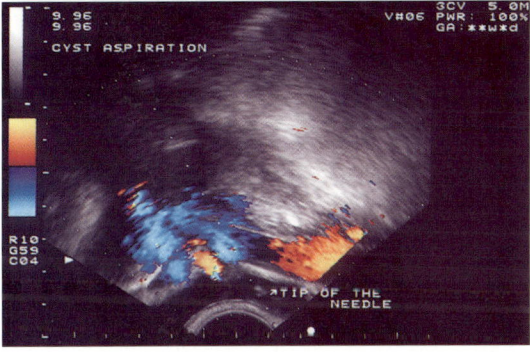

Figure 3 Demonstration of ovarian cyst aspiration. The dotted guideline passes through the cyst. (a) A needle is inserted with the needle tip in the central part of the cyst, and aspiration begins. The visualization of the needle tip is facilitated by color flow. (b) Half of the cyst has been aspirated. Note the color signals indicative of the needle tip within the central part of the cyst. The iliac vessels are mapped in color. (c) Note the complete shrinkage of the cyst

been correctly placed in the uterine cavity. This technique showed its efficacy in patients with submucous myomas or uterine anomalies. This ultrasound-guided procedure allowed patients to visualize the entire procedure on the screen which resulted in decreased anxiety. Lenz and colleagues[32] and Parsons and associates[33] used transvaginal ultrasound to direct the transfer of embryos through the uterine wall into the fundal endometrium. This may be an alternative to cervical transfer in patients with cervical stenosis, in whom it is difficult to pass the catheter through the cervix.

TUBAL CATHETERIZATION

Proximal obstruction of the Fallopian tubes accounts for approximately 15% of female infertility. This location of tubal occlusion is due to intraluminal debris, light adhesions or muscular spasms[34]. Transcervical Fallopian tube catheterization can be used for both diagnosis and treatment of the patients[35-40]. Patients are selected for this procedure on the basis of either bilateral tubal occlusion or obstruction of the remaining tube after unilateral salpingectomy[30]. The catheter serves as a dilator by its advancement over a guide wire that inserts it into the Fallopian tube. With fluoroscopy, tubal catheterization is successful in up to 98% of tubocornual occlusions but has only a 33% success rate when the occlusion is distal to the tubocornual junction[36]. Transvaginal sonographic guidance can also be used for tubal catheterization, although there is little experience with this technique. Lisse and Sydow[41] reported tubal catheterization under control of transvaginal ultrasound. Simultaneous laparoscopy confirmed the correct placement of the catheter within the proximal Fallopian tube (3–6 cm from the uterine cornu). They achieved tubal patency in 85% of patients with proximal tubal obstructions. Breckenridge and Schinfeld[42] and Thurmond and colleagues[43] suggest that transabdominal ultrasound is simpler than transvaginal sonography for guiding the tubal catheterization. They report that the full bladder which is required for transabdominal ultrasound straightens the uterus for a more direct approach. Potential complications of transcervical Fallopian tube catheterization are tubal perforation, vasovagal reactions during the procedure, and infection. The patients should be informed about the increased risk for ectopic pregnancy after the procedure.

OVARIAN CYST ASPIRATION

Transvaginal guidance permits direct visualization and aspiration of persistent follicular cysts[30]. Such cysts may impair folliculogenesis due to elaboration of hormones, or as a result of decreased perfusion by parenchymal compression. In the puncture of an ovarian or paraovarian cyst the center of the cyst is targeted and the needle is inserted (Figure 3). Such a procedure is highly debated in the literature. The concern of cell spillage from a potentially malignant ovarian cyst into the abdominal cavity prevents many from using it more frequently. Although the aspirated fluid is necessarily submitted for cytologic evaluation, a negative cytologic examination may sometimes represent a false-negative result. High sensitivity and specificity of transvaginal color Doppler in differentiation between benign and malignant adnexal lesions seems to increase the reliability in deciding which cysts should be aspirated (Figure 4).

Bret and colleagues[44,45] published two papers describing their experience using transvaginal sonography in the aspiration of ovarian cysts. They reported a 48% recurrence rate after cyst aspiration in premenopausal patients,

and an 80% recurrence rate in postmenopausal women. This group attempted to prevent cyst recurrence by injecting alcohol immediately after cyst aspiration, but this procedure was successful in only four of seven patients[45].

The aspiration of endometriomata is considered to be relatively contraindicated. Aboulghar and associates[46] studied 21 patients in whom transvaginal ultrasonically guided aspiration of pelvic and endometriotic cysts was performed. Re-accumulation occurred in only six cases during a 12-month follow-up. Certainly, the aspiration of endometriotic cysts is technically simple; however, its overall benefit and safety are still inconclusive due to the lack of experience obtained by evaluating larger series[47]. In an infertility program, Waegemaeker and colleagues[48] aspirated 32 unilocular anechoic cysts, with an average diameter of 45 mm, transvaginally. The authors concluded that ovarian cyst puncture in the early follicular phase could diminish the cancellation rate of *in vitro* fertilization cycles.

DRAINAGE OF PELVIC ABSCESSES

Infertility is attributed to tubal obstruction or dysfunction in 30–40% of patients. It is well known that tubal occlusion is a common sequela of pelvic inflammatory disease (PID). Since recurrent episodes of PID are frequent, one should expect a high incidence of this entity in the infertile population. In patients with a tubo-ovarian abscess, abscess drainage with sonographic guidance can hasten the recovery process and improve the efficacy of antibiotic therapy. Once the needle is placed into the abscess cavity, the fluid can be aspirated as completely as possible and the needle withdrawn, or an indwelling drainage catheter can be placed[30]. Teisala and associates[49] used transvaginal ultrasound-guided aspiration to drain 10 tubo-ovarian abscesses receiving antimicrobial treatment. Only light sedation was required, and the procedure was well tolerated by the patients. This technique is accepted as an alternative to open laparoscopy for treating tubo-ovarian abscesses.

MULTIEMBRYO REDUCTION

During the past 15 years, the increased use of ovulation-inducing drugs as well as the increased number of medically assisted reproduction procedures, has resulted in a large number of multiple gestations. Multiple pregnancy is associated with high mortality and morbidity and the probability of achieving a term pregnancy with healthy neonates is inversely proportional to the number of fetuses. Therefore, multiembryo reduction seeks to reduce the number of embryos to improve survival for the remaining ones[50]. Women with four or more embryos may be offered selective reduction, with the number of embryos usually reduced to two[30]. The procedure is normally delayed until after 8 weeks, when the spontaneous loss rate is relatively low. The transabdominal ultrasound-guided technique was first presented by Dumez and Oury[51], and has since been adopted by others[52,53]. With the developing use of transvaginal sonography this approach was attempted and successfully applied in multifetal reduction as well. Advantages of this technique are a shorter puncture route and more precise needle placement, reducing the risk of inadvertent injury to adjacent gestational sacs or other pelvic structures. A brief explanation of the technique for transvaginal multiembryo reduction is as follows: a baseline mapping procedure of the chorionic sacs and a detailed evaluation of the heartbeat of the targeted fetus are followed by placement of the needle and injection of 0.5–1 ml of 2-mEq/ml KCl solution. The heartbeat of each injected fetus is observed for 5–10 min to confirm cessation. The patients should be rescanned 3 h and then 1 week after the procedure for follow-up. The disadvantage of transvaginal fetal reduction is that at an early gestational age the final number of fetuses is not yet established[47].

CONCLUSION

Although ultrasound-guided procedures are most commonly used in the field of reproductive assistance, it is clear that similar techniques can be applied in other clinical situations as well. Most of the transvaginally performed procedures described in this chapter can be performed in an office setting, proving technical simplicity and low complication rate. More details about contrast hysterosalpingography can be found in a separate chapter.

References

1. Edwards, R. G., Steptoe, P. C. and Purdy, J. M. (1980). Establishing full-term human pregnancies using cleaving embryos grown *in vitro*. *Br. J. Obstet. Gynaecol.*, **87**, 737–41

2. Trounson, O. A., Leeton, J. F., Wood, C., Webb, J. and Wood, J. (1981). Pregnancies in humans by *in vitro* fertilization and embryo transfer in the controlled cycle. *Science*, **212**, 681–4

3. Jones, H. W. Jr, Jones, G. S., Andrews, M. D., Acosta, A., Bundren, C., Garcia, J., Sandow, B., Veeck, L., Wilkes, C., Witmyer, J., Wortham, J. E. and Wright, G. (1982). The program for *in vitro* fertilization at Norfolk. *Fertil. Steril.*, **38**, 14–19

4. Jones, H. W. Jr, Acosta, A. A., Garcia, J. E., Sandow, B. A. and Veeck, L. (1983). On the transfer of conceptuses from oocytes fertilized *in vitro*. *Fertil. Steril.*, **39**, 241–5

5. Lopata, A., Johnston, I. W., Hoult, I. J. and Speirs, A. I. (1980). Pregnancy following intrauterine implantation of an embryo obtained by *in vitro* fertilization of a preovulatory egg. *Fertil. Steril.*, **33**, 117–21

6. Riddle, A. F., Sharma, V., Mason, B. A., Ford, N. T., Pampiglione, J. S., Parsons, J. and Campbell, S. (1987). Two year's experience of ultrasound-directed oocyte retrieval. *Fertil. Steril.*, **48**, 454–7

7. Lenz, S., Lauritsen, J. G. and Kjellow, M. (1981). Collection of human oocytes for *in vitro* fertilization by ultrasonically guided follicular puncture. *Lancet*, **1**, 1163–4

8. Lenz, S. and Lauritsen, J. G. (1982). Ultrasonically guided percutaneous aspiration of human follicles under local anaesthesia: a new method of collecting oocytes for *in vitro* fertilization. *Fertil. Steril.*, **38**, 673–7

9. Sharma, V. (1993). Transabdominal oocyte recovery. In Chervenak, F. A., Isaacson, G. C. and Campbell, S. (eds.) *Ultrasound in Obstetrics and Gynecology*, pp. 1379–89. (London: Little, Brown and Company)

10. Wikland, M., Nilsson, L., Hansson, R., Hamberger, L. and Janson, P. O. (1983). Collection of human oocytes by use of sonography. *Fertil. Steril.*, **39**, 603–7

11. Lewinthal, D., Mahadevan, M., Pattinson, H. A., Taylor, P. J. and Persaud, D. (1987). Follicular factors, serum estradiol, and outcome of pregnancy following *in vitro* fertilization and embryo transfer. *Fertil. Steril.*, **48**, 840–5

12. Cohen, J., Avery, S., Campbell, S., Mason, B. A., Riddle, A. and Sharma, V. (1986). Follicular aspiration using a syringe suction system may damage the zona pellucida. *J. In Vitro Fertil. Embryo Transfer*, **3**, 224–8

13. Gleicher, N., Friberg, J., Fullan, N., Giglia, R. V., Mayden, K., Kesky, T. and Siegel, I. (1983). Egg retrieval for *in vitro* fertilization by sonographically controlled vaginal culdocentesis. *Lancet*, **2**, 508–600

14. Parsons, J., Riddle, A., Booker, M., Sharma, V., Goswamy, R., Wilson, L., Akkermans, J., Whitehead, M. and Campbell, S. (1985). Oocyte retrieval for *in vitro* fertilization by ultrasonically guided needle aspiration via the urethra. *Lancet*, **1**, 1076–8

15. Dellenbach, P., Nisand, I., Moreau, L., Ferger, B., Plumere, C. and Gerlinger, P. (1985). Transvaginal sonographically controlled follicle puncture for oocyte retrieval. *Fertil. Steril.*, **44**, 656–61

16. Booker, M. and Parsons, J. (1993). Ultrasound-directed follicle aspiration for oocyte collection by the perurethral technique. In Chervenak, F. A., Isaacson, G. C. and Campbell, S. (eds.) *Ultrasound in Obstetrics and Gynecology*, pp. 1391–6. (London: Little, Brown and Company)

17. Booker, M. W., Pampiglione, J. S. and Parsons, J. (1988). A prospective randomized comparison of the perurethral transvesical route with the transvaginal route for ultrasound-directed follicle aspiration. *Fertil. Steril.*, **50**(Suppl.), 120–5

18. Feichtinger, W. (1993). Transvaginal oocyte retrieval. In Chervenak, F. A., Isaacson, G. C. and Campbell, S. (eds.) *Ultrasound in Obstetrics and Gynecology*, pp. 1397–1406. (London: Little, Brown and Company)

19. Kemeter, P. and Feichtinger, W. (1989). Experience with a new fixed-stimulation protocol without hormone determinations for programmed oocyte retrieval for *in vitro* fertilization. *Hum. Reprod.*, **4**(Suppl.), 53–4

20. Kurjak, A., Kupesic, S., Schulman, H. and Zalud, I. (1991). Transvaginal color Doppler in the assessment of ovarian and uterine blood flow in infertile women. *Fertil. Steril.*, **56**, 870–3

21. Kupesic, S. and Kurjak, A. (1993). Uterine and ovarian perfusion during the periovulatory phase assessed by transvaginal color Doppler. *Fertil. Steril.*, **60**, 439–43

22. Kurjak, A. and Kupesic, S. (1995). Ovarian senescence and its significance for uterine and ovarian perfusion. *Fertil. Steril.*, **64**, 532–7

23. Feichtinger, W., Putz, M. and Kemeter, P. (1988). New aspects of vaginal ultrasound in an *in vitro* fertilization program. *Ann. N. Y. Acad. Sci.*, **541**, 125–30

24. Schwimer, S. R., Rothman, C. M., Lebovic, J. and Oye, D. M. (1984). The effect of ultrasound coupling gels on sperm motility *in vitro*. *Fertil. Steril.*, **42**, 946–50

25. Feichtinger, W., Putz, M. and Kemeter, P. (1988). Four years' experience with ultrasound-guided follicle aspiration. *Ann. N. Y. Acad. Sci.*, **541**, 138–45

26. Asch, R. H., Balmareda, J. P., Ellsworth, L. R. and Wong, P. C. (1986). Preliminary experience with gamete intrafallopian transfer (GIFT). *Fertil. Steril.*, **45**, 366–9

27. Marmar, J. L. (1988). Idiopathic male infertility. In Garcia, C. R., Mastroianni, L., Arnelar, R. D. and Dubin, L. (eds.) *Current Therapy of Infertility 3*, pp. 196–201. (Toronto: BC Decker)

28. Society for Assisted Reproductive Technology, The American Fertility Society (1993). Assisted reproductive technology in the United States and Canada: 1991 results from the Society for Assisted Reproductive Technology generated from the American Fertility Society Registry. *Fertil. Steril.*, **59**, 956–9

29. Speroff, L., Glass, R. H. and Kase, N. (1994). Assisted reproduction. In Speroff, L., Glass, R. H. and Kase, N. G. *Clinical Gynecologic Endocrinology and Infertility*, 5th edn., pp. 931–46. (Baltimore: Williams and Wilkins)

30. Hill, M. L. and Nyberg, D. A. (1992). Transvaginal sonography-guided procedures. In Nyberg, D. A., Hill, L. M., Bohm-Velez, M. and Mendelson, E. B. (eds.) *Transvaginal Ultrasound*, pp. 319–29. (St. Louis: Mosby Year Book)

31. Hurley, V. A., Osborn, J. C., Leoni, M. A. and Leeton, J. (1991). Ultrasound-guided embryo transfer: a controlled trial. *Fertil. Steril.*, **55**, 559–62

32. Lenz, S., Leeton, J., Rogers, P. and Trounson, A. (1987). Transfundal transfer of embryos using ultrasound. *J. In Vitro Fertil. Embryo Transfer*, **4**, 13–17

33. Parsons, J. H., Bolton, V. N., Wilson, L. and Campbell, S. (1987). Pregnancies following *in vitro* fertilization and ultrasound-directed surgical embryo transfer by perurethral and transvaginal techniques. *Fertil. Steril.*, **48**, 691–3

34. Sulak, P. I., Letterie, G. S. and Coddington, C. C. (1987). Histology of proximal tubal occlusion. *Fertil. Steril.*, **48**, 437–40

35. Confino, E., Friberg, J. and Gleicher, N. (1986). Transcervical balloon tuboplasty. *Fertil. Steril.*, **46**, 963–6

36. Rosch, J., Thurmond, A., Uchida, B. and Sovak, M. (1988). Selective transcervical Fallopian tube catheterization: technique update. *Radiology*, **168**, 1–5

37. Thurmond, A. and Rosch, J. (1990). Nonsurgical Fallopian tube recanalization for treatment of infertility. *Radiology*, **174**, 371–4

38. Kumpe, D. A., Zwerdlinger, S. C. and Rothbarth, L. J. (1990). Proximal Fallopian tube occlusion: diagnosis and treatment with transcervical Fallopian tube catheterization. *Radiology*, **17**, 183–7

39. Segars, J. H., Herbert, C. M. and Moore, D. E. (1990). Selective Fallopian tube cannulation: initial experience in an infertile population. *Fertil. Steril.*, **53**, 357–9

40. Deaton, J. L., Gibson, M., Riddick, D. H. and Brumsted, J. R. (1990). Diagnosis and treatment of cornual obstruction using a flexible guide wire. *Fertil. Steril.*, **53**, 232–6

41. Lisse, K. and Sydow, P. (1991). Fallopian tube catheterization and recanalization under ultrasonic observation: a simplified technique to evaluate tubal patency and open proximally obstructed tubes. *Fertil. Steril.*, **56**, 198–201

42. Breckenridge, J. W. and Schinfeld, J. S. (1991). Technique for ultrasound-guided Fallopian tube catheterization. *Radiology*, **180**, 569–70

43. Thurmond, A. S., Patton, P. E., Hector, D. M. and Jones, M. K. (1991). Ultrasound-guided Fallopian tube catheterization. *Radiology*, **180**, 571–2

44. Bret, P. M., Guibaud, L. and Atri, M. (1992). Transvaginal ultrasound-guided aspiration of ovarian cysts and solid pelvic masses. *Radiology*, **185**, 377

45. Bret, P. M., Atri, M. and Guibaud, L. (1992). Ovarian cysts in postmenopausal women: preliminary results with transvaginal alcohol sclerosis. *Radiology*, **184**, 661

46. Aboulghar, M. A., Mansour, R. T., Serour, G. I. and Rizk, B. (1991). Ultrasonic transvaginal aspiration of endometriotic cysts: an optional line of treatment in selected cases of endometriosis. *Hum. Reprod.*, **6**, 1408–10

47. Lerner, J. P. and Monteagudo, A. (1995). Vaginal sonographic puncture procedures. In Goldstein, S. R. and Timor-Tritsch, I. E. (eds.) *Ultrasound in Gynecology*, pp. 223–38. (New York: Churchill Livingstone)

48. Waegemaeker, C. T., Berg-Helder, A., Blankhart, A. and Naaktgeboren, N. (1988). Transvaginal ovarian cyst puncture in the early follicular phase of an IVF cycle: indications and results. *Hum. Reprod.*, **3**, 80

49. Teisala, K., Heinonen, P. K. and Punnonen, R. (1990). Transvaginal ultrasound in the diagnosis and treatment of tubo-ovarian abscesses. *Br. J. Obstet. Gynaecol.*, **97**, 178–80

50. Berkowitz, R. I. and Lynch, L. (1990). Selective reduction: an unfortunate misnomer. *Obstet. Gynecol.*, **75**, 873–4

51. Dumez, Y. and Oury, J. F. (1986). Method for first-trimester selective abortion in multiple pregnancy. *Contrib. Gynecol. Obstet.*, **15**, 50–3

52. Birnholz, J. C., Dmowski, W. P., Binor, Z. and Radwanska, E. (1987). Selective continuation in gonadotropin-induced multiple pregnancy. *Fertil. Steril.*, **48**, 873

53. Brandes, J. M., Itskovitz, J. and Timor-Tritsch, I. E. (1987). Reduction of the number of embryos in multiple pregnancy. *Fertil. Steril.*, **48**, 326–7

The evaluation of tubal patency by hysterosalpingo-contrast sonography (HyCoSy)

22

U. Deichert

HISTORICAL DEVELOPMENT

Ultrasound visualization of the internal genital tract using exogenous contrast media was first described by Nanini, Richman, Randolph and their colleagues[1–3] who performed abdominal sonography after intracervical injection of fluid. Following instillation of dextran or saline solution into the uterine cavity it was possible to visualize lesions, such as submucous myomas and polyps, by sonography and subsequently to confirm their presence by hysteroscopy[3–6]. Although lesions of this type, which project into the uterine cavity, are clearly delineated by poorly echogenic or anechoic media, very small hollow cavities, such as the lumen of normal tubes, are rarely visualizable with such techniques[2,7]. Their demonstration requires visualization of the movement of a fluid, which in turn requires the use of a highly echogenic medium[8–10]. An ultrasound contrast medium of this type was produced for use in echocardiography, making it possible for the first time to visualize blood flow as well as the anatomy of the heart. Gramiak and Shah[11] reported their observation of an echo cloud in the M-mode procedure following injection of indocyanine green into a peripheral vein. The reflective properties of gas microbubbles can be used for ultrasonography of blood flow. It has been shown experimentally that the contrast effect of various materials is attributable to microbubbles in injection solutions.

Echovist® (SHU 454; Schering AG, Berlin, Germany) is an ultrasound contrast medium

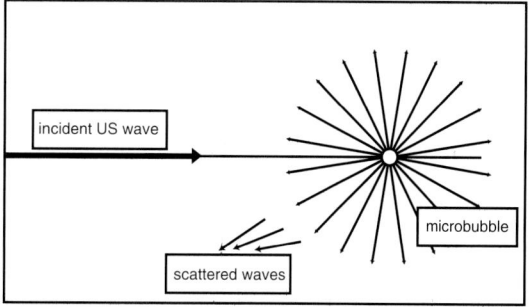

Figure 1 Scattering of ultrasound at a single bubble

consisting of a suspension of monosaccharide microparticles (50% galactose, 2 µm diameter), in a 20% aqueous solution of galactose (w/v). The echogenic suspension is reconstituted immediately before use from granules and a vehicle solution (200 mg microparticles in 1 ml of suspension)[12]. SHU 454 has been used for the ultrasound examination of uterus and tubes, as described below[13], and has been licensed for gynecological applications since 1991.

In October 1993, a number of European experts attended an Infertility Workshop in Las Vegas to evaluate all the available information on hysterosalpingo-contrast sonography (HyCoSy). The meeting has been fully reported elsewhere[14,15], however a brief summary of the most important information presented there and not covered in other sections of this chapter follows.

Results were presented from four clinical trials in 217 women whose tubal patency had bccn investigated by HyCoSy together with the echo contrast agent 'Echovist'.

Deichert assessed tubal patency using HyCoSy, conventional hysterosalpingography (HSG), or laparoscopy with dye in 76 women and visualized 152 Fallopian tubes (Table 1). In this study, HyCoSy showed 87.5% concordance with other techniques, predicted 100% of tubal occlusions and detected 86% of patent tubes. In a multicentre study, a further 224 women and 437 Fallopian tubes were investigated using HyCoSy alone; of the 437 tubes 410 were patent and 27 were occluded.

Degenhardt described his results in 77 women, again investigated with HyCoSy, HSG or laparoscopy with dye (Table 2). Reassessment of 14 of the 27 occluded tubes with HSG or laparoscopy and dye within 5 months of the HyCoSy investigation showed a concordance of 85% between results of HSG/laparoscopy and dye and HyCoSy.

Venezia investigated 41 women; HyCoSy was compared with HSG in 23 and with laparoscopy and dye in 15. HyCoSy showed bilateral tubal patency in 15 patents (37%), unilateral patency in 13 (32%), bilateral occlusion in three (7%) and failed to provide a diagnosis in 10 patients (24%). The degree of concordance between the methods is shown in Table 3.

Bourne compared HyCoSy with HSG in 23 women and classified the patients according to the number of tubes found to be occluded when assessed by either technique. Because patients found by HyCoSy to have occlusion of both tubes would automatically be investigated further using HSG, a false-positive result was defined as one of double occlusion detected by HyCoSy where subsequent HSG showed at least one tube to be patent (Table 4).

Overall, Bourne found a prevalence of 17% for blocked tubes, with a detection rate of 100% and a false-positive rate of 10.5%. The positive prediction rate was 66.7%, and concordance rate 91.3%. The sensitivity and specificity of HyCoSy using Echovist compared very well with those of HSG and laparoscopy and dye.

At the end of the Workshop the participants made an overall assessment of these benefits and limitations of HyCoSy (Table 5). The investigators concluded that: 'Combining these undoubted benefits with the clinical results obtained to date would indicate that HyCoSy has the potential to be employed as a reliable and well-accepted procedure for assessing tubal patency as part of the investigation of infertility'.

ULTRASOUND CONTRAST AGENTS BASED ON GALACTOSE

'Microbubbles', gaseous bubbles with microscopic diameters, are known to be extremely effective scatterers of ultrasound and because of their unique acoustic properties, they play a key role in the basic mode of action of ultrasound contrast media. However, single microbubbles with no protection against diffusion into, for example, carrier fluids, blood or serum exhibit a very short lifetime of only a few seconds[16]. This is one of the reasons

Table 1 Fallopian tubes classified as patent or not patent (Deichert study)

	HyCoSy		
	Not patent	Patent	Total
HSG or laparoscopy and dye			
Not patent	17	0	17
Patent	19	116	135
Total	36	116	152

Table 2 Tubal patency assessed by HyCoSy, laparoscopy (lap) and dye or conventional hysterosalpingography (HSG) (Degenhardt study)

	Agreed	Disagreed	Fallopian tubes	Patients	Concordance (%)
HyCoSy/lap and dye	100	10	110	57	90.0
HyCoSy/HSG	33	4	37	20	89.2

Table 3 Agreement between methods (Venezia study)

	HyCoSy/HSG	HyCoSy/laparoscopy and dye
Complete agreement	13 (57%)	8 (53%)
Partial agreement	7 (30%)	7 (47%)
No agreement	3 (13%)	0

Table 4 Tubal patency: HyCoSy versus HSG (Bourne study)

HSG/ HyCoSy	Both tubes blocked	At least one tube blocked	Total
Not patent	4	0	4
Patent	2*	17**	19
Total	6	17	23

*One tube patent by HSG; **Four patients with one tube patent by HSG and HyCoSy and one patient with one tube patent by HyCoSy alone

Table 5 Benefits and limitations of hysterosalpingo-contrast sonography

Benefits	Limitations
Reproducible and reliable assessment of tubal patency	Tubal spasm may lead to misdiagnosis of tubal occlusion (spasm also seen with other methods)
Avoids exposure to X-rays	
Avoids general anesthesia	In hydrosalpinx, tubal flow may give a false impression of tubal patency
Can be performed as an outpatient procedure	
Rapid	Cannot visualize intrapelvic pathology
Well tolerated: little discomfort and few adverse events	Requires a degree of technical competence
Avoids allergic reactions	10–20 investigations needed to acquire the new technique
Shows tubal patency to the patient in 'real time'	

for the frequently described problems of reproducibility and efficacy using self-made 'contrast agents', such as agitated saline or sonicated X-ray contrast media. After about 25 years of experimental work, there have been recent substantial advances, with the first industrial echocontrast agent being approved by health authorities.

This agent consists of galactose microparticles dissolved in a galactose solution. SHU 454 (Echovist) was introduced to the market in Germany in October 1991. Echovist is not stable enough to endure the transpulmonary passage and was developed for echocardiographic examination of right heart abnormalities (B-mode and color Doppler) as well as for the non-cardiac applications of phlebosonography and hysterosalpingo-contrast sonography (HyCoSy)[12,17]. The stabilized derivative of Echovist, a galactose-based agent, SHU 508 A (Levovist®) is able to pass into the lungs. Levovist is presently being evaluated in clinical trials in Europe for B-mode and Doppler blood pool echo enhancement[12,17].

Principles of echosignal enhancement

Basically, ultrasound contrast agents are media which when administered via the vascular system or into body cavities, change the acoustic properties of the body region under investigation. The acoustic parameters which contribute to tissue imaging by conventional sonographic units are backscatter, attenuation and velocity of sound. Of these, enhancement of backscatter is the most important contrast effect, since contrast agents introduce acoustic inhomogeneities caused by microstructures (scatterers) (Figure 1).

Image quality and contrast effects

The increase in echogenicity caused by ultrasound contrast agents can be exploited for B-mode scans as well as for Doppler examinations. When the baseline (precontrast) scan is of poor quality, the image quality and consequently the diagnostic improvement following contrast injection may be limited. Generally, the overall noise level in the B-mode image cannot be expected to change significantly following injection of a contrast agent. For Doppler sonography the situation is completely different. When signal intensity is sufficient, addition of the contrast agent is generally not required, but it may improve the diagnosis in patients in whom Doppler scans at baseline are suboptimal or non-diagnostic[17].

Characteristics of galactose-based contrast agents

With the help of a sophisticated sterile production process, special granules are produced consisting of numerous tiny galactose crystalline particles. In the case of Echovist, these microparticles consist of only galactose, which is a known nutritive monosaccharide. SHU 508 A (Levovist) microparticle granules contain in addition a very low concentration of physiological palmitic acid. A few minutes before use the granules have to be shaken vigorously for 5–10 s to be dissolved by an appropriate volume of aqueous galactose solution (Echovist) or sterile water (SHU 508 A). A milky suspension of galactose microparticles in a galactose solution is created after disaggregation of the microparticle 'snowball'. A proportion of the microparticles will dissolve until solubility equilibrium is reached: the remainder will be stabilized by that equilibrium. The air attached to and within the granules will produce a gas saturation of the liquid compartment: excess gas tends to form tiny bubbles, predominantly at the solid surfaces of the microparticles. It is a common experience that bubbles in an oversaturated liquid gas, such as champagne or carbonated mineral water, occur predominantly at certain sites on the glass. Similarly, the solid surfaces of the microparticles act as an origin for new bubble formation and stabilizing sites. The size of the microparticles helps to select bubbles of a certain diameter range: larger bubbles will disappear rapidly, like those in mineral water or shaken saline.

The suspension of Echovist is stable for about 5 min after preparation. Due to its extended stability, SHU 508 A may be administered up to 10 min after the suspension procedure. Figure 2 shows a vial containing Echovist, granules and the suspension fluid, 20% galactose solution, and the milky-white suspension containing scattering microbubbles which is ready for use. Different concentrations

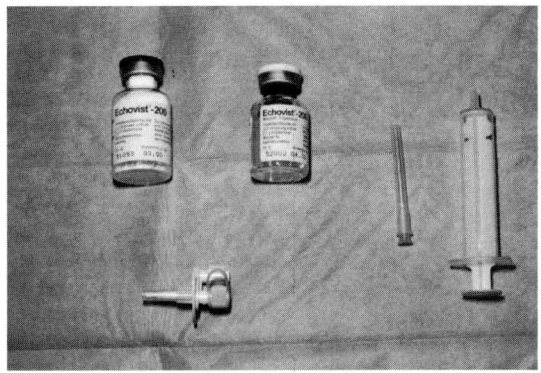

Figure 2 Echovist microparticle granules (left), Echovist suspension fluid (middle), mini-spike (below)

of scattering microbubbles can be obtained by varying the volume of the added suspension fluid. Depending on the indication and the imaging modality (B-mode or Doppler), clinically adequate suspensions of Echovist are with concentrations of 300 and 200 mg/ml. For SHU 508 A, the maximum concentration is 400 mg/ml. The predominant limitation at concentrations lower than 200 mg/ml is the decreasing suspension stability. Concentrations exceeding 400 mg/ml are limited by a rapid increase of viscosity[12,17,18].

Pharmacology and toxicology

Degradation

After intrauterine administration and emergence of Echovist from the fimbriae into the pelvis, the galactose microparticles dissolve. This progress is increased by warming to body temperature and dilution by the peritoneal fluid. In vitro, a rise in temperature of the Echovist suspension to 37 °C leads to complete dissolution within 30 min. The dissolved galactose is subsequently absorbed and metabolized.

Toxicology

Standard tests for assessing acute and subchronic toxicity, including local tolerance, embryotoxicity and mutagenicity, have been performed in several species. Even after repeated administration of diagnostic doses at short time intervals, there was no risk of acute intoxication from SHU 454 or SHU 508 A. Specially designed models were used to identify any potential risk from the injection of suspensions of microparticles and microbubbles. Vital microscopy for direct visualization of microcirculation and microbubbles was performed on the brain vessels of rabbits and cats, rat mesentery and hamster cheek pouch. No fluctuations in diameters of arterioles, density of perfused capillaries or any embolic events were observed[19].

TECHNIQUE OF HYSTEROSALPINGO-CONTRAST SONOGRAPHY (HyCoSy)

Requirements

Preparation

A case history must be obtained from women being considered for examination using this technique, to rule out the possibility of the rare condition of galactosemia, which is the only absolute contraindication apart from acute inflammatory diseases of the genital organs. Galactosemia is an autosomal recessive hereditary metabolic disorder, characterized by failure to metabolize galactose to glucose because of a deficiency of galactose1-phosphate-uridyl transferase 4. Newborn infants are initially normal, but suffer from loss of appetite, vomiting, hepatomegaly, jaundice, convulsions, proteinuria and aminoaciduria after only a few days of milk feeding.

These infants fail to thrive, develop edema and may die as a result of dystrophy. Surviving children exhibit growth retardation, brain damage, hepatic cirrhosis and cataracts. The early onset of the condition and the signs and symptoms of galactosemia are so distinctive that it is virtually impossible for the condition to go unrecognized.

Pertubal and periovarian adhesions are often present in patients with a history of pelvic inflammatory disease (i.e. fever associated with lower abdominal pain), or operations on the lower pelvis or appendectomy.

Such adhesions are likely to impair ovulation, but HyCoSy can only demonstrate tubal patency, and is not capable of detecting these types of lesions. The appropriate primary diagnostic procedure in these patients is diagnostic laparoscopy with chromopertubation, which can be combined with HyCoSy if extensive adhesions make it impossible to assess tubal patency. A gynecological examination and an ultrasound scan performed at the start of the menstrual cycle will detect prominent lesions such as uterine myomas and adnexal tumours. Again, the primary diagnostic procedure here is hysteroscopy and/or chromolaparoscopy or a combination of hysteroscopy with HyCoSy (see Applications).

HyCoSy should only be carried out after menstrual bleeding and in the first half of the menstrual cycle. Before any intervention, we perform a pregnancy test for legal reasons. The possibility of local or systemic infections is excluded by clinical examination (absence of elevated temperature), inspection of the genital tract, absence of signs of inflammation. The patients should be informed about the advantages and of the diagnostic capability of HyCoSy as compared with other methods. The risks of this procedure, which have been shown to be very small in previous studies, should be compared with those of other interventions for diagnosing uterine and tubal disorders.

Anesthesia

Unlike chromolaparoscopy, anesthesia is generally not required for HyCoSy, and the patient can follow the results of the examination herself on the monitor if she desires to do so (Figure 3). If HyCoSy is performed without anesthesia, patients occasionally report discomfort, especially if the tubes are occluded. The degree of discomfort experienced depends on the individual response of the patient. A premedication with 10 mg diazepam and 1 ml atropine 1 h before the intervention may ease the procedure. According to our experience, about 50% of patients tolerate the procedure without remarkable discomfort, about one-third report mild discomfort and the

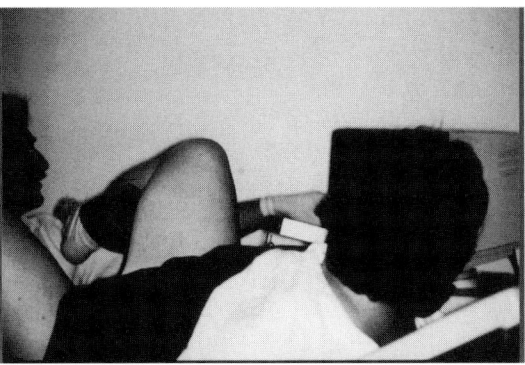

Figure 3 Demonstration of patient's finding of the Fallopian tubes on the monitor during the investigation

Table 6 Instruments required for HyCoSy

Sterile table with
Swabs in disinfectant solution
Speculum
Bullet forceps
Ringer's solution or NaCl solution in a kidney bowl
Two empty 20 ml syringes
Intrauterine catheter [bladder catheter (8 French)] with a guidewire (1 mm coarse wire) or other catheter (Ackrad, Bard, Cook, Zinnanti, see Table 7)
One empty 10 ml syringe (for Echovist)
Ultrasound contrast medium (not on the sterile table)
Vial containing galactose particles
Vial of diluent
Special filling connector with needle (package)

remainder require analgesia, or in a few cases anesthesia.

However, tubal spasm may occur if HyCoSy is performed without or even with anesthesia. This could mimic a tubal occlusion. For this reason, the diagnosis of a tubal occlusion should be confirmed by HSG or chromolaparoscopy under anesthesia before making a firm decision to perform microsurgery to clear obstructions.

In an analysis of the combined collectives of Hüneke *et al.*[20], and Böhmer *et al.*[21], 87 of 90 patients (97%) tolerated well the pertubation of the tubes by Echovist. By using hyporeflective contrast agents for pertubation, the analysis of a combined collective of 570 patients revealed 540 cases without severe discomfort (95%)[9,10,22–26]. By application of premedication this value could only be improved to 98%[27].

Instruments

To ensure that the procedure itself can be carried out without delay, a sterile set of all instruments required should be available in the examination room when the patient arrives (Table 6, Figure 4). The ultrasound equipment should be ready for use with the vaginal probe disinfected (for example in Cidex or prepared with a sterile cover).

If an HSG set is used instead of an intrauterine catheter, it is not advisable to use a standard condom because it is easily torn.

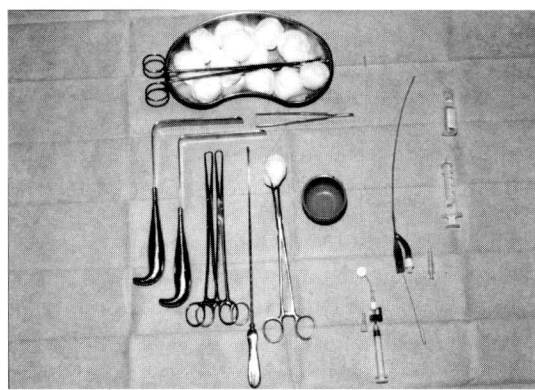

Figure 4 Instruments used for hysterosalpingo-contrast sonography

Special rubber covers are now available for the purpose.

The patient's identity may be entered into the computer before performing the procedure for documentation of the image. The findings of contrast medium pertubation should be documented by video, since motion or flow phenomena are the decisive features for making the diagnosis and if results are unclear the images can be re-examined after the end of the procedure or can be shown to the patient.

Procedure

Procedure up to injection of contrast medium

After the patient has taken the lithotomy position on the examination chair or the operating table, the external genitals and vagina have to be disinfected. The patient is asked to empty her bladder before examination, or alternatively she may be catheterized under anesthesia. During these preparatory steps, the patient should be kept informed about everything that is happening and should be told that she will shortly be able to follow the examination and the results herself on the ultrasound monitor. This information will contribute to the patient's sedation. The ultrasound equipment should therefore be placed to the right of the patient beside her right leg, to the left of the operator sitting between the legs of the patient. The instrument table should be adjacent and to the right of the operator. This arrangement is also to be recommended in other vaginal ultrasound procedures (Figure 3).

In anesthetized patients, after palpation of the genitals and insertion of the speculum, the cervix is clamped transversely with a small bullet forceps and the uterus is probed. If the patient is not anesthetized, it is usually possible to avoid clamping the cervix by using a balloon catheter, provided that the cervical canal readily admits passage of the catheter. However, clamping is required for passing the rigid HSG set (according to Cohen). If a balloon catheter is used, insertion of the tip of the catheter through the internal cervical os is easier if the cervix is gently pulled forward with the small bullet forceps, especially if the uterus is markedly flexed. This will make the procedure easier for those who are not yet entirely familiar with it. After inserting the catheter into the uterus, the balloon of the catheter is blocked with 1–2 ml of liquid (NaCl solution or water), the quantity depending on the width of the cervical os, or with an equal quantity of air. During this procedure, an awake patient sometimes experiences some pain and she should be warned to expect this. If a guidewire is used (with an 8 French urinary catheter, although with most other modern balloon catheters this is not necessary), this is then partly withdrawn. Gentle traction is then exerted on the distal end of the catheter to anchor the catheter to the internal cervical os.

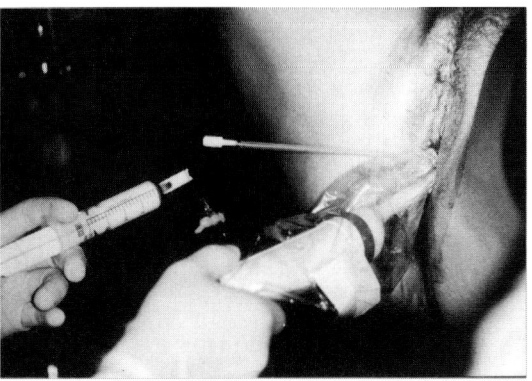

Figure 5 Positioning of the ultrasound probe and transcervical injection of the Echovist suspension

If the catheter is correctly positioned, the guidewire is withdrawn completely. If a double balloon catheter (Bard catheter) is used, after the first balloon has been blocked, the second balloon, positioned directly in the cervical canal and communicating with the outside via the external os, is filled with about the same quantity of liquid or air. This is then anchored in the cervical canal. If a simple balloon catheter is used, any subsequent examination is always performed while maintaining gentle traction on the distal end of the catheter. This seals the uterus while injecting fluid adds a slight excess pressure within the uterine cavity. The prepared vaginal ultrasound probe enters the vagina after lubrication with sterile gel or water. The internal genitals are inspected and the pouch of Douglas is tested for the presence of fluid. A syringe filled with 20 ml of Ringer's solution, attached to the distal end of the catheter, is held in the left hand ready for injection and the ultrasound probe is held in the right hand (Figure 5). Under vaginal ultrasound control, the uterine cavity is filled with fluid, and brief intermittent injections are made in a pulsatile fashion until the full contents of the syringe (10–20 ml) have been injected (in a few cases larger quantities may be needed). At the moment of injection the uterine cavity is most widely dilated and is thus well delineated for the assessment of intrauterine structures and the walls of the uterus (Figure 6). As the fluid is being injected, some patients report discomfort, especially if the outflow via the tubal ostia is blocked: although discomfort may indicate tubal occlusion this is not always the case.

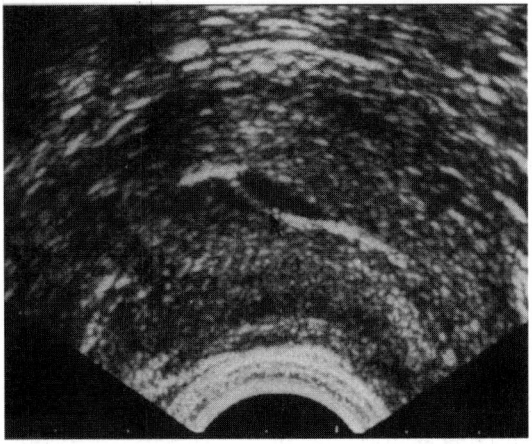

Figure 6 Intrauterine synechiae (arrow) confirmed by hysteroscopy, following abortion by curettage on three occasions. Longitudinal section evaluated by hysterosalpingo-contrast sonography with Ringer's solution

For precise differentiation of the uterine structures, systematic sections are made in the longitudinal ultrasound plane from the median to the lateral aspect and back again, then repeated on the other side of the pelvis. The catheter balloon or the cone of the HSG set is considered, then the normally smooth contour of the endometrial layers is followed from the anterior and posterior wall to the fundus, and structures projecting into the cavity are noted. Sweeping from the median to the lateral aspect reveals any increase or decrease in the thickness of the myometrium in the fundus: any raising or lowering of the upper margin of the uterine cavity indicates possible malformations (Figure 7). Finally, the pouch of Douglas is examined for any increase in retrouterine fluid, which may in itself be sufficient evidence that at least one of the tubes is patent[9,28]. An examination is also carried out for the formation of cystic structures such as hydrosaplinges (Figure 8).

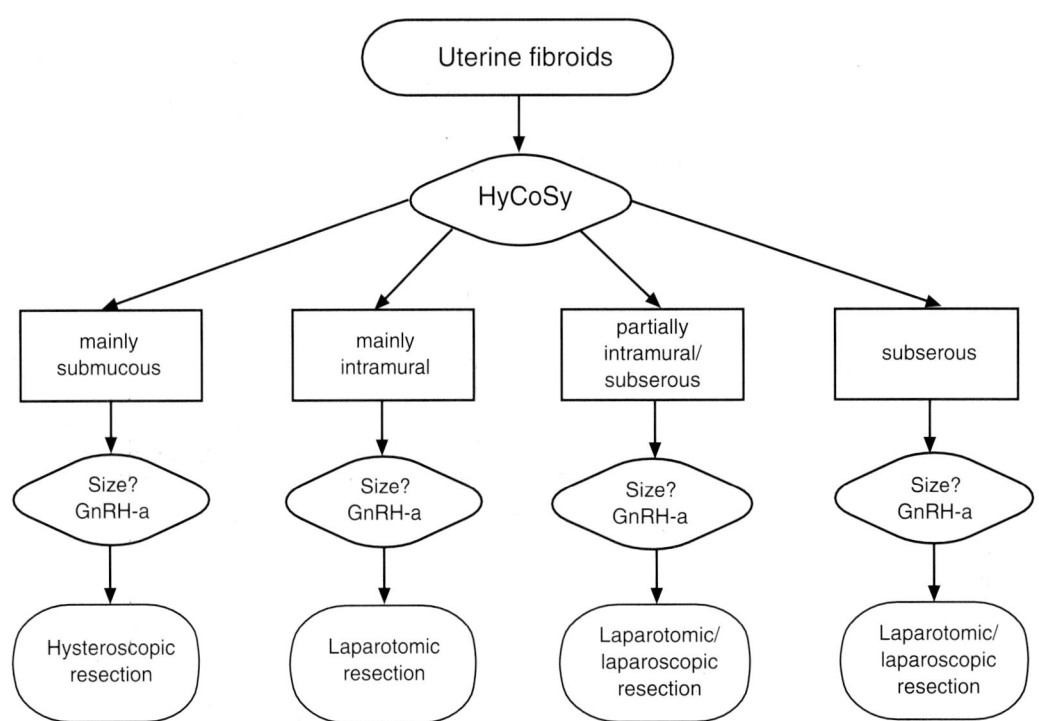

Figure 7 Schematic diagram to decide the optimal treatment of uterine fibroids on the basis of hysterosalpingo-contrast sonography (HyCoSy) findings

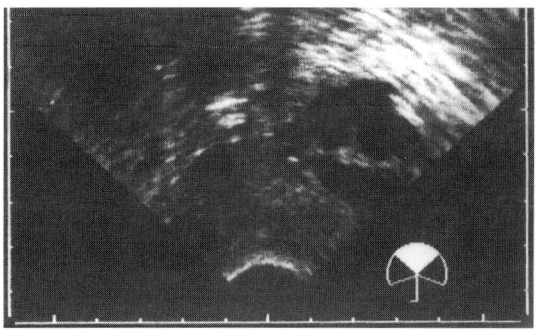

Figure 8 Hydrosalpinx filled with fluid (in transverse section) in a conglomerate tumor of ovary and uterine tube. The ultrasound signals characteristic of a thick-walled sometimes fleshy hydrosalpinx are the rigid mucosal fold projecting into the lumen

Examination of the uterus is now continued in the transverse plane. To ensure that the ultrasound probe is positioned as close to the fundus as possible, it is moved into the anterior fornix if the uterus is anteflexed and into the posterior fornix if the uterus is retroflexed. Ultrasound sections are scanned from the cervix to the fundus and back with further pulsatile injections of fluid. The examinations made in the longitudinal plane are now repeated in the transverse plane. The fundus region is again examined for the presence of uterine malformations and associated features (see below). Finally, a section of both tubal angles is scanned to visualize the perfusion of triangular filling pattern of the tubal angles. This is not always possible depending on the position of the ultrasound probe in relation to the uterine fundus. The findings, whether normal or abnormal, are documented on a video printer, polaroid camera or video tape.

Visualization of the uterine tubes using echogenic contrast agents

During the last stages of the examination the ultrasound contrast medium, SHU 454, is prepared by the operating theatre nurse or by an assistant. Diluent (9 ml of solvent) is placed into the vial containing galactose particles using a minispike inserted into the filling port. The suspension is shaken vigorously for about 5 s and then drawn up into a 10 ml syringe (see Figure 2). The uterine tubes are then visualized by contrast ultrasonography. After attaching the syringe with the contrast medium to the intrauterine catheter as described above, the injection is made with the left hand and the ultrasound probe is guided with the right hand (Figure 5). Again, the examination starts in the median longitudinal plane. The uterine cavity, which in most cases will still be dilated by the Ringer's solution instilled previously, is slowly filled with the echogenic ultrasound contrast medium. When the contrast medium reaches the fundus, the ultrasound probe is swept in the longitudinal plane to the right via the tubal angle and the pars intramuralis. If the tube is patent, constant flow in a pattern resembling a point, spot or streak is seen. Further intermittent injections of volumes of 1–2 ml, given slowly and continuously, with further lateral sweeps of the ultrasound probe, allow visualization of intraluminal or intratubal flow under normal anatomical conditions via the pars intramuralis into the medial and distal segments of the tubes. Depending on the course followed by the tubes, the tubal lumen is examined in the transverse plane, oblique plane or longitudinal plane. If, for example, the tube runs steeply into the pouch of Douglas, a longitudinal ultrasound scan shows a relatively long segment in one plane, possibly extending to the end of the fimbriae (see also Figures 9–11).

After reaching the distal segments, the ultrasound probe is guided back to the median aspect following the intratubal flow, and longitudinal scans are made of the other side via the same segments, noting the characteristic flow dynamics. If the anatomical structures are normal and if the operator has some experience of the procedure, about half the contrast medium will have been used at this stage in the examination (some 3–5 ml).

The examination is continued in the transverse plane. The fundus uteri is visualized, with both intramural segments if possible. As before, small volumes of contrast medium are injected and the flow patterns are observed. The contrast medium usually continues to flow

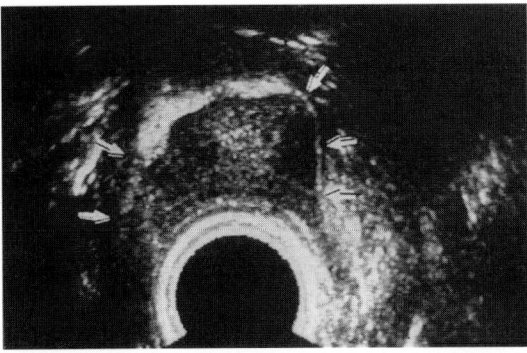

Figure 9 Fallopian tubes patent bilaterally. Frontal section in the fundus region, intraluminal flow (arrows), the proximal third of both tubes is passed by the contrast agent

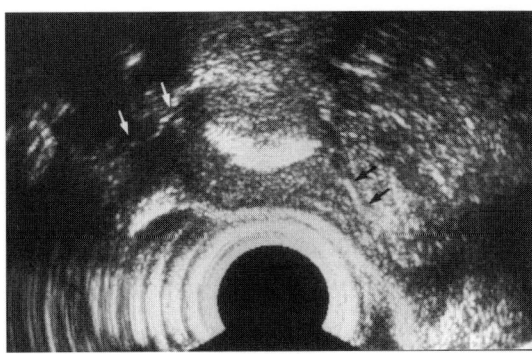

Figure 11 Frontal section showing broad flow of contrast medium (Echovist) in the tubal ampulla (arrows) and at tubal fimbriae

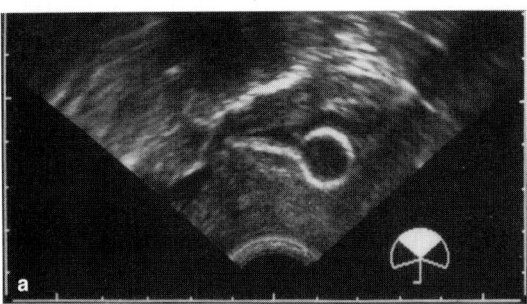

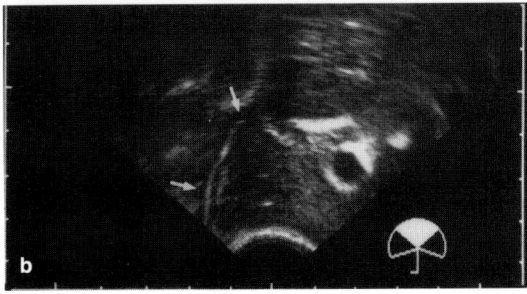

Figure 10 (a) The tip of the balloon catheter with side opening, displaced into the right tubal angle, occludes the tubal ostium. Uterine fundus in transverse section. (b) If the catheter is withdrawn slightly, the tip of the catheter no longer obstructs the tubal ostium, and contrast medium flows through the right tube (arrows), showing that the tube is patent. Transverse section

through the tubes for a short time, even immediately after the injection. Simultaneous visualization of the left and right proximal segments of the tubes in one plane is possible, but is not always achievable (Figure 9). In this case, the side which is thought to be easier should be examined first. This is mostly the

side on which at least one proximal tubal segment can be visualized (it may be apparent only as a point or a spot). This is examined as peripherally as possible in the longitudinal or transverse plane; the ultrasound probe is then held at the point of flow and is no longer swept in the longitudinal or transverse plane but is simply carefully rotated about its own long axis (i.e. the long axis of the ultrasound probe). In this way it is often possible to visualize even the medial and distal tubal segments in a longer section. The same procedure is repeated on the other side, starting from the pars intramuralis. Generally, for diagnosis of tubal patency, two or three observation phases per tube are needed, with an observation period of continuous flow of about 10 s (while the contrast medium is slowly injected). Although visualization of a longer segment of the tube beyond the pars intramuralis is more convincing, in our experience the part of the tube which is selected for following the flow of contrast medium does not seem to be particularly important provided that the flow is visible over a distance of more than 2 cm. The longest possible tubal segment left and right and simultaneous visualization of the proximally perfused tubes in the transverse plane are documented as confirmation of tubal patency and are later shown to the patient (see Table 5).

Finally, the adnexal regions are examined for filling of the distal segments of the tubes,

Table 7 Advantages and disadvantages of different instruments and catheters

Instrument/catheter	Advantages	Disadvantages
Schultze instrument	Fixed position, good seal, no retrograde leakage of fluid, good visualization of cavity, re-usable	Considerable problems with limited space in nulliparous and women with narrow vaginas, two bullet forceps needed for clamping cervix. Large dead space
Cohen instrument	Good visualization of cavity, re-usable	Possible problems with limited space, one forceps for cervical clamping. Moderately large dead space, may not give good seal with cervix in multiparas
8 French bladder balloon catheter with guidewire (disposable)	No problems with space, cheap	Possible guidewire problems, balloon limits evaluation of cavity, balloon and catheter tip may lodge in the tubal angles (in this case, withdraw a few centimeters), possible problems with anchoring, pain may occur on inflating the balloon
Zinnanti catheter (disposable, 2 mm, Zinnanti Surgical Instruments, Chatsworth, California)	No problems with limited space, stopcock	Possible pain on anchoring, balloon limits evaluability of cavity somewhat. Outlet tip often becomes blocked during injection of SHU 454. In this case, must be rinsed with Ringer's solution before the next injection of contrast medium
Bard catheter (disposable, C.R. Bard. Inc., Billerica, Massachusetts)	Optimal positioning because of the double balloon system, stopcock, extra channel for tube sound	Possible pain on anchoring, especially in cervical canal, intrauterine balloon limits evaluability of cavity slightly
Ackrad catheter (disposable, Ackrad Laboratoria Inc., Cranford, New Jersey)	No problems with limited space, very flexible catheter (although this is a disadvantage in cervical stenosis)	Possible slight pain on anchoring

indicating sactosalpinx. Examination of the pouch of Douglas for any increase in retro-uterine fluid, compared with the picture at the start of the examination, completes the examination procedure.

Special features of the use of the technique with an intrauterine catheter

In principle, there is no reason why contrast ultrasonography of the uterus and tubes cannot be performed using a standard HSG set after Schultze or Cohen (Table 7). However, the size of this apparatus makes it difficult to guide the vaginal ultrasound probe during the examination.

Hence, we prefer to use intrauterine catheters with inflatable balloons at the catheter tip. Modern catheters are simple to insert into the uterus, make a good seal with the cervix after anchoring and thus allow a good overview of features close to the fundus and the cervix, an advantage in the simultaneous diagnosis of uterine septae and submucosal myomas. A simple balloon catheter may become displaced cranially, leading to retrograde leakage of contrast medium through the cervix into the vagina. Moreover, the catheter tip may become lodged in a tubal angle. If the catheter has side holes the outflow of contrast medium may be blocked; if the catheter hole is at the tip only one tube may be filled (Figure 10). For this reason, the position of the catheter tip and the catheter balloon should be checked when injection of contrast medium is started.

Simple catheters (especially the 8 French bladder catheter) should be held under gentle caudal traction in the uterine cavity after anchoring and during the injection of contrast medium. This helps to ensure that the cervix is sealed and also that the fluid (contrast medium) is able to disperse freely into the tubal angles.

HyCoSy in combination with pulsed wave Doppler

If the examination reveals evidence suggesting tubal occlusion or if it is only possible to visualize a segment of tube of less than 2 cm in length, it is advisable to confirm the findings using pulsed wave Doppler scanning (Figures 12 and 13). Initially at least, this investigation is easier if a second ultrasonographer makes the adjustments to the ultrasound machine, so that the position of the ultrasound probe does not change, especially if the tubal segments are only partially visualized.

The perfused tubal segment is first examined in B-mode. The Doppler gate is placed over the perfused pars intramuralis or, if possible, over a distal tubal segment, which can be identified by the echogenicity of the contrast medium flowing through it (Figure 12). After the Doppler gate has been positioned over the area to be examined, the gate width is reduced to measure only the flow noise from the pertubation and not vascular or other noise. The apparatus is now switched to Doppler registration, and brief (about 5 s) injections of contrast medium are made again. The sounds heard, which are long, drawn-out and initially hissing, and the simultaneous visualization of a broad noise band on the monitor, the width of the band which slowly decreases after injection, indicate that the tube is patent. Thus unobstructed flow is characterized by a short filling phase with a rapid, steep increase in Doppler shift and a slow, uniform fall in Doppler shift along the time axis, indicating unobstructed free distal outflow (Figure 13).

The absence of these acoustic signals or optical tracings indicates obstruction of tubal flow or tubal occlusion. In this case there is only a short, steep Doppler shift with no subsequent noise signals (see below and Figure 14). This indicates an absence of outflow of contrast medium distal to the Doppler gate[5,20].

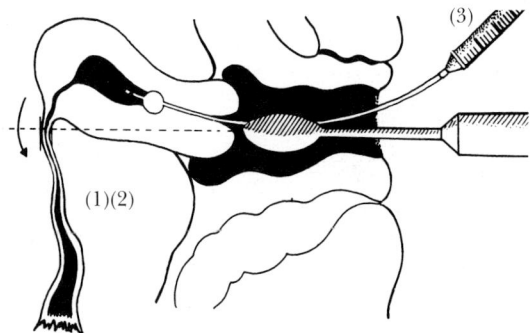

Figure 12 Schematic diagram of hysterosalpingo-contrast sonography with pulsed wave Doppler: (1) Positioning of the Doppler gate over a (perfused) segment of the tube; (2) Setting switched to Doppler recording; (3) Injection of contrast medium

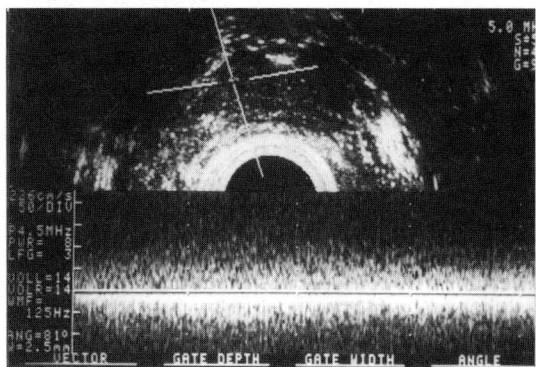

Figure 13 The pars intramuralis perfused with contrast medium (Echovist) in longitudinal section shows focusing of the Doppler gate. Positive Doppler signal during the free passage of contrast medium of the Fallopian tube is shown

HyCoSy with color Doppler

The essential feature of color-coded duplex sonography is the black and white or grey scale visualization of static structures and the color visualization of flowing reflective fluids. Flows towards the ultrasound probe appear red and flows away from the probe appear blue. Experience with color Doppler sonography confirmed the value of this technique for contrast sonography to investigate tubal patency[29,30]. The perfused tubes are shown in color (Figures 15–17). Because the color Doppler apparatus is set to pick up very small

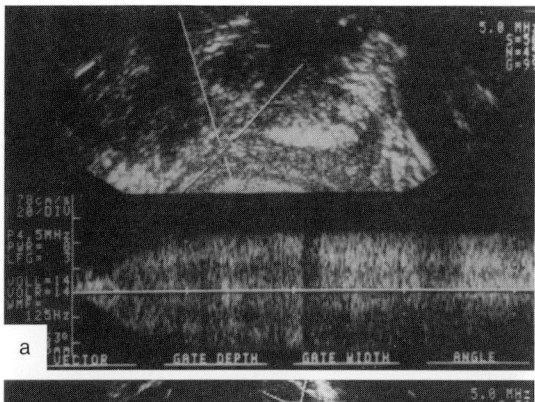

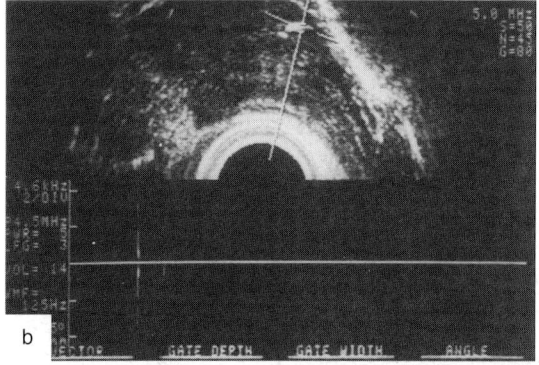

Figure 14 (a) Unobstructed tubal flow in pulsed wave Doppler hysterosalpingo-contrast sonography. (b) Proximal tubal occlusion (left side) with a patent right tube on hysterosalpingo-contrast sonography with pulsed wave Doppler. The Doppler gate is over the left pars intramuralis. After switching to Doppler recording and simultaneous injection of contrast medium (Echovist) only a short steep Doppler shift is seen instead of the broad Doppler band seen with patent tubes

signals from blood flow, use of the highly echogenic contrast medium SHU 454 may give rise to color artefacts. These can be controlled, however, by reducing the sensitivity (color gain) and thus limiting the color-coded flow image to the tubal lumina.

It is doubtful whether intratubal flow can be evaluated directly using non-echogenic saline solution with color Doppler[25,26]. At the very least this would make it more difficult to visualize the flow of a contrast medium, since *a priori* there are no echo dispersants in the pertubed fluid. Unfortunately, the cited papers do not give examples of ultrasound images, which would provide some idea of whether this is the case or not.

APPEARANCE OF THE NORMAL UTERUS AND IN THE CASE OF LESIONS VISIBLE ON HyCoSy

On longitudinal ultrasound section, the contour of the uterine cavity filled with Ringer's solution or with ultrasound contrast medium is normally spindle- or club-shaped and smooth. This applies to both anteflexed and retroflexed uteri if the ultrasound probe is positioned at the level of the uterine convexity. If the ultrasound probe is swept from the right to the left tubal isthmus in longitudinal section, the margin of the fundus is at the same level, i.e. visually it is not significantly higher or lower (see Figure 7). If it is not at the same level, it is a sign of malformation of the uterus. In the frontal section, the upper part of the uterine cavity is elliptoid to dumb-bell in shape, with a restriction of the smaller diameter toward the cervix (see Figure 6).

In many cases, thin structures projecting from the endometrium into the lumen and floating in the fluid stream are visible during injection of the contrast medium. These are detached strips of mucosa, produced by previous manipulation (e.g. hysteroscopy) or arising independently. These are normally of no pathological significance. They lie loosely in the uterine cavity and can easily be collected for histological examination using a curette. The uterine musculature exhibits uniform echogenicity without thickenings and a uniformly smooth external contour.

Appearance of the uterus with lesions visible on ultrasound in HyCoSy

Uterine cavity

Any non-motile large structures detected in the fluid stream of the injected contrast-medium are suspect. Rigid, slender connections between the anterior and posterior walls of the uterus may represent synechiae. Round, hyporeflective, broad-based structures represent uterine polyps or submucosal myomas: hysteroscopy is helpful for differential diagnosis. The correctness of contrast sonographic diagnoses of intrauterine myomas, polyps,

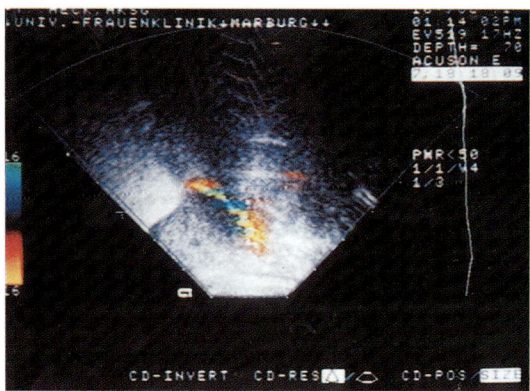

Figure 15 Color coded Doppler sonography shows the frontal section of the uterine fundus. The uterine cavity and the first one-third of the left tube is filled with contrast medium. The color marking demonstrates the unobstructed intratubal flow of the left tube

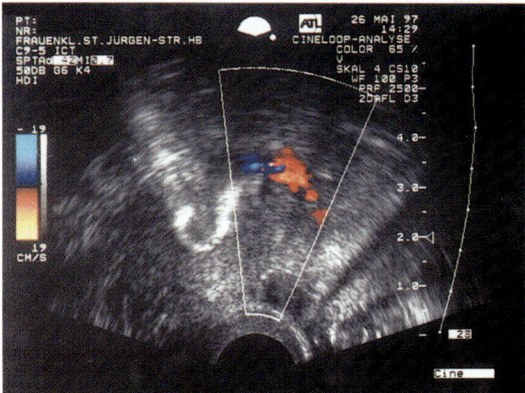

Figure 16 Color-coded Doppler sonography shows the frontal section of the uterine fundus. The uterine cavity is filled with the white contrast medium. The first part of the left Fallopian tube is shown to be patent by red spots

and synechiae has been confirmed by hysteroscopy[3] (Table 8).

Uterine walls in cases of myoma

If the uterus in palpably enlarged, abdominal or even vaginal ultrasound examination alone does not always permit an unequivocal assessment of the mass of myometrium and myoma. However, when a myomatous uterus is generally enlarged, filling the uterine cavity with fluid usually allows the proportion of the

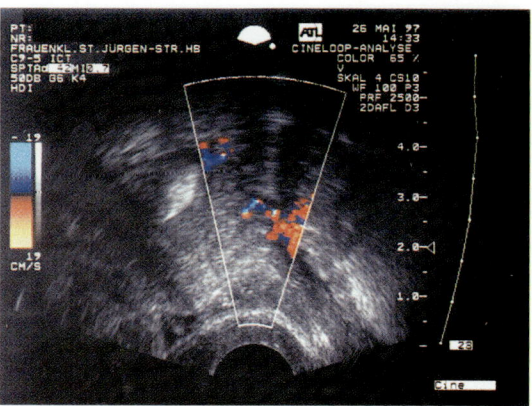

Figure 17 The color marking demonstrates the open pars intramuralis of the left side and the more peripheral flow in the middle of the left tube in the same patient as Figure 16

Table 8 HyCoSy findings in the uterine cavity

Structures	Indicates
Floating, thin strips	Parts of endometrium
Rigid, thin strips, stretched obliquely from the anterior to the posterior wall (Figure 6)	Adhesions
Round, narrow- or broad-based structures seated on the myometrial wall or stretching into the myometrium (Figure 18)	Polyps, submucosal to intramural myoma

endometrium to myomatous tissue to be determined (see Figures 6 and 18). The localization and differentiation of intramural and submucosal myomas and determination of the distance of the myomas from the uterine cavity may be better assessed with HyCoSy than with other techniques[5,6,31]. This technique can be used to decide whether patients with large myomas very close to the uterine cavity should initially be treated conservatively with a gonadotropin-releasing hormone (GnRH) analog to reduce tumor size before the myoma is removed. The HyCoSy results provide information on whether an adequate distance between the myoma capsule and the uterine cavity or endometrium is present for surgical removal of intramural myomas, and whether surgical intervention is likely to result in perforation of the uterine cavity. If myomas are sited submucosally, contrast sonography can be used to assess how deep the nodes extend into the myometrium (Figure 18). This technique for visualizing the layers of the uterine wall makes it easier to plan a therapeutic strategy and to decide between pharmacological and surgical treatment or alternatively between endoscopic surgery and laparotomy (Figures 1, 6 and 7).

Malformations

The value of ultrasound screening (in the case of abdominal ultrasound) for detecting uterine malformations has been discussed[32,33] (Table 9). High grade malformations such as uterus bicornis are strikingly evident in an ultrasound scan and are usually diagnosed correctly[32]. On the other hand subtle uterine malformations, such as an arcuate or subseptate uterus, are rarely if ever recognizable on ultrasound scan, unless HyCoSy is used. In these cases, radiological HSG formerly offered advantages. Distension of the uterine walls, caused by the fluid or contrast medium injected into the uterine cavity allows similar conditions to those obtained with X-ray HSG. The ultrasound anatomy of uterine malformations in HyCoSy, in comparison with the anatomy of the normal uterus, is shown in Figure 19.

In the normal uterus, the cranial margin of the uterine fundus is raised only slightly if the ultrasound probe is directed from the medium longitudinal plane laterally, and the thickness of the myometrium in the fundus remains about the same. In cross-section, the uterus from caudal to cranial normally exhibits a narrow longish cleft leading to the club-shaped cavity, terminating in the comma-shaped echoes of the lateral angle of the cavity (tubal angle).

In the arcuate uterus, the uterine fundus shifts cranially if the ultrasound probe is moved in the longitudinal plane from the median to the lateral position, and vice versa. The cross-sectional image reveals two spindle-shaped hyporeflective structures close to one another, described as the 'cat's eye phenomenon' (Figure 20).

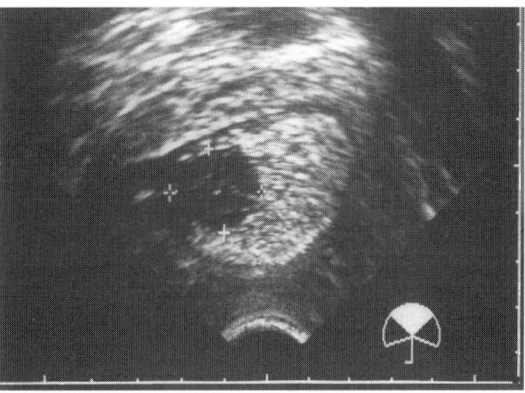

Figure 18 Submucosal myoma shown by hysterosalpingo-contrast sonography with Echovist (transverse section). The myoma was resected hysteroscopically

Table 9 Uterine malformations in hysterosalpingo-contrast sonography (HyCoSy)

	HyCoSy findings	
Malformation	Longitudinal plane	Transverse plane
Arcuatus (Figure 20)	Slight upward shift of fundus laterally	'Cat's eye phenomenon'
Subseptus (Figure 1)	Thickening of the 'musculature' at the fundus level from lateral to median; external border of fundus same	Figure of eight, broad median septum
Bicornis, duplex (Figure 21)	Deepening of external border of fundus from lateral to median (thickness of myometrium about same in contrast to uterus subseptus)	Appreciable distance of cavity echo
Unicornis unicollis with rudimentary cornus on the other side (Figure 22)	Cavity and tubes can be visualized only on one side	Drop-like cavity echo up to the patent tube, on the other side hyporeflective projection with endometrial echo

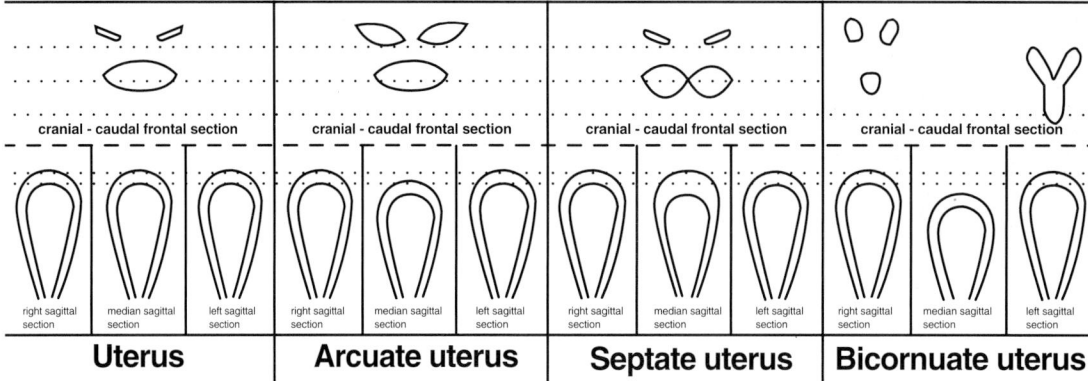

cranial - caudal frontal section	cranial - caudal frontal section	cranial - caudal frontal section	cranial - caudal frontal section
right sagittal section / median sagittal section / left sagittal section	right sagittal section / median sagittal section / left sagittal section	right sagittal section / median sagittal section / left sagittal section	right sagittal section / median sagittal section / left sagittal section
Uterus	**Arcuate uterus**	**Septate uterus**	**Bicornuate uterus**

Figure 19 Schematic overview of uterine malformations seen on transvaginal hysterosalpingo-contrast sonography, comparing the sonographic findings in frontal and sagittal sections at the plane of the uterine fundus, in the normal uterus and malformed uteri

In the subseptate uterus, lateral movement of the probe in the cross-sectional view shows no appreciable lowering or raising of the external border of the fundus, although there is an increase in the thickness of the uterine wall towards the median aspect. The cross-sectional view resembles the 'cat's eye phenomenon', with the single exception that the hyporeflective areas are more oval in shape and are broader in the anterior–posterior direction (Figure 1).

In high grade malformations, such as uterus bicornis unicollis or duplex uterus, palpation or inspection alone are often sufficient to make the diagnosis. The shift of the fundus when the probe is swept laterally is even more evident (Figure 21). In the frontal section, when a uterus bicornis unicollis is extended, a Y-shaped structure is visible. On transverse section of an anteflexed uterus, a star-shaped contrast figure represents the echo from the uterine cavity. On cross-section of the uterus, the shadows of the cavity are widely spaced. Uterus bicornis, as a high grade malformation, may be apparent even on basic ultrasound from the median indentation and, especially in the luteal phase, from the typical hyperreflective (secretory) endometrial echo, seen as the principal structure.

Uterus bicornis unicollis with a rudimentary cornus uteri on one side is a rare special case. If the connection between the two corni

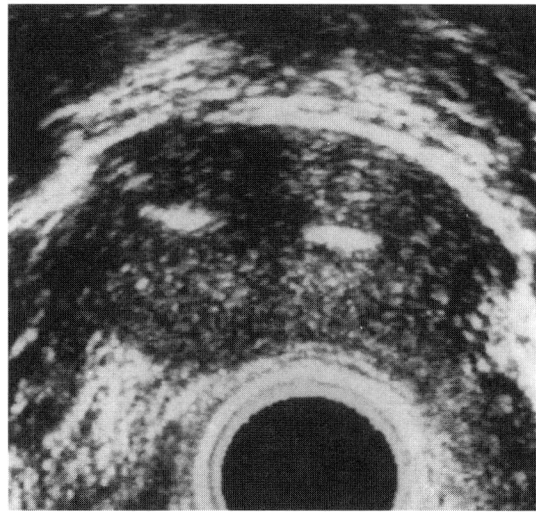

Figure 20 Transverse section of the uterine fundus showing the 'cats eye phenomenon', using hysterosalpingo-contrast sonography with Echovist

is absent, only the principal cornus or only one cavity is filled and only one tube can be visualized.

Evidence of a second cavity is provided by the endometrial echo of the rudimentary cornus (Figure 22). Hysteroscopy reveals on one side a smooth uterine wall without a tubal angle. Over a period of 1.5 years, we found significant abnormalities (myoma, septae, malformations, synechiae) in the uteri of 30 of 80 patients with fertility problems. Five cases

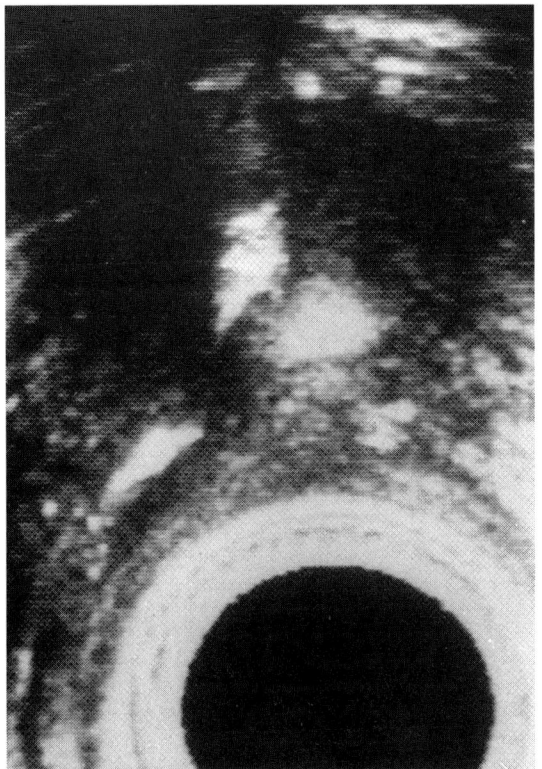

Figure 21 Uterus bicornis unicollis; frontal section of the extended uterus using hysterosalpingo-contrast sonography with Echovist

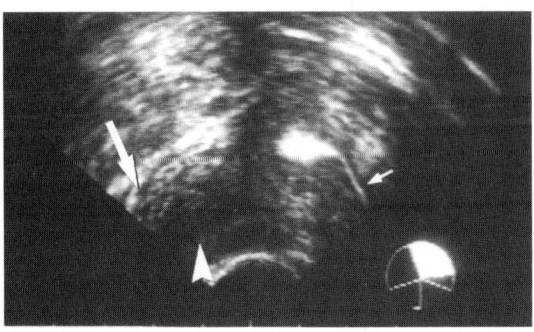

Figure 22 Transverse section showing uterus bicornis unicollis with a rudimentary right cornus uteri (large arrow); right cavity (arrowhead) with small serometra unconnected to the cavity of the left uterine cornus. The left cavity is filled and the left Fallopian tube is perfused (small arrow)

of malformations, two of which had been suspected beforehand, were recognized on contrast sonography and confirmed by HSG carried out subsequently under the same

anesthesia. Although three small malformations (arcuate uterus) were overlooked on HyCoSy in the early phase of the study, this type of malformation was discovered later when the described ultrasound appearance was taken into consideration.

APPEARANCE OF NORMAL TUBES IN HyCoSy

Because of the different courses and localization of the tubes it is advisable to carry out a systematic procedure in the ultrasound examination, as described previously in this Chapter. In schematic terms, three main directions of the tubes can be distinguished (Table 10).

B-Mode

To confirm patency in a tube in B-mode, it is necessary to visualize the intratubal fluid flow via the pars intramuralis into the isthmus or the ampulla (see above). The following descriptive criteria apply to the individual segments of the tubes:

(1) Contrast medium filling and flow in the pars intramuralis;

(2) Filling and flow in the isthmus and/or beyond this (Figure 23);

(3) Filling and flow in the ampulla with outflow of contrast medium from the end of the fimbria (Figures 11 and 25);

(4) Additional criterion: absence of elongated cystic structures in the adnexal region (these would suggest sactosalpinges) (Figure 3).

According to our experience, there is adequate evidence of tubal patency if a perfused tubal segment can be visualized over a minimum length of 2 cm. Even flow in the pars intramuralis, confirmed by a positive Doppler signal (see below), observed for an adequately long period (at least two observation periods over 10 mins) and with the absence of elongated cystic structures in the adnexal region, is sufficient to indicate that the tubes are patent. However, the recommended quantity of fluid should still be used to indentify any obstruction

Table 10 Principal directions of tube in patients in lithotomy position

Anatomical	HyCoSy findings
Running by the shortest route into the pouch of Douglas, parallel to the uterus	According to the position of the uterus, long tubal segments in longitudinal or frontal section (Figure 23)
Initially laterally, medially around the ovary, then to the pouch of Douglas	Proximal tubal segments in frontal or cross-section, possible peripheral segments in longitudinal section (Figure 24)
Cranial, parallel to the pelvic wall with the fimbriated end cranial. Often seen in patients with large tumors filling the pouch of Douglas, ovarian cysts, posterior wall myoma or as a result of fixation of tubes by adhesions to the pelvic wall	Difficult: proximal tubal segments in longitudinal and cross-section, no visualization distally (distant from ultrasound probe) (Figure 23)

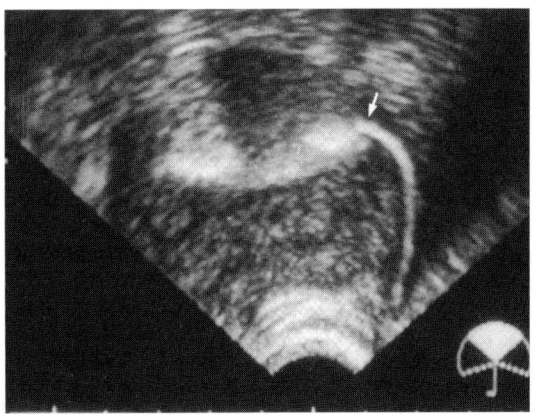

Figure 23 Frontal section showing flow of contrast medium in the left tube, proximal third. Tube runs by the shortest route into the pouch of Douglas. The pars intramuralis is arciform (arrow)

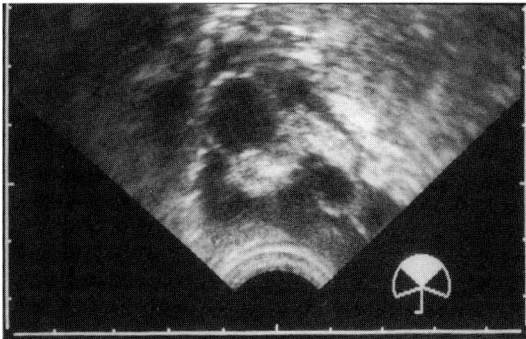

Figure 25 Broad flow of contrast medium (Echovist) through the tubal ampulla, the three fairly large hydatid cysts protruding into the fluid in the pouch of Douglas

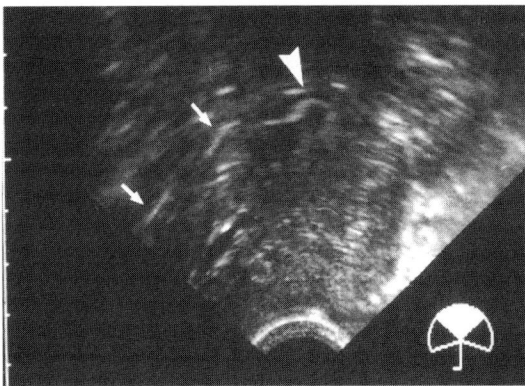

Figure 24 Flow of contrast medium (Echovist) in the left tube of a subject with a retroflexed uterus. S-shaped pars intramuralis (arrowhead) and view of the tubal isthmus (arrows)

of intratubal flow in thin sactosalpinges and to identify accumulations of fluid in the tubal ampulla if thick sactosalpinges are present.

In pulsed Doppler scanning

HyCoSy using pulsed wave Doppler scanning has been described earlier in this Chapter. Unobstructed flow through the tubes is indicated by a rapid, steep rise in the Doppler shift in the initial phase of the contrast medium injection (Figure 14a). This is apparent acoustically as a high frequency noise rising to a crescendo, and is visible on the ultrasound monitor as a 'noise band' rapidly becoming wider then remaining constant, during injection of the contrast medium. After the injection there is a long drawn-out noise, the frequency of which becomes narrower. Depending on the setting of the high-pass filter, the flow phase may be represented on the monitor chiefly by a thick white band of noise with parallel edges (Figure 14) or by a more jagged pattern which does not currently provide any information on the flow rate in the segment of the tube being examined.

In color Doppler

If the tubes are patent, a flame-red or mixed coloration – as aliasing – is seen during pulsatile injection of the ultrasound contrast medium. Depending on the intensity setting, this may appear either as a spot-like cloud, or at low intensity as a narrow luminous band of color along the perfused tubal segment (Figure 15).

Comparison of methods

A sonographic finding of unobstructed tubes on the basis of the noise band in pulsed wave Doppler or on the color in color-coded Duplex sonography is without doubt more impressive than that of a shorter segment of tube in standing B-mode. This is convincing evidence to place in the case records. Nevertheless, video recording of unobstructed intratubal flow in black and white in B-mode is of equal value for demonstrating intraluminal fluid flow, if this can be visualized over a sufficient length of tube (more than 2 cm).

APPEARANCE OF TUBAL LESIONS ON HyCoSy

Those who are familiar with the technique of contrast sonography can use this method as a tool for the differential diagnosis of the localization of tubal obstruction and the differentiation of cystic adnexal masses and endometrial pathology (Figure 26).

Proximal tubal occlusion

In B-mode, after the patent pars intramuralis has filled, the flow of contrast medium is interrupted after only a few milliliters have been injected. In the cross-sectional view of the uterus, the normal appearance of narrow filling of the pars intramuralis with continuous intraluminal flow is not present. Instead, at the point at which the flow of contrast medium is obstructed there is a broader area of filling of the patent proximal tubal segment (Figures 27 and 28). A further sign of obstructed tubal flow is interruption of the stream of contrast medium by poorly echoic lacunae (Figure 29). In B-mode, a proximal tubal occlusion exhibits a short, steep Doppler shift on the monitor and is confirmed acoustically by the absence of the typical Doppler signal (Figure 14b).

Distal occlusion and sactosalpinx

Proximal tubal occlusion may be easily diagnosed alone or by a combination of B-mode scanning and pulsed wave Doppler, because of its proximity to the easily recognizable uterine cavity. Contrast sonographic visualization of a distal obstruction may be more difficult. In the case of distal tubal occlusion, initially there is continuous flow of contrast medium in the proximal tubal segments, which is primarily a sign of unobstructed intratubal flow. Intratubal flow is then interrupted antegradely, at a point in time which depends on the size of the sactosalpinx. Thus, intraluminal flow should, as previously recommended, be observed for a suitable period and should be followed into the distal tubal segments as far as possible. A thin sactopsalpinx will cause interruption of contrast medium flow to become apparent earlier than with a thick sactosalpinx. If there is any doubt, the obstruction of flow should be confirmed with pulsed wave Doppler.

If basic ultrasound has not already given cause for suspecting sactosalpinx, on the basis of elongated, cystic, para- or retrouterine formations, the diagnosis will be confirmed by pronounced and progressive accumulation of fluid in a recognizably preformed, smoothly outlined oval structure, in contrast to the fluid in the pouch of Douglas (Figure 8). A further sign is the occurrence of fluid turbulence during the injection of the contrast medium. When Echovist is injected into a previously NaCl-filled hydrosalpinx the 'snow flurry' sign can be demonstrated (Figure 30).

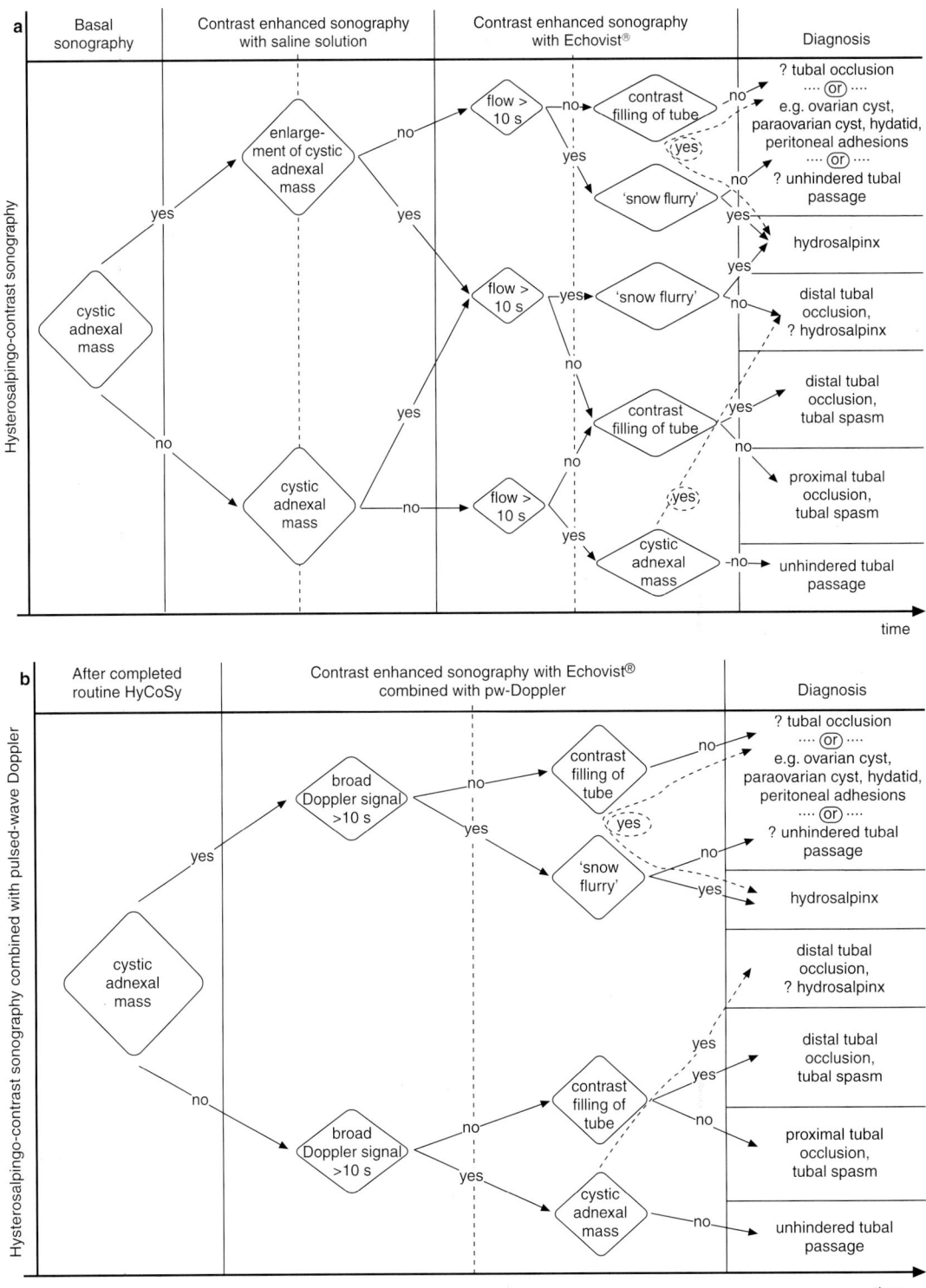

Figure 26 Flow diagrams for clinical diagnosis of tubal state by (a) hysterosalpingo-contrast sonography (HyCoSy); (b) hysterosalpingo-contrast sonography with pulsed-wave (pw) Doppler

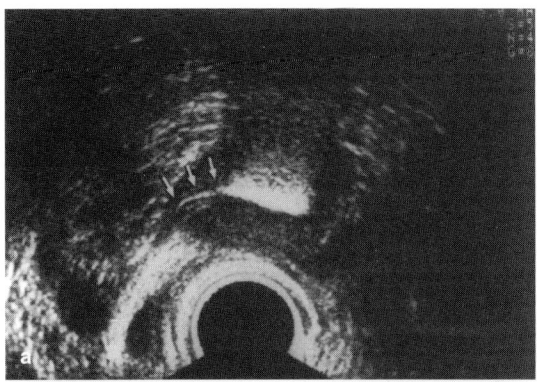

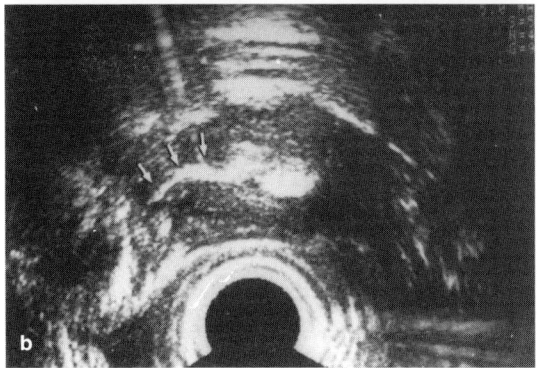

Figure 27 Artificially produced tubal occlusion on hysterosalpingo-contrast sonography. Transverse sections of the uterine fundus. (a) Thin flow of contrast medium (Echovist) in the pars intramuralis of a patent tube. (b) Absence of flow after broad filling of the pars intramuralis. Occlusion of the isthmus following sterilization by tubal coagulation

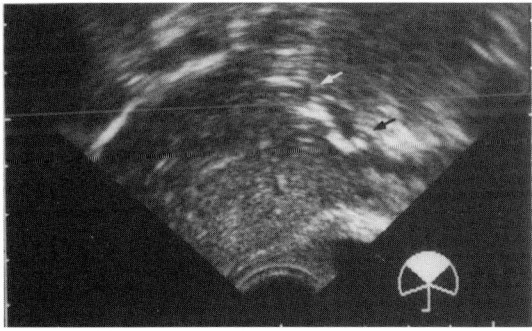

Figure 28 Post-inflammatory proximal tubal occlusion on hysterosalpingo-contrast sonography in a patient with a history of salpingitis. Transverse section of the uterine fundus after broad filling of the pars intramuralis and the start of the tubal isthmus (black arrow); there is no further flow of contrast medium

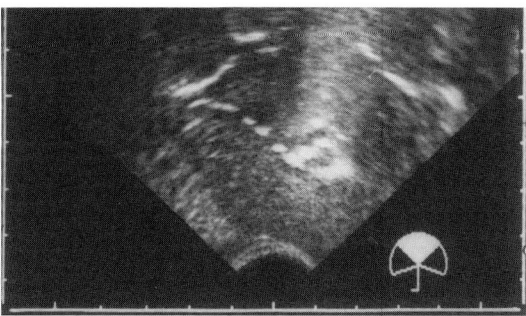

Figure 29 Proximal tubal occlusion (right tube) in the same patient as shown in Figure 28. Hysterosalpingo-contrast sonography shows the pars intramuralis filled with contrast medium (Echovist); flow is absent. The contrast medium is interrupted by poorly echoic lacunae. The phenomenon may arise as a result of some retrograde flow of contrast medium after further injection of contrast medium against resistance (bilateral tubal occlusion)

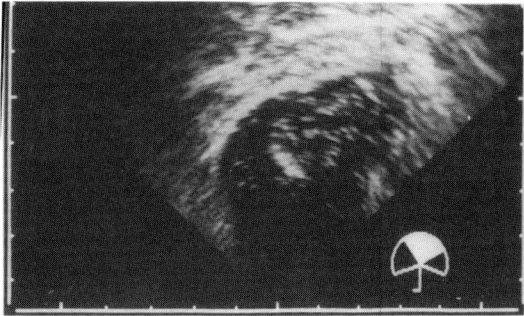

Figure 30 Distal tubal occlusion in a subject with sacto-salpinx with a broad lumen: inflowing contrast medium (Echovist) in the sactosalpinx previously filled with Ringer's solution produces turbulence

To rule out the possibility of distal tubal occlusion, after tubal patency has been demonstrated bilaterally, before concluding the procedure and before using all the contrast medium (10 ml), continuous intratubal flow should be observed again bilaterally in B-mode over a period of 10 s. Sometimes flow will continue without needing to give a further injection. Finally, the adnexal regions should be examined.

Contrast sonography therefore allows sacto-salpinges to be differentiated from other cystic structures in the adnexal region (e.g. ovarian cysts) or in the pouch of Douglas (i.e. cystic formations on the basis of peritoneal adhesions).

COMPARISION WITH CONVENTIONAL METHODS OF DIAGNOSING TUBAL DISEASE

Compared with the findings obtained by hysterosalpingography or chromolaparoscopy, the results of HyCoSy are in good agreement with those of conventional diagnostic techniques. The findings of B-mode ultrasound are in agreement with those of conventional methods in 65–93% of cases[13,18,34]. In a clinical study of 120 female patients, the sensitivity of HyCoSy compared with conventional tubal diagnosis was 88% for the right tube and 90% for the left tube; the specificity was 100%: i.e. in this group of patients the diagnosis of tubal patency made by HyCoSy was always confirmed by subsequent conventional diagnosis, HSG or chromolaparoscopy. However, the diagnosis of tubal occlusion by HyCoSy was correct in only 50% of cases (see also Tables 1–4).

A different study of color Doppler and HyCoSy found 70% agreement between ultrasound findings and those of conventional methods[29]; the additional use of pulsed Doppler scanning, with a total agreement of 95–100%, appears to be promising. The use of pulsed wave Doppler helps to clarify the tubal findings, particularly when B-mode results are doubtful. The following recommendations on the procedure may be made:

(1) Initial scanning in B-mode: patency is evidenced by throughflow of 2 cm or more over two or more observation phases of 10 s each.

(2) Pulsed Doppler should also be used if there is a suspicion of tubal occlusion in B-mode (or an absence of constant intratubal flow) or if flow is only demonstrable over a short segment, e.g. only the pars intramuralis or flow over a short distance in a peripheral (tubal) segment.

APPLICATIONS

Screening of uterus and tubes in infertility

Impairment of tubal function accounts for 30–45% of all causes of female infertility. Because of the known risks (Table 11), it is not advisable to use HSG or chromolaparoscopy until at least 6 months after the start of treatment for infertility; HyCoSy can be used, however. In B-mode (possibly supplemented with pulsed wave Doppler) and in color Doppler, transvaginal HyCoSy allows a preliminary investigation of the uterus and tubes to be performed using a method which is less invasive than those used hitherto. Because HyCoSy is not very invasive, has a low risk of side-effects and requires no special equipment, it is, with due observance of sterile precautions, suitable for use in the early stages of infertility diagnosis, after endocrinological, andrological and immunological assessment and before expensive and time-consuming hormonal treatment is started. In practice, at present we proceed as follows:

(1) Recording of case history:
   Lower abdominal inflammatory disease;
   History of operations on the lesser pelvis.

(2) Monitoring during one cycle (basal infertility diagnosis) with:
   Recording of basal temperature curve;
   Sonographic examination of ovulation;
   Postcoital test and examination of ejaculate (and if required endometrial biopsy on day 12 after ovulation after a negative human chorionic gonadotropin test).

(3) HyCoSy in the first half of one the subsequent cycles (Figure 31).

If HyCoSy reveals abnormal features, more invasive diagnostic methods, such as hysterosalpingography for more precise localization of an obstruction or chromolaparoscopy for additional investigation of the ovum pick-up mechanism, should be used, possibly leading to corrective endoscopic surgery or to planning of microsurgical intervention. If the patient has a history of pelvic inflammatory disease or operations on the lesser pelvis, there is a higher probability that tubal function is impaired, leading to impairment of the ovum pick-up mechanism. It is then more appropriate to use chromolaparoscopy, since this provides more information on tubal function than HyCoSy.

Table 11 Comparison of risks and diagnostic value with respect to uterine and tubal factors of hysterosalpingo-contrast sonography (HyCoSy), hysterosalpingography (HSG), chromolaparoscopy and hysteroscopy

	HyCoSy	HSG	Chromolaparoscopy	Hysteroscopy
Risks				
Infection	+	+	+	+
Injuries				
Intestine	−	−	+	(+)
Blood vessels	−	−	+	(+)
Perforation of uterus	−	−	−	+
Radiation load	−	++	−	−
Wound infection	(+)	(+)	+	(+)
Iodine allergy	−	+	−	−
Galactosemia	+ (rare)	−	−	−
Anesthesia	−	−	++	±
Diagnostic value with respect to:				
Uterus				
Malformations	++	++a	++b	−c
Myoma/ polyps	+d	−e	−f	+ (submucosal myoma only)
Intrauterine synechiae	+	(+)	−	++
Tubal angle (polyps)	+	(+)	−	++
Tubes	+	+	++	−
Patency				
Location of tubal occlusion	−g	++	(+) h	−
Ovum pick-up mechanism	−	−	++	−

Risks: ++ present; + possible; (+) conceivable; − unlikely
Diagnosis: ++ very good; + good; (+) not certain; − not possible
a, differentiation of uterus subseptus and uterus bicornis only possible using laparoscopy or HyCoSy; b, for differential diagnosis of uterus bicornis and duplex uterus; c, differentiation of uterus subseptus and uterus bicornis necessary using laparoscopy or HyCoSy; d, especially sub-mucosal and intramural, with large pedunculated myomas laparoscopy may be needed to dif-ferentiate from ovarian tumor; e, submucosal/calcified myoma, according to experience. Visualization in two planes may be necessary; f, chiefly pedunculated and subserosal myoma; g, further experience is needed to attain the same diagnostic value as HSG; h, may be discernible from translucent blue solution

Since the ultrasound contrast medium SHU 454 is rapidly absorbed after injection, it can also be used during courses of treatment. Our own experience with conceptions (and gesta-tion to term) in the cycle during which HyCoSy was performed or in a subsequent cycle, and similar experience reported by other workers[21] indicate that the epithelial tolerability of the contrast medium is good.

Examination of uterus and tubes before treatment

Before conservative treatment of myoma

If uterine myoma is suspected, and uterus-sparing surgery is indicated, the precise site of the tumor can be established by hysteroscopy, contrast sonography and laparoscopy, its mar-gins can be delineated from the myometrium

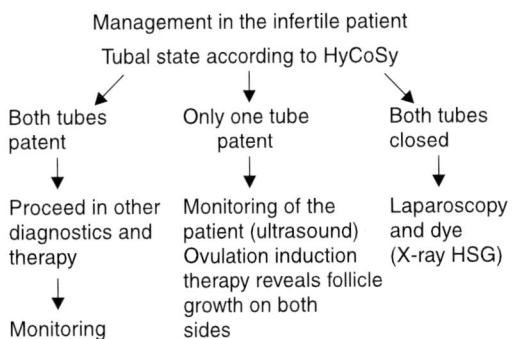

Figure 31 Management of the infertile patient depending on tubal patency

and subsequent treatment can be planned according to these findings.

Intrauterine lesions such as submucous myomas and small polyps, up to about 1 cm in diameter, diagnosed by HyCoSy and hysteroscopy, can be removed by curettage. If necessary, the myoma can be removed under abdominal ultrasound control. Larger myomas are resected by hysteroscopy, which may need to be performed in two stages. After resection of the most accessible part of the myoma, the remaining basal parts are removed after about 8 weeks, when these will have migrated towards the cavity. Predominantly intramural or large, intramural-subserosal myomas can be enucleated by laparotomy, after attempts to reduce the tumor size and to induce degeneration and a reduction in blood flow by treatment with a GnRH analog (response rate approximately 70%) (Figure 14). HyCoSy provides information on:

(1) The distance between the uterine cavity and the myoma, to indicate the probability of perforating the uterine cavity during enucleation, and to provide information for deciding whether or not pretreatment with a GnRH analog will improve the situation before surgery;

(2) The patency of the tubes, the pars intramuralis of which may be displaced by compression. It is advisable to check this immediately preoperatively after treatment with GnRH analog, since hormonal reduction of myoma size may free a previously blocked tube.

Laparoscopically, it is not possibly to 'see through' the layer of the uterine wall, but subserosal myomas, especially pedunculated tumors, can be delineated with certainty and distinguished from ovarian tumors before treatment is started. Smaller subserosal or pedunculated myomas can be removed laparoscopically.

Before adnexal operations

Adnexal operations in young girls and in women who have not yet attained their desired family size should be as tissue-sparing as possible; if at all possible they should be performed using microsurgical techniques, to ensure that they do not cause adhesions, which might impair ovulation. It may also be advisable to investigate tubal patency in women of childbearing age before adnexal operations for treatment of ovarian cysts, so that if necessary tubal cleaning can be performed at the same time. With ovarian cysts, this may be done either laparoscopically or by laparotomy. HyCoSy without anesthesia in such cases allows simple and rapid preoperative assessment. Pathological findings on HyCoSy require further diagnostic investigation mostly by chromolaparoscopy.

During surgery

Intra-abdominal adhesions or large tumors, such as ovarian cysts or large subserosal myomas, may make it difficult or impossible to assess tubal function using chromolaparoscopy. Hitherto, the alternative method of assessment was HSG, usually performed at some later time. Using HyCoSy, tubal patency can be assessed under the same anesthesia after chromolaparoscopy has been performed, assuming that the ultrasound apparatus is ready.

When adnexal lesions have been discovered during previous gynecological examinations or on the basic ultrasound scan, or if the history suggests adhesions, HyCoSy should initially be combined with chromolaparoscopy. In this case, contrast sonography is performed first, since intra-abdominal filling with CO_2 gas at subsequent laparoscopy may make it difficult to visualize the adnexae sonographically.

SUMMARY

Transvaginal HyCoSy is a diagnostic technique for the investigation and differential diagnosis of intrauterine and myometrial lesions and can reliably assess the site and extent of these legions. HyCoSy is an adjunct to conventional techniques such as hysteroscopy, HSG and laparoscopy, and thus helps in planning treatment.

Transvaginal HyCoSy is a reliable technique for demonstrating tubal patency in B-mode ultrasound, and combination of this technique with pulsed wave Doppler sonography improves the diagnostic effectiveness.

There is little risk of side-effects if sterile conditions are maintained, the technique is simple and can be performed as an outpatient procedure. These features make HyCoSy a suitable screening method for assessing uterine and tubal factors in the first phase of infertility diagnosis, to ensure that appropriate therapy is instituted as promptly as possible.

During organ-sparing adnexal operations in young women, HyCoSy allows a preliminary assessment of the condition of the uterus and uterine tubes. Further clinical studies are needed to improve the visualization of pathological findings, e.g. the localization of tubal occlusions. Improvements in ultrasound techniques which may prove useful include:

(1) A small ultrasound probe with a wide-angle image;

(2) A color Doppler technique adapted to the requirements of contrast sonography;

(3) Small ultrasound probes which could be used intraoperatively to locate tubal obstructions at an exposed site;

(4) Special software programs for selective identification of contrast medium which has flowed into an occluded tube but which is now stagnant.

ACKNOWLEDGEMENTS

I would like to thank Dr M. van de Sandt for assistance and Mrs H. Strunk for secretarial assistance.

References

1. Nannini, R., Chelo, E., Branconi, F., Tantini, C. and Scarselli, G. F. (1981). Dynamic echohysteroscopy. A new diagnostic technique in the study of female infertility. *Acta Europ. Fertil.*, **12**, 165–71

2. Richman, T. S., Viscomi, G. N., deCherney, A., Polan, M. L. and Alcebo, L. O. (1984). Fallopian tubal patency assessed by ultrasound fluid injection. *Radiology*, **152**, 507–10

3. Randolph, J. R., Ying, Y. K., Maier, D. B., Schmidt, C. L. and Riddick, C. H. (1986). Comparison of real-time ultrasonography, hysterosalpingography and laparoscopy/hysteroscopy in the evaluation of uterine abnormalities and tubal patency. *Fertil. Steril.*, **46**, 828–32

4. Deichert, U., van de Sandt, M. and Daume, E. (1987). Die vaginale Hysterokontrastsonographie-Ersatz oder Ergänzung zur Hysterosalpingographie und Chromo-Laparoskopie. *Ultraschall Klin. Prax. Suppl.*, **1**, 48

5. Deichert, U., van de Sandt, M. and Daume, E. (1987). Vaginale Hysterokontrastsonographie zur differentialdiagnostischen Abklärung eines Pseudogestationsacks. (Vaginal hysterocontrast sonography for differential diagnosis of a pseudgestational sac.) *Ultraschall Klin. Prax.*, **2**, 245–8

6. Deichert, U., van de Sandt, M., Lauth, G. and Daume, E. (1988). Die transvaginale Hysterokontrastsonographie (HKSG). Ein

neues diagnostisches Verfahren zur Differenzierung intrauteriner und myometraler Befunde. *Geburtsh. Und Frauenheilk.*, **48**, 835–44

7. Davison, G. B. and Leeton, J. (1988). A case of female infertility investigated by contrast-enhanced echogynecography. *J. Clin. Ultrasound*, **16**, 44–7

8. Allahbadia, G. N. (1992). Fallopian tubes and ultrasonography. The Sion experience. *Fertil. Steril.*, **58**, 901–7

9. Bonilla-Musoles, F., Simòn, C., Sampaio, M. and Pellicer, A. (1992). An assessment of hysterosalpingosonography (HSSG) as a diagnostic tool for uterine cavity defects and tubal patency. *J. Clin. Ultrasound*, **20**, 175–81

10. Broer, K. H. and Turanli, R. (1992). Überprüfung des Tubenfaktors mittels Vaginalsonographie. *Ultraschall Klin. Prax.*, **7**, 50–3

11. Gramiak, R. and Shah, P. M. (1968). Echocardiography of the aortic root. *Invest. Radiol.*, **3**, 356–66

12. Schlief, R. (1991). Ultrasound contrast agents. *Radiology*, **3**, 198–207

13. Deichert, U., Schlief, R. van de Sandt, M. and Juhnke, I. (1989). Transvaginal hysterosalpingo- contrast-sonography (Hy-Co-Sy) compared with conventional tubal diagnostics. *Hum. Reprod.*, **4**, 418–24

14. Bourne, *et al.* (1994). *Int. J. of Obstet. Gynecol.*

15. Campbell, S., (ed.) (19). *Viewpoints in Medicine: Infertility Investigation in Europe and the Future Role of Hysterosalpingo Contrast Sonography (HyCoSy).* (Worthing: Cambridge Medical Publications)

16. de Jong, N., Ten Cate, F. J., Lancèe, C. T., Rodand, J. R. T. C. and Bonn, N. (1991). Principles and recent developments in ultrasound contrast agents. *Ultrasonics*, **29**, 324–30

17. Schlief, R., Schürmann, R., Balzer, T., *et al.* (1993). Saccharide based contrast agents. In Nanda, N. C., Schlief, R. (eds.) *Advances in Echo Imaging Using Contrast Enhancement.*, pp. 71–96. (Dordrecht, Bosten, London: Kluwer)

18. Schlief, R., Schürmann, R. and Niendorf, H. P. (1991). Saccaride-based ultrasound contrast media. Basic characteristics and results of clinical trials. In Katayama, H., Brash, R. C., (eds.) *New Dimensions of Contrast Media*, pp. 141–6. (Tokyo: Excerpta Medical Ltd.)

19. Fritzsch, T., Maass, B., Müller, B., Schöbel, C., Siegert, J. and Stevens, K. (1991). Composition and tolerance of galactose-based echo contrast media. In Katayama, H., Brash, R. C. (eds.) New Dimensions of Contrast Media, pp. 156–62. (Tokyo: Excerpta Medica)

20. Hüneke, B., Lindner, Chr. and Braedle, W. (1989). Untersuchung der Tubenpassage mit der vaginalen gepulsten Kontrastmittel-Doppler-Sonographie. *Ultraschall Klin. Prax.*, **4**, 192–8

21. Böhmer, S., Degenhardt, F., Gohde, M. and Schneider, J. (1992). Ambulante vaginosonographische Durchgängigkeitsprüfung der Eileiter mit der Hysterosalpingokontrastsonographie (HKSG). Vaginal sonographic testing of tubal patency as an outpatient procedure using hysterocontrast sonography (HCSG). *Fertilität*, **8**, 62–5

22. Henkel, B. and Schlief, R. (1987). Transvaginal contrast-sonographic assessment of Fallopian tube patency. Presented at *The Euroson 1987, Proceedings of the Sixth Congress of the European Federation of Societies for Ultrasound in Medicine and Biology, Helsinki, Finland*, June 14–18, No. 223

23. Maroulis, G. B., Parsons, A. K. and Yeko, T. R. (1992). Hydrogynecography. A new technique enables vaginal sonography to visualize pelvic adhesions and other pelvic structures. *Fertil. Steril.*, **58**, 1073–5

24. Mitri, F. F., Andronikou, A. D., Perpinyal, S., Hofmeyr, G. J. and Sonnendecker, E. W. W. (1991). A clinical comparison of sonographic hydrotubation and hysterosalpingography. *Br. J. Obstet. Gynaecol.*, **98**, 1031–6

25. Stern, J., Peters, A. J. and Coulam, C. B. (1992). Colour Doppler ultrasonographic assessment of tubal patency. A comparison study with traditional techniques. *Fertil. Steril.*, **58**, 897–900

26. Yarali, H., Gurgan, T., Erden, A. and Kisnisci, H. A. (1994). Colour Doppler hysterosalpingosonography. A simple and potentially useful method to evaluate Fallopian tubal patency. *Hum. Reprod.*, **9**, 64–6

27. van de Sandt, M. (1997). Die Hysterosalpingokontrastsonographie (HKSG) – eine kontrastmittelunterstützte sonographische Untersuchungsmethode von Uterus und Tuben in der Sterilitätsdiagnostik. Thesis, Marburg

28. Allahbadia, G. N., Nalawade, Y. V., Patkar, V. D., G. M. and Shah, P. K. (1992). The Sion Test. *Aust. NZ J. Obstet. Gynaecol.*, **32**, 67–70

29. Deichert, U., Schlief, R., van de Sandt, M., Göbel, R. and Daume, E. (1990). Transvaginal Hysterosalpingo-Kontrastsonographie (HKSG) im B-Bild-Verfahren und in der farbkodierten Duplexsonographie zur Abklärung der Tubenpassage. *Geburtsh. und Frauenheilk.*, **50**, 717–21

30. Fobbe, F., Becker, R., Koch, H.-Ch., Hammerstein, J. and Wolf, K.-J. (1991). Nachweis der Durchgängigkeit der Tuba uterinae mit der farbkodierten Duplexsonographie in

Kombination mit Ultraschallkontrastmittel. *Fortschr. Röntgenstr.*, **154**, 349–53

31. Cicinelli, R., Romano, F., Anastasio, P. S., Blasi, N. and Galantino, P. (1995). Transabdominal sonohysterography, transvaginal sonography, and hysteroscopy in the evaluation of submucous myomas. *Obstet. Gynecol.*, **85**, 42–7

32. Nicoloni, U., Belotti, M., Bonazzi, B., Zimberletti, D. and Candiani, G. B. (1987).

Can ultrasound be used to screen uterine malformations? *Fertil. Steril.*, **47**, 89–93

33. Valdes, C., Malini, S. and Mallnak, L. R. (1984). Ultrasound evaluation of female genital tract anomalies: a review of 64 cases. *Am. J. Obstet. Gynecol.*, **149**, 285–92

34. Schlief, R. and Deichert, U. (1991). Hysterosalpingo-contrast sonography: results of a clinical trial with a novel US contrast medium in 120 patients. *Radiology*, **1788**, 213–5

Index